PRIMARY CARE ORTHOPEDICS

Royce C. Lewis, Jr., M.D., F.A.C.S.

Clinical Professor
Departments of Orthopedic Surgery and
General Surgery (Plastic)
Chief of the Hand Surgery Service
Texas Tech University Health Sciences Center
School of Medicine
Lubbock, Texas

Churchill Livingstone
New York, Edinburgh, London, Melbourne 1988

Library of Congress Cataloging-in-Publication Data

Lewis, Royce C.
    Primary care orthopedics.

    Bibliography: p.
    Includes index.
    1. Orthopedia.   2. Family medicine.   I. Title.
[DNLM: 1. Orthopedics. WE 168 L675p]
RD732.L49   1988   617'.3   87-15854
ISBN 0-443-08356-8

© Churchill Livingstone Inc. 1988

All rights reserved. No part of this publication may be reproduced, stored in a retrieval
system, or transmitted in any form or by any means, electronic, mechanical,
photocopying, recording, or otherwise, without prior permission of the publisher
(Churchill Livingstone Inc., 1560 Broadway, New York, N.Y. 10036).

Distributed in the United Kingdom by Churchill Livingstone, Robert Stevenson House,
1-3 Baxter's Place, Leith Walk, Edinburgh EH1 3AF, and by associated companies,
branches, and representatives throughout the world.

Accurate indications, adverse reactions, and dosage schedules for drugs are provided
in this book, but it is possible that they may change. The reader is urged to review the
package information data of the manufacturers of the medications mentioned.

Production Designer: *Angela Cirnigliaro*
Production Supervisor: *Jocelyn Eckstein*

Printed in the United States of America

First published in 1988

To
Ruthie

PREFACE

It is the basic intent of this book to provide information for the management of musculoskeletal conditions when seen by the primary care physician. An attempt has been made to discuss these conditions from a rather unique standpoint. To this end, the book is written on the premise that all orthopedic patients seen by the primary care physician fall into three categories.

The first category consists of those patients with some type of musculoskeletal complaint in which there is little question that the primary care physician can treat the patient himself. A large segment of the orthopedic problems seen in family practice are of a nonacute nature, with patients coming into the office for diagnosis and treatment. In most instances the primary contact physician is likely to be the *only* treating physician. Thus, the establishment of a diagnosis and points concerning treatment of these often perplexing therapeutic problems are discussed. A wide variety of conditions are covered, such as minor foot deformities in children, tendinitis, bursitis, low back pain, and similar static conditions that are seen with considerable frequency in family practice. For each anatomical area these various conditions are discussed in regard to aid in establishing a diagnosis, differential recognition from similar conditions, and proper management.

The second group consists of those patients in whom the situation is marginal; the primary care physician institutes treatment and closely monitors the patient. If progress is not satisfactory, or if some dangerous signs begin to indicate an impending complication, the patient can be referred to the specialist for more expert care. It is in regard to these patients that this book probably has its greatest value. Many times the primary care physician will institute treatment for a condition that appears to be relatively routine, and it is not until matters have progressed further that he realizes referral to a specialist is needed.

It is hoped that this book will make it easier for the primary care physician to decide whether or not he is capable of providing treatment and will help him refer those patients that pose special problems before these problems become great. Included is a description of certain warning signals that should alert the physician to seek help. In the discussion of each anatomical region those areas that are most likely to give trouble are pointed out as are certain types of cases in which the chances of developing complications are extremely high. As an example, this dilemma of "whether or not to refer" exists no more acutely in any area than in the treatment of trauma. For this reason a section on fracture treatment and complications is included, which describes the best methods of preventing these complications when the fracture is first treated.

The third category consists of those patients for whom there is no question from the onset that referral to an orthopedist is needed. In the chapters dealing with the various anatomical regions the features that help to identify the cases that need specialty care are pointed out. An example might be the interarticular fracture of one of the phalanges in the hand in which open reduction is almost invariably necessary if one is to restore a good joint surface and adequate joint function. Often these seemingly trivial injuries are not recognized as being as serious as they are, and the practitioner will attempt to treat them until it becomes obvious that he should have referred the case in the very beginning. In addition, some general information is included about what most likely will be done by the specialist after the patient is transferred, so that the physician can relate to the patient and his family the most likely course of treatment that will be recommended and administered by the consulting specialist. Most practitioners enjoy being able to accurately explain what will be done and most of the time this is a great aid in maintaining rapport with the patient and his family.

Chapters 1 and 2 contain information on general concepts particularly with respect to orthopedic evaluation of the injured patient. Chapters 3 and 4, on fractures, include the principles of healing of fractures as well as those events that keep fractures from healing satisfactorily. Of particular interest to most practitioners is Chapter 4, on fracture complications, which includes basic concepts rather than treatment of any specific fracture per se.

Following these introductory chapters, the various specific conditions are discussed by anatomical regions rather than by diagnostic category. This allows for greater readability and reference possibilities for the busy practitioner. Each of these chapters presents an overall picture of the area including anatomical considerations, conditions unique to that area, and treatment of injuries. Also included for each area are conditions that are more common in children.

In summary, *Primary Care Orthopedics* is written in an effort to present the management of musculoskeletal conditions in a rather unique light. Most orthopedic books for primary care physicians try to keep the discussion of orthopedics simple and uncomplicated; this book, however, is dedicated more to helping the practitioner to treat cases that he is capable of treating and to identify those cases that he should not attempt to treat but should monitor for signs of impending complications. This would seem to be a new concept that should be very inviting to the primary care physician, and, it is felt that if this approach can instill in the reader an expertise in decision making, then its purpose will have been accomplished.

Royce C. Lewis, Jr., M.D., F.A.C.S.

CONTENTS

1

ORTHOPEDIC EVALUATION: GENERAL PRINCIPLES

General Observation
Attitude
Deformity
Gait
Obvious Functional Loss
Emotional Stability or Secondary
   Gain
Pain
Location, Distribution, and Radiation
Associated Signs
Tenderness
Pain at Rest
Pain on Motion
Precipitating Factors
Specific Areas
Obvious Deformity

Swelling
Ecchymosis or Bruising
Heat
Muscle Atrophy
Trophic Changes
Stability
Musculature
External Support
Function
Locomotion
Muscle Action
Sensation
Joint Contractures
Autonomic States
Summary

GENERAL OBSERVATION

Attitude

The important thing when seeing an individual for the first time is to determine the extent of his problem and incapacities. The observation of his attitude is extremely important: whether he can stand up and walk or whether he must lie down because of weakness or pain. These are all important considerations. He may come in with a complaint in only a specific area, such as the hand or wrist, in which case the examination may well be more limited. However, it is important to note that in many cases the localization of symptoms and signs to a single part is but a manifestation of a more generalized systemic disease; one must be careful to notice anything in the patient's demeanor or his functional capacities as a whole individual. If the patient is lying down when first seen, notice whether he can move comfortably about the bed or lies rigidly in one position. Notice whether he protects or guards a single area; his general demeanor is often a key to the underlying problem.

Deformity

The observation of deformity is likewise important when you are first seeing the patient. Of course, with fractures or injuries the deformity may be obvious. However, the patient who first enters for examination should again be seen as an entire individual. Notice whether he stands erect or has a list to one side. Notice whether he has a deformity of his spine and the general alignment of his trunk in relationship to the head and pelvis at either end. Deformities of the extremities are often easier to see. These include even swelling and loss of motion in joints, particularly flexion contracture of joints of the extremities, and should be viewed as "deformities," which add to the overall picture of the patient's condition.

Gait

The evaluation of a patient's gait will often give very valuable information about the cause of his major complaint. Watch for list or limp and note whether or not the patient has the ability to walk with a normal stride or, instead, exhibits an antalgic-type of gait due to pain in his lower extremities. The patient with a painful extremity will guard this extremity and step on this side for a brief time until he can get the sound leg out in front of him again when taking a step. Note whether or not the limp, if it occurs, appears to be related to some obvious deformity such as shortening of the extremity or whether it might be due to a flexion contracture of the hip or knee thus rendering the entire extremity shorter than the opposite side. Gait will often also indicate muscular deficiencies, whether related to weakness, atrophy, or spasm, and one should be alert to changes in the gait related to the muscle imbalances.

Obvious Functional Loss

Obvious functional loss can often be seen when first observing the patient in the examining room. Of course, it is not difficult to see major functional losses such as a hemiparalysis or the various manifestations of cerebral palsy at the original examination. However, the more subtle functional losses sometimes will be missed by the examiner until pointed out by the patient himself during the examination. The type of injury or the nature of his major complaints could lead one to suspect functional loss. For example, in the patient who has a laceration or gunshot wound in the midportion of his arm in the region of the musculospiral groove, the examiner would, of course, immediately suspect the possibility of a radial nerve paralysis with loss of extensor power in the forearm and the hand. Other obvious functional loss will occasionally not be noted by the patient. It is interesting to note that a patient with a recent foot-drop due to pressure on the fifth lumbar nerve root will walk into the office with a slapping sort of gait without actually realizing that he has lost the ability to dorsiflex his foot. The experienced examiner, however, should pick up these various functional losses immediately. Careful attention to detail and time spent in thorough observation of the patient will often reward the examiner with a proper diagnosis even at the beginning of the examination.

Emotional Stability or Secondary Gain

One would be remiss, I think, to leave out the obvious modifying effects of emotional instability and secondary gain, which often so cloud the objective findings that it becomes difficult to establish a true diagnosis.

The patient with emotional instability will be somewhat easier to recognize since the other manifestations of depression or anxiety will be obvious and the implications of bizarre physical findings can be recognized. On the other hand, even though one suspects exaggeration or falsifying of response during the examination in individuals who have litigation pending or who are covered by worker's compensation claims and merely do not wish to return to work, one should guard against the tendency to discredit all physical findings. In individuals suspected of emotional instability or secondary gain problem often, even though they have obviously modifying situations, they still can have true disease that manifests objective findings and should not be overlooked by the examining physician. As a matter of fact, it has often been said that a patient with these obvious psychosomatic overlays requires even a more careful examination to be certain that nothing is being missed from an objective standpoint. In his efforts to mislead the examiner the patient will often make it very difficult to recognize the very obvious positive organic findings; these people require a special skill in examination to separate the "wheat from the chaff."

PAIN

Pain, of course, is the presenting and major complaint of many patients seen with orthopedic problems. There is no question that pain as a symptom is greatly modified by the patient's own perception of the pain and ability to withstand it. Some individuals have a very high pain tolerance and the examiner may be misled into believing that a situation is not serious because of the patient's unwillingness to admit that he has a great amount of pain. On the other hand, patients with extremely low thresholds of pain or those who are exaggerating their pain for emotional or secondary gain reasons often make it extremely difficult for the physician to evaluate the true magnitude of the pain present. Experienced examiners have come to recognize that various conditions are likely to cause varying types and degrees of pain. They have also come to recognize that the extent and the magnitude of the pain are more or less characteristic of the condition seen.

Some conditions cause pain that is out of proportion to what one would expect from the nature of the underlying pathology, while other conditions may be quite severe but cause relatively little pain. For this reason the pain itself must be carefully evaluated in making the final assessment of the diagnosis and planning the treatment for the patient.

Location, Distribution, and Radiation

The area in which the pain occurs is of paramount importance. One must determine from the history the location, distribution, and radiation of any pain the patient notes. The patient should be questioned not so as to lead him into giving an answer that seems appropriate but to make it possible for him to relate facts concerning his pain so that one can fully evaluate their importance. It is altogether too easy, when examining a patient with median nerve entrapment at the wrist, to tap over the volar aspect of the wrist and ask if this creates an "electric shock type of pain out into the index or middle fingers." This leading of the patient may evoke some irresponsible answer in the patient's effort to try to comply with what he feels the examiner is looking for. On the other hand, tapping over the volar aspect of the wrist in a patient with true median nerve compression will promptly cause the patient to complain of the lanceting type of pain characteristic of a neuropathy. One does not really need to lead him to describe the pain as "electrical" or "shooting" since he will volunteer this information. Of course, a knowledge of anatomy is imperative for the examiner since the distribution and radiation of the pain should correspond to the anatomical location of the nerve distally in order for the symptoms to have much meaning.

Associated Signs

The fact that an area has the presenting symptom of pain may direct the examiner to this location and to the observation of other associated features of which the patient may not even be aware. One of the typical examples, of course, is muscle spasm associated with pain. This is particularly apparent in conditions involving the low back and cervical area. In these instances even simple sprains of the vertebral joints often result in a massive protective spasm in the paravertebral musculature that itself may be one of the major causes of pain. Associated signs may take any form and are often related to the primary disease causing the pain rather than to the pain per se.

Tenderness

Tenderness probably is the best single indicator of the exact *location* of the pain and, often, the exact *cause* of the pain. Even though a patient may have marked pain and swelling of the lateral aspect of the ankle the finding of generalized tenderness may lead the examiner to believe that there probably is not a torn ligament present. By the same token, if at examination one finds point tenderness over the lateral collateral ligament of the ankle that far exceeds the tenderness anywhere else over the swollen painful area, one is lead to believe that a tear of this ligament probably has occurred even though the two ankles may look very similar. Tenderness may also be an indication of the true nature of a painful condition as contrasted to pain, which is magnified, or even entirely fabricated, by the patient. Pain in an area, particularly in the extremity, not associated with any tenderness is usually suspect as objective pain. On the other hand the patient may come in complaining of severe pain in the elbow without any known cause, and the examiner may find a point of exquisite tenderness over the lateral epicondyle that may not be larger than 1 cm^2 but still represents the area of the tendinitis of the extensor musculature attaching to the lateral epicondyle. In such cases, the rather generalized nature of the pain may not lend a clue to the diagnosis. Areas of tenderness are also important in examination of the low back, for instance, in which the painful areas are expected to overlie anatomical features rather than being in random locations throughout the low back and buttocks. For example, a very tender area just over the sciatic notch has much more serious diagnostic implications than pain in an area of the buttocks that does not overlie any important anatomical structures. By the same token, a patient may complain of back and leg pain and the examiner find a severely tender area over the trochanter, which indicates a trochanteric bursitis as being the cause of the patient's pain that may mimic clinically a herniated intervertebral disc with radicular pain. The examiner, therefore, must always palpate the area of complaint and should produce localized pressure over anatomical structures in the area to see if the pain can be elicited over an area that may provide a clue to the diagnosis.

Pain at Rest

Pain at rest is an important finding since this relegates the cause to a category sometimes quite separate from that present on pain with motion. Infections occurring within the musculoskeletal system usually cause severe pain even at rest. An example is the anterior close space of the finger (the so-called bone felon) in which the pain may be excruciating even though the patient is doing everything that he can to decrease its severity. Bone tumors often cause pain that occurs at rest and may even wake the patient up at night. Osteoid osteomas are often characterized by nocturnal pain as are many types of bone malignancy. This type of complaint, particularly pain that wakes the patient up from a sound sleep in the middle of the night, should be thoroughly investigated by the examiner.

Nocturnal pain or pain at rest is likewise characteristic of median nerve compression syndromes at the wrist. The edema that occurs at rest at night magnifies the compression of the nerve with symptoms severe enough to waken the patient from a sound sleep. If the patient does complain of pain at rest, and particularly if it wakes him up at night, the examiner should classify that type of pain within the proper areas of possibility such as the examples given.

Pain on Motion

Pain on motion, on the other hand, may be merely an aggravation of pain already present at rest but often denotes a more characteristic type of pain following injury or related to joints. A knee joint filled with fluid or blood may cause severe pain even at rest. However, a knee that has only minimal effusion can be made quite comfortable by resting it, particularly in a slightly flexed position. The movement of the joint causes the pain and weight-bearing in particular tends to accentuate the pain quite markedly. The patient's admission that his pain is present basically on motion or weight-bearing should lead the examiner to suspect the conditions related to this type of stress or strain on the skeleton.

Precipitating Factors

One should question the patient at length concerning "what makes the pain worse" and, "what can you do when the pain is occurring to make it better." Since the two factors are interrelated, it is important to ascertain both. Many times the patient can tell you exactly the types of motion, positions, or circumstances that tend to make his pain quite severe and also the position that he must get into or the circumstances he must create to relieve the pain. Pain of an extremity is commonly improved by elevation, though this may not be true if the pain is of vascular origin. Pain, however, that is due to muscular injury or strain, will usually be improved by heat. However, pain due to a hemangioma in the soft tissue or knee joint, for instance, will almost invariably be made worse by heat since this tends to dilate the vessels and increase the engorgement in the tumor. One should try to be realistic and analyze the precipitating factors that will often help to point the finger to the definite cause of the pain.

SPECIFIC AREAS

Most of the time the patient who is examined by the physician for an orthopedic problem will be able to direct his attention to a specific area. Whether the area represents the area of an injury or a localization of the pain, he is usually able to point out the area that should be examined most thoroughly.

Obvious Deformity

Obvious deformities usually point to the cause of the trouble and the patient with a list or a limp usually will have an obvious cause for it. Deformities that have occurred from the gradual subluxation of joints, such as in an arthritic, will usually direct the attention of the physician to that area for his examination. For example, a patient may come to the physician with severe pain in the radial aspect of the hand, extending down into the thumb and palm. However, on examination one can readily see a partial subluxation of the first metacarpal base from the trapezium, indicating a degenerative arthritis in this joint with the resulting deformity. One should be careful, however, not to assume that a deformity is caused by a certain condition but one should evaluate the deformity and think of all of the possibilities before settling on a single idea.

Swelling

Swelling is the most obvious result of inflammatory reaction and its absence often makes one wonder about the presence of the pain at all, or at least about the localization of the condition where the pain exists. An example, of course, is the pain experienced down in the lateral aspect of the leg due to nerve root pressure in the lower lumbar area. The patient will usually swear to pain in his calf but the absence of swelling or any other localizing feature should make the examiner turn to an area higher up to determine the cause of his pain, which must be assumed to be radicular. Likewise, a joint that is the site of severe pain usually will be associated with marked swelling. When that swelling is not present the examiner's suspicions as to the cause of the pain should be raised, since almost all conditions involving the synovial membrane cause an outpouring of fluid that is readily visible. Swelling may also be present over a rather generalized area, particularly in a dependent part of the body even with a rather localized injury. The sprained ankle, as mentioned previously, is often characterized by severe swelling of the ankle area even though the tender area over the torn lateral collateral ligament may be relatively small.

The examiner should always be cautious in evaluating an area of swelling that seems out of proportion to what he would expect from the condition he believes to be present. Patients will occasionally aggravate swelling on purpose to impress the examiner with the severity of the disease. Occasionally a patient will be seen who has even applied a tourniquet surreptitiously to his upper extremity to create marked swelling of the hand and wrist to convince the examining physician that a serious malady exists. The practitioner should not be hesitant to ask the patient directly if he is contributing to this swelling by some mechanism, if he feels that this is a possibility. Swelling, of course, is almost always more severe in dependent parts of the body and this should be recognized.

Finally, swelling of a lower extremity that does not subside when the part is elevated leads one to suspect some type of interruption of venous return such as with a thrombus, since most other types of edema will improve markedly with elevation of the part.

Ecchymosis or Bruising

Ecchymosis or bruising should indicate the extravasation of blood from the area's vessel. This may occur from injury or from abnormal capillary or small vessel fragility. Usually the latter factor is determined by a correlation of the amount of soft tissue bleeding with the severity of the injury. Bleeding in the soft tissues will be usually more severe in the dependent part of the body, due to the higher vascular pressure there. By the same token, any type of bleeding in the soft tissue will be greatly aggravated by dependency and improved by elevation. Areas of bruising in the lower extremity are particularly likely to gravitate downward; bleeding that might occur from an injury in the popliteal area often will result in an ecchymosis in the toes. The patient may become quite alarmed about this phenomenon and should be reassured by the practitioner that this is related to the pull of gravity bringing the extravasated blood into the most dependent area.

Heat

Heat is one of the major signs of inflammation and can usually be so considered by the examining physician. On the other hand, heat may also be caused by conditions such as sunburn or increased vascularity over a huge hemangioma and should not be taken unequivocally as a sign of an inflammatory reaction. Heat over a joint or an area that is painful and tender tends to bear out the presence of inflammatory reaction in the underlying tissue and usually is merely an adjunct to the other physical findings. The absence of heat over an area of complaint makes one wonder about the validity of the complaint or diagnosis. The supposed site of an acute inflammatory reaction (such as infection) that does not have increased local temperature should raise the suspicion of the examiner as to the presence of infection or at least about the type of organism that might be involved. Many organisms do not cause an increased local temperature and the presence of a "cold abscess" in an area with no increased local temperature, but other signs of an abscess formation, should not be overlooked.

Muscle Atrophy

Muscle atrophy may occur from one of two causes. The muscle may have lost its innervation and therefore undergone atrophy because of its lack of muscular tone due to this loss of nerve supply, or it may be related to disuse due to immobilization in a cast, related to loss of function in the part served by these muscles, or caused by pain. The patient with an acute knee injury with pain and effusion in the knee often develops a profound quadriceps atrophy in a relatively short time. It is likewise common for a patient with a stiff painful shoulder to develop marked atrophy of the periarticular muscles due to disuse. A patient who has some numbness of the little finger associated with tenderness over the medial side of the elbow should be suspected of having a compression of the ulnar nerve in the cubital tunnel. However, muscular atrophy in the intrinsic musculature of the hand makes this diagnosis much more certain. Muscular atrophy, if due to nerve injury should, of course, follow the anatomical distribution of that nerve and should not be generalized in the extremity unless all nerves are involved. Conditions that do result in a functional loss of an extremity with resulting disuse atrophy will usually manifest a more diffuse type of atrophy involving muscles from all innervations, since the atrophy is related not to nerve supply but to lack of use.

Trophic Changes

Trophic changes should also be observed and are usually related to loss of either vascularity or innervation. The diabetic patient, for instance, may have trophic ulcers on his foot. Since he may have either a diminished blood supply due to athrosclerosis or a loss of sensation due to neuropathy, the trophic change's cause is often hard to identify. Likewise, the presence of trophic changes in an area that has functionally diminished sensation is usually a sign that the sensory loss is relatively profound. It is often difficult to evaluate sensory loss, since it requires a subjective response on the part of the patient during the testing procedure. However, if trophic changes are seen such as pulp atrophy of a digit, or, occasionally, the development of trophic or ulcerative areas in the part, one can be certain that the sensory loss is profound. Trophic changes should lead one to investigate the adequacy of the circulation to the part and of the sensory innervation.

STABILITY

Stability should be ascertained at the original examination. Often the presence or absence of stability in a part will materially influence the type of treatment necessary. Lack of stability in the site of an interphalangeal joint following injury will most likely point to the likelihood of a tear of the collateral ligament. However, loss of stability in the knee may be related to a severe atrophy of the quadriceps musculature even when the ligamentous structures are normal and intact. The examiner will have to analyze the amount of instability and the area of instability to determine the cause.

Musculature

Supporting musculature that has undergone atrophy from either loss of nerve supply or disuse is one of the most common causes of instability. As indicated previously, the patient with marked quadriceps atrophy will show instability of the knee even though the knee joint per se is otherwise normal. X-ray examinations of the patient with severe muscular atrophy of the shoulder area will often show subluxation of the humeral head from out of the glenoid fossa. This is quite frightening when visualized on the radiograph, but if the patient has marked atrophy of the shoulder girdle musculatures one can be certain that a strengthening of these muscles, if this is possible, will result in a return of the glenohumeral joint to its normal relationship. Lack of support in the quadriplegic or paraplegic patient results in periodic strains of the extremities' joints due to pressure against them without the normal protection of the supporting musculature. On the other hand, long bone fracture in paralyzed patients usually will heal without the need for immobilization, since loss of position of the fragments usually is not severe without the associated effect of muscle pull.

External Support

External support may have previously been ordered by another physician or may have been devised by the patient himself on a need basis. If these external supporting structures are present, one should determine if they are necessary, and if they provide comfort or merely stability for weight-bearing. The patient with severe low back pain who comes in using two crutches is sometimes suspect since crutch-walking does not tend to relieve low back pain to any great extent. Likewise, the patient who comes into the office using a single crutch or cane for pain in the hip or knee and who uses that support in the ipsilateral hand will have a very strange and awkward gait due to improper use of the supporting device. One cannot really evaluate the gait he has developed until the cane or crutch has been moved to the opposite hand to obtain maximal support from the device. Also, external supporting devices result in a considerable amount of muscular atrophy relatively early. The patient who has been using some sort of external supporting device should be expected to have a degree of muscular atrophy in the extremity.

FUNCTION

Function in an area that has otherwise abnormal structures, or the absence of function in an area that should be expected to work properly, is important in making a diagnosis. The examiner should be realistic in his analysis of the functional loss and determine whether it is appropriate from the condition he sees. Often the patient who comes in with an extremity such as a hand and wrist that he claims to be unable to use because of pain can be coaxed by an expert examiner into demonstrating its use. Therefore, one should temper the analysis of function with judgement and a realistic approach to the possibility of this type of functional loss rather than assuming from the beginning that the functional loss is organic.

Locomotion

Locomotion is the responsibility of the lower extremities; a loss of function in the lower extremities will result in the loss of that ability to locomote. However, conditions involving the spine may result in such painful spasm that the patient is not able to walk. These factors all should be evaluated when evaluating the patient's ability to walk properly.

Muscle Action

Muscle action, as indicated previously, may be varied by several factors. Obvious loss of muscle function from disruption of innervation should raise no problem in diagnosis except in the determination of the cause of loss. Loss of ability to move a muscle that should otherwise be functioning poses a considerably greater task for the examining physician. The second cause of muscular weakness is disuse atrophy but this should be relatively easy for the examiner to determine on the basis of the description given earlier. The third cause of diminished muscle action is voluntary, and may be due to pain caused by use of this musculature, or to a hysterical type of inability to move the part, or to a voluntary lack of effort in the person with secondary gain motives.

Testing grasp, for instance on a dynamometer, will indicate a marked diminished grasp in the involved hand of an individual who wants to impress the examiner with the severity of his condition. However, by varying the settings on the dynamometer as far as the width of the two handles on the apparatus, the astute examiner can get some idea as to whether the patient is giving maximum effort. This is difficult to ascertain when the patient is voluntarily not contracting his muscles maximally and it takes an experienced examiner to evaluate this type of patient. The primary care physician is advised to seek the help of the specialist and relieve himself of the responsibility of making these judgements if the patient seems to have physical findings out of proportion to what he would expect.

Sensation

The same recommendations for the loss of muscular power apply to the loss of sensation. The patient with sensory loss or diminution should have some obvious anatomical distribution to back up the subjective failure to admit sensation over an area. When there is no anatomical distribution to the sensory loss (such as the stocking or glove type of loss in the hysterical patient), full evaluation probably should be left to one more experienced in proving the authenticity of these findings.

Sensation can be very important in establishing a diagnosis when it does follow the anatomical distribution expected. An insensible little finger and ulnar half of the ring finger are classic in true lesions of the ulnar nerve and make the establishment of this diagnosis easy. Sensory loss of the entire palmar aspect of the hand is suspect, since this would require loss of function in both the ulnar and median nerves simultaneously. When the patient has loss of sensation over the dorsum of the entire hand as well as the palmar surface one adds an additional nerve to the ones that must have functional deficit; the likelihood of this happening to this degree with sensory loss at a given level around the extremity is very remote. Sensation should be tested with a sharp pin, as mentioned in the section on hand evaluation. The earliest sensory modality to be returned is that of moving touch, so stroking the touch pad with the pin is much more accurate early than the Weber two-point discrimination or the single static pin prick.

Joint Contractures

Joint contractures may be caused by a number of factors and require individualization to establish a diagnosis. However, in the absence of any other external factors that might result in joint contracture one must remember that contractures of the volar plate of joints or of the capsular structures of other joints result in joint deformities without many external signs. Evaluation of joint contractures often requires more expert judgement. If there is any question, these patients should be referred to the orthopedist for evaluation.

Autonomic States

The autonomic state will often influence the entire physical appearance of an extremity. Vasomotor stability should be evaluated since this makes a considerable difference in the treatment and eventual outcome. The patient with a mottling discoloration or triphasic color change in the hand should be suspected of having vasomotor instability or lability, which will have a considerable impact on the other findings. Vasomotor problems are often related to stiffness of joints and related to severe types of pain associated with those losses of joint motion. The patient with a full-blown reflex sympathetic dystrophy will usually manifest a severe "touch me not" attitude of the extremity (usually the upper extremity). The hand will be slick, shiny, somewhat swollen, and usually stiff. The hand will feel cold to the touch and the pseudomotor activity will be abnormal. The evaluation and treatment of the various autonomic imbalance states require a certain amount of expertise both in diagnosis and management. These cases should be referred to the specialist if there is any degree of severity or resistance to therapy.

SUMMARY

These recommendations comprise guidelines for examination. Each subsequent chapter will point out specific and individual findings in each area and will emphasize the general points that have been made here. However, the general outline created above should be used to monitor the usual orthopedic examination. The practitioner might do well to use this as a checklist to be certain that he has not neglected any of these features in his regular examination.

2

ORTHOPEDIC EVALUATION OF THE INJURED PATIENT

Closed Injuries
Extent of Injury
Structures Involved
  Bone
  Nerves
  Vessels
Open Injuries
Extent of the Wound
  Location
  Contamination
  Deep Structure Involvement

Age of the Wound
Tissue Viability
  Cut/Crush/Tear Ratio
Unique Features
  Bone
  Blood Vessels
  Quality of Distal Circulation
  Nerves
  Tendons
  Muscles
  Joint Coverings

This chapter deals with the musculoskeletal system in the patient who has been injured and is being evaluated for the first time. It is obvious that there are many other factors in dealing with the acutely injured patient that are not within the scope of this chapter. There is, first, the obvious possibility of injury to other systems, particularly in the patient with a suspected or obvious head injury, which requires complete evaluation probably on a higher priority basis than the evaluation of most musculoskeletal injuries unless generalized and severe. Likewise, the patient with possible abdominal injury will require evaluation of that along with the musculoskeletal injury. The second obvious exclusion is the need for evaluation of the general state with respect to shock, blood loss, volume control, and the like. These have the highest priority and will require attention before one begins with the musculoskeletal system, unless it is obvious that multiple fractures with gross instability are contributing to the blood loss and shock. Finally, there is an obvious need for evaluation of medical problems such as diabetes, heart disease, hypertension, and other conditions that will affect the patient's response to treatment. The general evaluation of the acutely injured patient will therefore require a concomitant evaluation and treatment of his entire condition, including the musculoskeletal system. The following discussion centers on the musculoskeletal system but is not meant to exclude or diminish the urgency of the need for evaluation and treatment of the patient as a whole.

13

Orthopedic injuries can be roughly classified into those associated with open wounds and those that are closed injuries. However, the extent of exterior wounds does not in any way indicate the magnitude of the underlying musculoskeletal injury. Severe pelvic fractures, or fractures of the long bones particularly in the lower extremity, will result in marked alteration in the patient's physiology since they ordinarily are associated with massive blood loss. The patient without external wounds will bleed into the soft tissue and the extent of the blood loss may not be appreciated because it is not visible.

CLOSED INJURIES

Extent of Injury

The first procedure in the examination of the injured patient is to determine the extent of injury. If a youngster has fallen off of a swing set at school and hurt his elbow, the extent is obvious. However, individuals in motor vehicle accidents are sometimes so severely injured in some areas that significant injuries are not seen in others. A good example is also the patient who falls from a height and suffers fractures of the os calcis of both feet. The pain and deformity are severe and all attention is directed toward the feet. It may not be for a day or so that one finds that he also has a fracture of his pelvis or perhaps a compression fracture of one of his vertebral bodies. For this reason the examiner must be certain of the extent of the injuries before any type of treatment is begun. One should anticipate the possibility of other injuries based on the nature of the injury and look for these "hidden injuries" when the patient is first evaluated. At this point the involvement of other organ systems can be ascertained as well as the state of shock, blood loss, and other systemic problems.

Structures Involved

In closed injuries the possibility of damage to structures must be evaluated clinically since there is no chance to visualize them. There may be massive damage to any structure in the area. However, the important components of the evaluation of the musculoskeletal system are the condition of bony structures, the peripheral nerves and blood vessels of the extremities, as well as injuries to the torso in general.

Bone

Identification and treatment of mild compression fractures of the vertebral bodies are covered in Chapters 5 and 7. Severely displaced fractures of the spine are diagnosed principally by x-ray examination and by clinical findings of neurologic deficit. Patients with such findings should be transferred immediately to the care of a physician experienced in their management. The greatest care should be taken to maintain strict immobilization on a flat surface that can be transported, to prevent accentuation of the neurologic deficit during transportation.

Other than fractures of the spine and pelvis, discussion of structures involved will be limited here to the extremities.

Location: Amount of Displacement.   It should be possible to ascertain the location of the fracture in the bone itself by x-ray examination. This information should then be relayed to the specialist if the patient is to be transferred. If the patient is to be treated by the primary care physician, the amount of displacement present in the fracture should be ascertained and the difficulty in reduction should be anticipated to know whether this falls within the capacities of the practitioner.

Communition of the Fracture.   Comminution of the fracture is an important feature from the standpoint of stability. Comminution or "shattering" of the bone at the fracture site renders the fracture extremely unstable in most instances and make the maintenance of position, once it has been restored, very difficult.

Joint Involvement.   Determining the involvement of joint surfaces in the fracture process is extremely important since it is mandatory in all cases to secure anatomical alignment of the joint surfaces if one is to avoid degenerative changes within the joint once healing has occurred. Cases with joint involvement should be referred if there is any displacement at all. Patients without a great amount of displacement can be evaluated by the primary care physician. Periodic radiographs should be taken, however, to be certain that alignment is maintained.

Stability.   The stability of the fracture usually indicates the mechanism by which position must be maintained once reduction is accomplished. A fracture that is quite unstable will require more sophisticated mechanisms for maintaining position. Once the fracture that is stable has been reduced, it can usually be quite easily held by external fixation. Follow-up studies should ascertain that the position has been maintained and that healing is progressing satisfactorily. Patients with fractures that are quite unstable should probably be referred for expert management.

Epiphyseal Involvement.   Epiphyseal involvement is an extremely important finding since complete anatomical reduction of the epiphyseal plate should be done with reduction of the fracture lines on either side of the plate. This often requires pin fixation. However, if the displacement is very slight at the time of the injury, holding with a simple external fixation will accomplish healing and the patient can be cared for by the primary care physician. If there is significant displacement of the fractures involving the epiphysis, the patient should be referred to the specialist for expert management (see Ch. 18).

Nerves

When the patient is examined the presence or absence of motor and sensory deficits should be ascertained. It is important to do this early in the course of the examination to be certain that any change in the amount of neurologic deficit can be seen. It is important to know the anatomy of the extremity well enough to anticipate the nerve that might be injured in the process and enough about the motor and sensory distribution of this nerve to determine whether or not it is functioning. Complete records should be kept of the examination to document the changing picture. Particularly in cases with medicolegal possibilities, early recording of nerve function is mandatory.

It is important to ascertain, if possible, whether the nerve has been completely divided or whether it has been injured but is still intact. This is often very difficult to ascertain and only time may provide the full answer. If one can determine that the nerve has been divided, such as by piercing with adjacent bone, early operative restoration of continuity should be performed and the patient referred for specialized care. If, however, it appears that the nerve has only been bruised or is bleeding due to the nature of the wound, careful observation and evaluation of the amount of neurologic deficit are permissible. If in doubt, however, the primary care physician should most likely refer this patient to one experienced in treating nerve injury.

Vessels

Determining the sufficiency of the circulation is important when the patient is first seen. Mechanisms that interfere with venous return result in a cyanosis of the part if the arterial circulation is still present. The veins, of course, are much more easily compressed than arteries. If tamponade is occurring from swelling or bleeding within a fixed compartment in the extremity, the venous circulation is lost first but is soon afterwards followed by loss of arterial circulation. The loss of arterial supply leaves the part completely white or cadaveric in Caucasians and various degrees of pallor can be seen in the skin or the nail beds of people with pigmented skin. Obviously the patency of vessels should be evaluated to determine whether the vessels have been sectioned, impaled on a spicule of bone, or thrombosed by severe damage to the vessel wall or whether encroachment by other structures has resulted in occlusion. It is often impossible to determine this in the beginning, but if the patient develops acute vascular insufficiency in the extremity operative intervention is indicated to prevent circulatory damage that cannot be repaired. The patient should be referred to a specialist as soon as possible. The same is true for tamponade by acute swelling, particularly in fascial compartments of the extremity, where occlusion of otherwise normal vessels results from the increased extrensic pressure. Such cases are also surgical emergencies and should be referred to a specialist as soon as possible.

OPEN INJURIES

The acute orthopedic injury with an open wound often appears more serious than the closed wound, but may have some advantages over the closed injury. The extent of bleeding can be ascertained more adequately, tamponade from a compartment syndrome is less likely, and the open wound allows better visibility in determining the amount of damage to deep structures. There is also sometimes less likely to be prolonged damage to structures since bleeding into the soft tissues does not occur to as great an extent because the blood is not trapped. The structures are not damaged to as great a degree and do not become the site of such an intense inflammatory reaction because of the retained blood, and the prognosis for restoration of function may be better. However, open wounds always provide open access to bacteria and may be the site of gross contamination that greatly increases the likelihood of infection. Also, open wounds usually signify a greater amount of trauma so that the entire injury is likely to be more severe. Finally, open wounds require immediate surgical treatment for cleansing and debridement along with any definitive care that can be carried out. Open wounds will reflect different indications and aims of treatment and will be discussed more or less along the same lines as were closed injuries.

Extent of the Wound

The magnitude of the open wound signifies the extent of the injury in most, but not all, cases. All physicians have seen relatively small puncture wounds from a knife that has lacerated the femoral artery. On the other hand a mammoth wound with a 20 or 30 cm laceration may not have resulted in any damage other than to the superficial tissues and muscle. The extent of the wound is important from the standpoint of the magnitude of the injury but does not necessarily interpolate into the gravity of the situation. Several factors are important in evaluating the open wound.

Location

Location of the wound is a guide to the possibility of damage to underlying structures. Once again it becomes important for the physician to visualize the deep anatomy to determine the possibilities for injury to deep structures from any single wound. A puncture wound in the palm of the hand has serious implications even though it is relatively small because of the great many of important structures there. Such wounds cause the examiner to evaluate distal function since most of the structures running through the palm act on the digits. It is important to reiterate the admonition to examine function distal to the wound before injecting local anesthetic. The anesthetic will cause sensory loss to common digital nerves; and if the examination is done after the anesthetic has been injected the examiner will not be able to determine whether sensory loss is due to the injury or to the anesthetic. Wounds in other locations require a similar careful evaluation, and functional evaluation distal to the point of the wound is always the key to determining structures that may be damaged.

Contamination

The amount of contamination is of great importance and should be noted at the original examination. Massively contaminated wounds will require a much more thorough operative procedure, including debridement and cleansing. Even with this, massively contaminated wounds will have a greater chance of postinjury infection. Usually they should be left open and packed for a later secondary closure. Even small wounds should be carefully examined for gross contamination if the wound is made by a penetrating object since that object may be grossly contaminated and inoculate the wound.

Deep Structure Involvement

Although deep structure involvement has been discussed previously, it should be reiterated that the path of a penetrating projectile is often difficult to ascertain from clinical examination. The examiner must not necessarily assume that the object penetrates at right angle to the skin surface. Angulation of the path of the object may result in involvement of structures at some distance from the entrance wound and should be taken into account. Early in the examination it may be possible to palpate gently the depths of a wound to determine its course and the possibility of damage to underlying structures.

Age of the Wound

The age of the wound when first examined is important since wounds seen after the traditional 8-hour period required for colonization of injected bacteria are much more likely to become infected than wounds seen and cleansed immediately. Wounds that have been opened after 8 or 10 hours, even though relatively clean, should be treated as contaminated since bacteria injected into the wound at the time of injury have had ample time to begin colonization and multiplication in the excellent natural incubator afforded by the deeper structures of the extremity. Antibiotic coverage almost routinely given to patients with open injuries will extend this period considerably. If the patient has been given appropriate prophylactic antibiotics relative early, so that a blood level has been present, one can often assume that bacterial growth has been impeded and the time for successful debridement significantly extended.

Tissue Viability

Tissue viability is often difficult to determine in treating open wounds. If there is considerable mangling of soft tissue, small islands and pedicles of soft tissue are likely to be present since these have been detached superficially but may still have an adequate blood supply from intact deeper vessels.

While it is important to adhere strictly to the rules of debridement (resection of obviously dead, dirty, and devitalized tissue), determining what tissue has become devitalized is often difficult. The experience and judgement of the operator will then be the primary indicator. As a general rule, if there is adequate soft tissue in the area and a small island of tissue appears to be badly damaged, it is probably better not to take the chance on the tissue subsequently dying and it should be removed. On the other hand, if the area of questionable tissue is relatively vital for coverage of important structures or for maintenance of function, one can gamble somewhat on leaving the tissue in the hope that a considerable amount of time will have been saved when reconstructive procedures are begun. Since partially devitalized tissue has a much greater susceptibility to infection, excision of this questionable tissue is much more likely to be necessary if there is gross contamination of the wound. The judgement call should probably favor excision.

Cut/Crush/Tear Ratio

The cut/crush/tear ratio is of considerable importance in many parts of the body but particularly in the hand. Cleaned incised wounds usually heal without difficulty and with minimal scarring. However, crushing usually results in damage to soft tissue structures including capillaries. This results in an outpouring of inflammatory edema fluid soon after the injury, which evokes a fibrocytic response and results in greater scarring. Two wounds with the same obvious damage to structures will have completely different postoperative courses if one is a cleanly incised wound and the other is a result of crushing that "pinches" the structures rather than merely cutting them.

The latter will have a much greater chance of intense fibrocytic response and a much greater amount of scarring. While nothing much can be done about this at the original surgery, recognition of these factors should be recorded so that the prognosis can be more readily determined.

Unique Features

As with closed injuries, unique features of open injuries relate to the specific structure involved.

Bone

In cases of open wounds near a fracture, one must assume that the fracture has communicated with the outside and should be treated accordingly. Even though a fragment of bone may not be seen protruding from the wound, careful palpation of the wound will reveal communication with the fracture in most instances, particularly if the fracture is comminuted with many smaller spicules of bone. It is also important to determine whether a wound overlying a fracture is caused by a portion of the fractured bone protruding from the skin or whether the object that caused the fracture penetrated through the soft tissue to the bone. The implication of each possibility is immediately obvious. Bone that protruded from the skin may have been contaminated and then been withdrawn back into the wound as the fracture was reduced, possibly at the scene of the accident. The penetrating wound will therefore have been contaminated with foreign material as the object passed through the soft tissue. Bone that has been exposed, particularly if it has protruded, must be meticulously cleaned and any small fragments that are likely to become nonviable should be completely removed. Once again, the extent of the debridement is relative to the amount of contamination and the time since the injury.

Blood Vessels

Blood vessels are somewhat easier to identify through open wounds and the extent of the injury to the vessel is more easily determined than in closed wounds. Although there is not the accumulation of extravasated blood seen with closed wounds it is often difficult to determine the exact amount of blood loss in an open wound. The blood may have been shed at the scene of the accident and its amount not fully appreciated once the patient is seen in the emergency room. If the vessels can be visualized in an open wound, one can be more certain that considerable blood loss has occurred. Immediate evaluation of the blood count as well as the blood volume is necessary.

Quality of Distal Circulation

The quality of distal circulation should be ascertained. If there is massive injury with complicated fractures of the bones of the extremity, circulation distal to this can be expected to be poor.

This is particularly true if there is considerable shortening of the extremity with kinking and twisting of the vessels. Once the extremity has been brought out into its proper length and better alignment of the vessels accomplished, a much better chance for function may exist and the circulation will often improve considerably. This is probably more true of venous than arterial function since the former is a lower-pressure system with thinner-walled vessels. Often the circulatory loss seen immediately following severe injury to an extremity is due in part to vasospasm. If the extremity has been restored to its approximate normal length and there is still marked vascular insufficiency with intact vessels present, consideration should be given to the means of relieving this arterial spasm.

Nerves

Evaluation of the status of peripheral nerves distal to the injury is of utmost importance and should be done early in the initial evaluation. The original evaluation should be recorded so that subsequent examinations can be compared with it. In most instances recording of a complete motor or sensory deficit at the time of the original evaluation is important. Much more important than this, however, is when one finds an intact motor and sensory component to a nerve and a deterioration of the neurologic status on subsequent examinations to the extent that the motor or sensory function is lost. This indicates progressive damage to the nerve, such as by swelling, bleeding, or subsequent impaling, and is usually an indication for exploration.

The nerve should be inspected (if it is easy to do without a great amount of dissection) to note whether the injury is from actual division or merely from contusion and/or intraneural bleeding. Most investigators' treatment of choice today for a massive open wound with contamination is to clean out the wound, close or pack in whatever manner is necessary, and return to do a delayed primary repair when the tissue balance has been established, usually in a week or 10 days. If a segmental loss of the nerve occurs, complete wound healing can be established first since a nerve graft will be necessary. This can be done within the first 2 or 3 months with an equal prospect of recovery. There is no real objection to a primary repair of severed nerves at the time of the original debridement, if time permits and the facilities are adequate. However, when the patient is seen in one emergency setting but transferred to another for subsequent care there is no harm in leaving the nerve repair to be done on a delayed primary basis after several days, since statistics show that the results of this procedure are at least equal to those of primary neurrophaphy at the time of the injury.

Tendons

Tendons are ordinarily repaired at the time of the original injury if they occupy an area of the extensive open wound that makes them accessible and if there is time following completion of debridement and repair of other structures. As with nerves, there is no harm in suturing a primary wound and returning in 7 to 10 days for a delayed primary repair of the flexor tendon.

As in the case of lacerated nerves, results have been shown statistically to be as good with a delayed primary repair of tendons as with a repair done at the time of the original injury. A laceration across the volar aspect of a finger that sections the flexor tendons can well be treated by the primary contact physician with simple cleansing, debridement, irrigation, and primary closure of the skin wound. The hand and finger should then be splinted in flexion to prevent retraction of the proximal end of the tendon and the patient should be referred to a specialist for subsequent delayed primary repair. Splinting of the wrist and finger in flexion is important to prevent retraction of the proximal end as much as is possible. More discussion of this subject is given in Chapter 11, The Hand.

Muscles

Muscle tissue has excellent blood supply and healing usually occurs without much difficulty. Scarring may occur, but muscle elasticity can usually be restored with time and proper therapy. Muscles should be debrided adequately to remove all dead, dirty, and devitalized tissue. However, muscle has a much better resistance to infection because there is a great degree of vascularity. Wounds involving primarily muscle bellies can usually be debrided and closed well without much fear of poor consequences.

Joint Coverings

Joints should always be covered if at all possible. If an open wound extends into a joint, the joint should be opened wide enough for inspection to be certain that no contaminated material is included. Once this has been ascertained, the joint should be thoroughly lavaged and closed primarily to restore its integrity as quickly as possible. In some instances there may be a loss of some capsular material, so complete closure is not possible. If this occurs, adjacent soft tissue should be pulled over the joint to try to close the wound as well as possible over the joint. In the case of larger joints such as the knee it is wise to use, in conjunction with primary closure of the joint, a continuous wound drainage tube within the joint so that accumulation of blood and fluid will not destroy the capsular repair during the immediate postoperative period. This can be removed in 24 to 48 hours. Otherwise, always attempt to establish joint coverings as much as possible with the materials at hand. Ligaments should likewise be restored as much as possible at the time of the original repair. Splinting should then be used to allow complete healing of the ligamentous or capsular repair before motion is started.

3

FRACTURES: GENERAL PRINCIPLES

HEALING

Cortical Bone

A discussion of fracture healing must be divided into two parts since there is a tremendous amount of difference in the healing of fractures that occur in cortical bone and those occurring in cancellous bone.

In a fracture with minimal separation in cortical bone the callus that forms around the fracture usually begins in two different areas. First it begins as external callus that occurs by proliferation of the osteophytes along the periosteum. These are stripped up from the end of the bone with periosteum. As the cells begin to form bone matrix they begin to build up on the end of each of the bones that will bridge across, much as a suspension bridge does from points on either side. Of course, this occurs circumferentially around the bone so that an actual knob is formed at the end of each bone.

At the same time external callus is forming, an internal callus forms from osteophytes that line the inner surface of the bones. Around the margins of the medullary canal certain cells have the property of becoming osteophytes under specific conditions: these cells become osteophytes if provoked by the stimulus of an injury.

Endosteal callus is not nearly as important as external callus, but it does allow for some increase in the amount of new bone mass that forms. Because there is both internal and external callus, there is a much greater amount of callus formation in this weld and healing occurs more rapidly. Cells that change into osteophytes are what early investigators called "cells of the terrain." These

23

nonspecific cells suddenly gain the function of osteophytes and begin to form osteoid tissue. Once formed, osteoid tissue gradually fills in with mineral salts to become mature bone.

When much comminution occurs there is a greater stimulus to the formation of osteoid tissue. This may partially be due to subperiosteal hemorrhage, because we know that stripping or irritation of the periosteum provokes a response to form osteoid. Comminution may merely increase the amount of periosteal reaction and thereby create more new bone. Direct trauma to the midshaft of a bone such as the tibia will result in a periosteal lifting that will allow for bone formation underneath. Periosteum that has been lifted up by hematoma, even without fracture, will form a prominence on bone by much the same process that we see in healing fractures.

Cancellous Bone

Cancellous bone consists of a labyrinth of trabeculae lined by osteoblastic cells. New bone is created in all areas of cancellous bone simultaneously. All the bone spicules are covered with osteoblasts that begin to form bone when stimulated. Healing in cancellous bone is therefore usually much more rapid, much more complete, and much more certain.

Cancellous bone such as is found in the upper tibia has one undesirable feature: it tends to compress because it is spongy. Therefore, a fracture of the tibial plateau that compresses down on one side of the plateau will result in an actual condensation of bone underneath. When the articular surface is lifted back up into position, a large defect in the bone occurs because this bone is compressed. Bone grafting will be necessary to fill this void.

When cancellous bone does heal it is much more difficult to evaluate by x-ray studies because it does not tend to build up external callus. Therefore, watching a fracture healing across the tibial plateau usually is a matter of waiting until the fracture line has disappeared in order to determine whether or not it is healing. Because of this a timetable of the length of time necessary for these various fractures to heal is established. They are usually considered to be healed if enough time has elapsed, almost regardless of what the radiograph shows.

Radiographs are taken to see if the fracture line has disappeared. A fracture, for instance, in cancellous bone in the superior part of the tibia usually requires a minimum of 10 to 12 weeks to heal well enough for pressure to be allowed on it. Weight-bearing is usually begun at that time purely on the basis of time elapsed. A bone that has healed by external callus, on the other hand, will demonstrate callus formation, and bridging will be seen. Healing is not considered to be solid in these fractures until this bridging can be demonstrated on the x-ray examination.

The carpal navicular bone is entirely cancellous but in spite of this the percentage of nonunion of fractures in this bone is relatively high. This is true because this bone has a unique blood supply and many times the fracture itself destroys the blood supply in one of the fragments. Therefore, in spite of the fact that it is cancellous and should heal in 6 weeks, this bone usually takes a minimum of 12 weeks to heal because of the poor blood supply.

DEFORMING FORCES

When a fracture occurs in a long bone, three primary forces result in the loss of position of the fracture.

Force of Injury

The most common factor is the force of the injury itself. It is a deforming factor because the amount of injury necessary to break a bone is that amount necessary to overcome the physical structure of the bone and result in disruption of its continuity. There is no way, however, to apply that amount of pressure and suddenly stop as soon as the bone breaks. The force that breaks the bone carries on through and separates the parts once they are broken. An example of this is the bumper fracture of the tibia. The bumper breaks the tibia by contact but the pressure is not suddenly withdrawn: the force of the car still goes on through so the deforming factor is usually what causes the injury.

Effect of Gravity

The deforming effect of gravity is important and easier to understand when one thinks of it in terms of a long bone. For instance, consider the femur of a person lying on a stretcher. The bone is more or less suspended because it is supported at its two ends, plus whatever intervening support the muscle gives. If the bone is broken in the center there will still be suspension at the hip area and at the knee, so bowing occurs in the middle because of the effect of gravity. One must overcome the pull of gravity if this fracture is to be reduced with the patient in this position. This best can be done by traction.

When a fracture is caused by direct trauma, the fracture occurs and the force that created it suddenly is withdrawn. The effect of gravity, however is continuous and must be overcome by internal fixation, traction, or other methods. As long as the fracture is in a position not longitudinal to the pull of gravity, the factor of gravity will be working continuously unless counteracted.

Muscle Pull

Probably the most important factor is that of muscle pull. The fracture that occurs in an extremity with flaccid paralysis will usually not be deformed because it has no muscle pull. In a paralyzed extremity, the deformity of the fracture is minimal and is usually only that of gravity since gravity is still functional. The person who does have muscle pull presents a completely different problem because the muscles themselves tend to cause deformity. The first thing that happens following a fracture is that the muscles surrounding the bone go into spasm and deformity occurs because they act as a bowstring. The bowstringing effect causes the loss of position of fractures. Though all three factors must be taken into consideration, the most important in many fractures is muscle pull.

METHODS OF TREATMENT

The basic aims of treatment of fractures are (1) to restore the alignment of the fracture and remove deformities in the extremity, (2) to secure apposition of fractures so that healing may occur, and (3) to obtain union of the fragments and healing of the fracture. Any mechanism for treating fractures must take these factors into account; not addressing any one of these three factors will often result in failure. If alignment is not obtained, of course, deformity results; if apposition does not occur, union is likely to be faulty; if union does not occur, of course, the whole project has been of no avail.

The treatment of fractures must therefore include the restoration of position and then some means of maintaining that while healing occurs. There are three primary methods of reduction—traction, closed reduction, and open reduction—and all have their inherent requirements for immobilization once the fracture has been reduced.

Traction

Skin traction per se has very little place in the treatment of fractures and is useful only for temporary immobilization, perhaps as a means of getting the patient ready for transportation. Skeletal traction is, therefore, the only mechanism that has any merit. This requires drilling a pin or wire through the bone and the application of traction utilizing this point.

The theory of traction is relatively simple. As described previously, one of the main mechanisms of displacement of fractures is muscle pull. If one considers that the bones are maintained in a soft tissue tube, it is easy to visualize that stretching the extremity by traction reestablishes that tube. The soft tissues, particularly the muscles, act as a means of immobilizing the bones once this soft tissue "tube" has been reestablished by the traction. This is particularly true in comminuted fractures, where the multiple small pieces are extremely hard to approximate by any other mechanism.

However, if it is to be effective traction must also include a mechanism to prevent the effects of gravity and its action on the segments being treated.

Consider a fracture of the femur. A pin is drilled through the distal femur to set up longitudinal traction. If this is done with the extremities lying on the bed, the proximal fragment will still be pulled against the bed by the effect of gravity and the distal fragment will be mobile, even though reduction has been established. It would follow, then, that any type of motion through the distal portion of the set-up will cause motion at the fracture site. The establishment of nonunion in this instance would be very likely.

If a mechanism such as a sling totally suspends the extremity so that there is no effect of gravity on any portion, the entire extremity including the fracture is

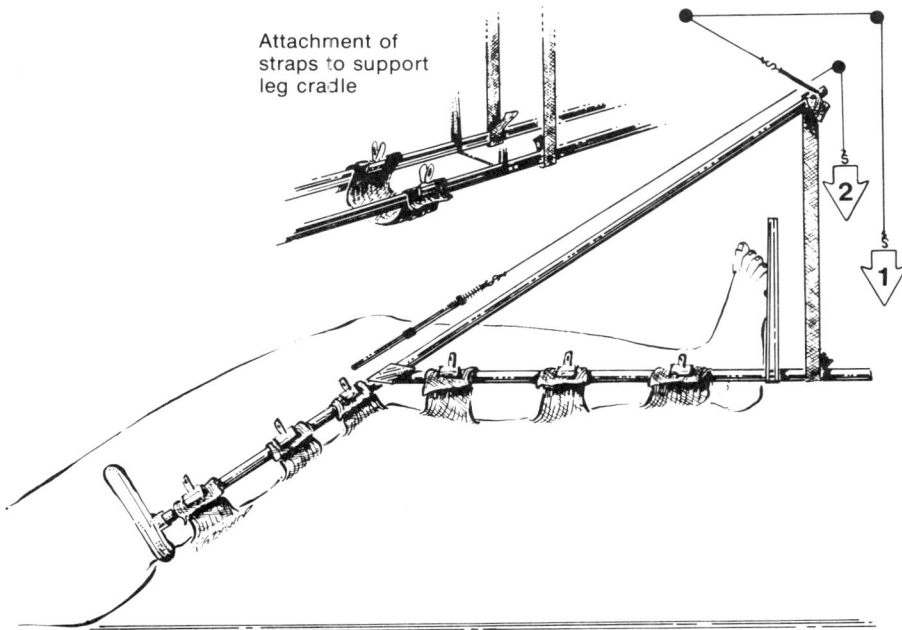

Attachment of
straps to support
leg cradle

Fig. 3-1. The typical balanced traction setup for the lower extremity. The basic suspension unit is composed of some type of traction frame, such as the Thomas traction ring or one of the various modifications. To this is attached an out-rigger that can be moved up or down the long axis of the basic traction frame so that the length of the femur can be accommodated. This small out-rigger, then, allows for the support of the extremity below the knee. The distal portion of the out-rigger is attached to the distal end of the main frame by means of tape or straps (*inset*). These may be adjusted to allow for variations in the amount of flexion at the knee, but as a general rule, approximately 45 degrees of flexion is desirable and is most comfortable. The amount of flexion at the knee does not materially influence the traction that occurs through the distal femur, proximal to the knee joint itself. The frame is suspended by a rope (1) that is attached to the distal end of the frame and passed through a pulley. The pulley is placed proximally, in order to support the frame in the elevated position. The rope then runs to a distal pulley and over to a weight. The amount of weight is that just sufficient to create a weightless condition in the extremity, so that the frame, being precisely counterbalanced, will stay in almost any position in which it is placed. A second line is then attached to the traction bow (2) and is brought either over or under the distal portion of the main traction frame. It is attached to a single pulley bearing the amount of weight that is deemed desirable for traction to the femur. It should be noted that the two weights have entirely different responsibilities, that through line (1) having the function of supporting the frame against the pull of gravity, and that of (2) furnishing the actual traction through the femur (Lewis RC, Jr: Handbook of Traction, Casting and Splinting Techniques. JB Lippincott, Philadelphia, 1977.)

transformed into a single segment, with motion occurring only at the hip joint. By maintaining length with the traction and maintaining reduction by the "soft tissue sleeve" concept, the fracture will be very likely to heal since motion will occur only at the hip joint and not at the fracture site.

The usual mechanism for suspension of the extremity in traction is shown in Figure 3-1, in which a Thomas traction ring is used with a Pierson attachment so that the extremity can be held with the knee flexed and traction at the distal femur. This allows for traction without any interference from gravity through the fracture site itself and transforms the entire extremity into a single unit. The Thomas traction ring and Pierson attachment sling are then set up with a system of ropes, pullies, and weights so that they are exactly "counterbalanced" and assume a condition of weightlessness. In this position the effect of gravity has been completely overcome: the extremity swings weightless in the sling and the effects of traction work on the fracture site unimpeded.

Variations of this type of balanced traction are used in the "90–90" type of traction in children. The extremity itself is put in a cast and the traction can be placed at right angles to the bed. Therefore, longitudinal pull is along the lines of the effects of gravity. Gravity is overcome and the extremity is still held in a relatively weightless condition so that the effects of traction are exerted along the long axis of the femur.

These basic principles of traction can be altered slightly to accommodate any situation in any extremity. One is referred to textbooks on this subject, one of which is written by the author.

Closed Reduction

Reduction of the fracture without an open operation is the procedure of choice when possible; when acceptable, reduction with adequate fixation can be established by this means. The treatment of fractures by traction is, as a concept, a method of closed reduction and immobilization being maintained by the traction itself. However, the term "closed reduction" implies reduction of the fracture by manipulation and some type of anesthesia is, therefore, required. If the fracture is in such a location that muscle pull is not a great factor (such as in the hand), local infiltration or at least regional block anesthesia is adequate and usually the most feasible. If the fracture occurs in such a location that muscle pull is a major factor in the creation of the deformity, the anesthetic must also induce muscle relaxation so that the deforming factor may be overcome. A fracture of the midshafts of both bones of the forearm, for instance, is extremely difficult to reduce without some type of anesthesia that affords muscle relaxation. The general anesthetic, therefore, is usually much preferable, though a block anesthesia will afford enough muscle paralysis for reduction to be done. In the author's experience, complicated or badly comminuted fractures of the distal radius, as seen in some types of Colle's fractures, are much easier to reduce and maintain with the patient anesthetized. One will find the anesthetized patient much easier to manage and reduction will be much easier to maintain.

The second point of importance in the nonoperative treatment of fractures concerns the adequacy of reduction. While some fractures will "fall back into place" by closed manipulation it is usually very difficult to secure a 100 percent anatomical reduction using closed methods.

The operator must therefore decide whether the reduction he can obtain by closed means is acceptable. A complete discussion of the points involved in ascertaining the adequacy of reduction is included in Chapter 4, Complications of Fracture Treatment. It should be emphasized, however, that the decision to leave the fracture in a less than anatomical reduction is easy for the primary care physician to make. If he considers that he has done the best that he can in securing this reduction, the immobilizing apparatus can be applied and the patient referred to the orthopedic surgeon. This decision is not irrevocable at the time the original manipulation is done; the fracture can be remanipulated or treated by open means and internal fixation any time within the first week or so after the fracture has occurred, if the orthopedic surgeon feels that it should. When a fracture has initially been reduced and the decision is not clear as to whether the reduction is acceptable, the patient can be referred and the responsibility of that decision turned over to the specialist.

Following completion of the reduction by closed means, the acceptable method of immobilization must then be determined. It should be pointed out that a fracture that is not relatively stable in the reduced position cannot be held by external fixation, such as a splint or casting. A position favorable to maintenance of reduction, of course, is of great value. The Colles fracture that may be unstable in the straight or slightly extended position of the wrist may be quite stable with the wrist flexed. The cast or splint can be applied, but serial radiographs should be taken at relatively short intervals to be certain that reduction is being maintained.

The use of undue pressure from an external splinting device, in an effort to maintain reduction of a relatively unstable fracture, is to be avoided. These mechanisms not only cause pressure phenomena within the cast, or circulatory embarrassment by being too tight, but also are not adequate to hold the fracture and result only in unwanted complications. A cast or splint created in a ridge to maintain pressure over a fracture so that its reduction can be maintained usually will not be successful. Such practices are extremely dangerous since they almost invariably result in a soft tissue damage from pressure necrosis. Of course, the joint above and below the fracture site should be immobilized in the splint or cast and the favorable position for maintaining stability should be recognized, as already mentioned.

Other than this attention to details, however, the primary care physician should attempt to reduce and maintain the fracture under a suitable anesthesia by relatively standard measures and then take frequent postreduction radiographs to determine the stability of the fracture. If it can be maintained in this manner, the patient can remain under his care only for the time required for adequate healing. If, however, these repeated radiographs do show some shift or change in position of the fragments in the immobilization mechanism the patient should be referred for consultation with the orthopedic surgeon. It is not worth the risk of creating soft tissue damage or circulatory embarrassment by more heroic means. Most of the time, referral of the patient with questionable position or stability is the ''better part of valor.''

Open Reduction

Use of an open operation to reduce and stabilize a fracture is to be reserved for instances in which these cannot be done by closed measures. Open reduction, of course, has the advantage of allowing a more nearly anatomical reduction of the fracture along with removal of intervening soft tissue and the retrieval of important structures such as nerves or vessels from the fracture. Once the fracture has been reduced by open means some type of internal fixation can usually be applied so that the fracture is much easier to manage and the type and degree of immobilization becomes most critical postoperatively. This is not to say that most fractures that undergo open reduction and internal fixation do not require further immobilization. Most of them do. However, it makes the maintenance of position dependent not only on the internal or external fixation mechanisms alone but on a combination of the two so that external immobilization particularly is not as critical.

There are certain disadvantages of open reduction treatment of fractures however. An open operation involves all of the inherent dangers of anesthesia and infection through the open wound. Of increasing importance in these days of high medical costs is that open reduction is often more expensive. Finally, the chances of nonunion or delayed union of fractures are thought by many to be increased by open reduction. Stripping of soft tissue from the bones will often interfere with blood supply, so healing may be impaired. In addition, the fixation device may be inappropriately applied so that the fracture ends are slightly distracted, resulting in the obvious increased chance for problems in healing of the fracture.

For these reasons the physician must very carefully weigh all factors before recommending open reduction treatment of any fracture. Most open reduction procedures do not fall within the realms of the primary care physician unless he has had considerable experience. The physician must evaluate his own experience and ability in deciding whether the patient should be referred to the specialist.

It is not within the scope of this book to evaluate the various means of internal fixation. Various fractures will be stable with only the use of transfixing screws whereas others will require bone plates and screw fixation to maintain adequate stability. Intermedullary rods and fixation devices have become quite popular in the past several years. These techniques, for the most part, are dependent on a greater amount of expertise in their use and should be reserved for use by the specialist.

Among the simplest and most frequently used methods of internal fixation are percutaneous pins. With the wide availability of facilities for image intensifying, many fractures, particularly in the small bones of the hand and upper extremity, may be very adequately treated by closed reduction with percutaneous pinning under image-intensifier control.

Likewise, even when fractures are subjected to open reduction, percutaneous pins can be used for internal fixation. This seems to have particular merit since these pins can be left protruding or can be buried just under the skin for subsequent removal with very little difficulty once the fracture has healed. As with open reduction techniques, the use of percutaneous pinning depends upon a certain level of expertise and the availability of equipment that allows better visualization. The primary care physician must evaluate the availability of this level of expertise and specialized equipment before making a final decision.

4

COMPLICATIONS OF FRACTURE TREATMENT

Failure of Recognition
Loss of Position
Apposition
Angulation
Loss of Length
Rotation
Causes
Vascular Complications
Immediate
Delayed
Treatment
Neurologic Complications

Immediate
Delayed
Reflex Sympathetic Dystrophy
Persistent Swelling
Joint Stiffness
Contractural Phenomenon
Muscular Atrophy
Vasomotor Phenomena
Pain
Treatment
Pressure Phenomena

While having certain rules and guidelines, the treatment of fractures still is relatively arbitrary in some cases. Opinions vary among even expert orthopedic surgeons concerning the proper treatment. The treatment of fractures, however, no matter how good, is occasionally associated with various complications. It is important for the primary care physician to recognize, evaluate, and treat these complications.

FAILURE OF RECOGNITION

Failure to recognize fractures, of course, is the one feature that haunts many primary care physicians, since all have been confronted with occasions in which the fracture was very difficult to visualize on the original film. It is always advisable to have quality radiographs before attempting to evaluate the presence or absence of a fracture. Many times, however, films taken in the emergency department are of relatively poor quality, not only in their exposure and development but also their positioning. Quite often also, an inadequate number of views are taken. This makes it impossible to evaluate the presence or absence of a fracture properly. While there are many instances in which the fracture is very difficult to visualize, several are relatively common and bear mentioning (Fig. 4-1).

It is sometimes quite difficult to determine whether or not a subcapital fracture of the hip exists. The patient is brought into the emergency department with pain in the hip but x-ray evaluation does not allow the physician to make a definite diagnosis. The features pointed out above are very important in the recognition of hip fractures. To start with, a spot film should be taken. Many times a simple anteroposterior (AP) view of the pelvis is taken, which does not give true projectional information about the hip. The spot film should be taken with the central beam directly over the hip for better evaluation. A lateral film should also be taken. This can generally be done by "across the table" technique with the plate impinged upon the iliac crest on the same side with the tube at table level, and the opposite or normal leg elevated so that the beam shoots underneath it. A true lateral view can thus be obtained and many times the very

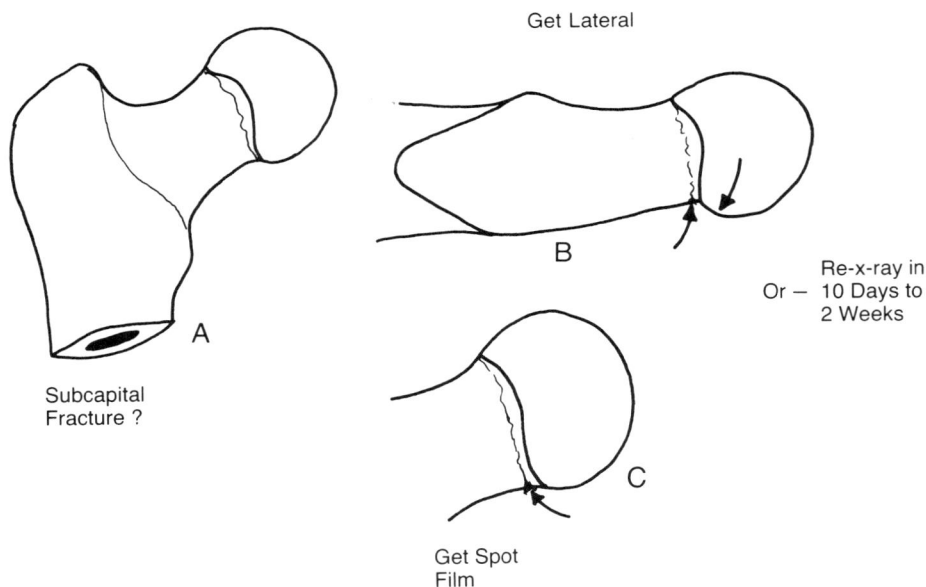

Fig. 4-1. Examples of the methods used to identify the subcapital fracture of the hip when it is difficult to see on the plain anteroposterior (AP) film. **(A)** This drawing indicates the normal film with a possible crack in the subcapital view. **(B)** The same hip in a lateral projection is represented. This must be taken as an "across the table lateral" with the tube tilted horizontally underneath the opposite or sound leg and the plate placed across the opposite hip, with the hip held in a completely neutral rotational position (toes up). The film should be at approximately 45 degrees to the long axis of the femur in order to obtain a true lateral picture. Note the small amount of posterior displacement of the head fracture and wrinkling of the cortex on the posterior margin of the fracture. **(C)** Often a simple spot film taken directly over the fracture site will show evidence of wrinkling or breaching of the cortex that can not be seen on a plain film. If a fracture still cannot be determined, new radiographs should be taken 10 days to 2 weeks after the first set. Demineralization around the fracture site will make it show up more clearly.

subtle changes present at the cortical margins can be picked up on lateral films only.

If it is still impossible to ascertain whether a fracture is present, the best policy is to have the patient not bear weight, ambulating on crutches, and repeat the radiographs in 2 weeks. At that time enough demineralization should have occurred around the fracture site to allow positive identification of the fracture line. The patient should be informed that it is difficult to make the diagnosis and that additional films will be taken in 2 weeks.

Fractures of the carpal scaphoid are often extremely difficult to identify. When the proper candidate (usually a young man in his late teens or early 20s) has fallen on the outstretched arm with the wrist in extension and has pain and swelling over the anatomical snuff box, the index of suspicion should be great. Once again it is impossible to tell without adequate x-ray examination and multiple films should be taken. These should include a "scaphoid series," which takes AP films in both the ulnar and radial deviation position as well as oblique and true lateral film. Again, if it is still impossible to tell for certain whether a fracture exists, the patient should be immobilized in a gauntlet type cast that includes the thumb for 3 weeks and the cast removed at that time for reexamination by x-ray. Enough demineralization should have occurred that the fracture will be easily identifiable. If none is seen at that time one can be relatively certain that none exists. The 3 weeks of immobilization should be considered as excellent treatment for the sprained wrist, which, of course, is the alternative diagnosis if no fracture exists.

Fractures of the elbow in children are often difficult to evaluate because of the considerable variation in the presence of the epiphyseal centers around the elbow. In this instance, as in many other instances, particularly in children with unusual epiphyseal center presentations, x-raying the opposite normal joint will often give an excellent model with which to compare the questionable side.

LOSS OF POSITION

Often when a fracture has been reduced and additional radiographs are taken in a short period of time the position will be found to have changed. The physician is confronted with the question of whether this fracture remains in an acceptable position. There are four considerations from the standpoint of position.

Apposition

Figure 4-2 demonstrates the great latitude acceptable from the standpoint of apposition, since the development of callus will invariably remodel the bone and allow for any offset in position, as long as the patient has (1) no angulation at the fracture site and (2) no shortening. Otherwise, even relatively large percentages of degrees of apposition may be acceptable, particularly in younger patients.

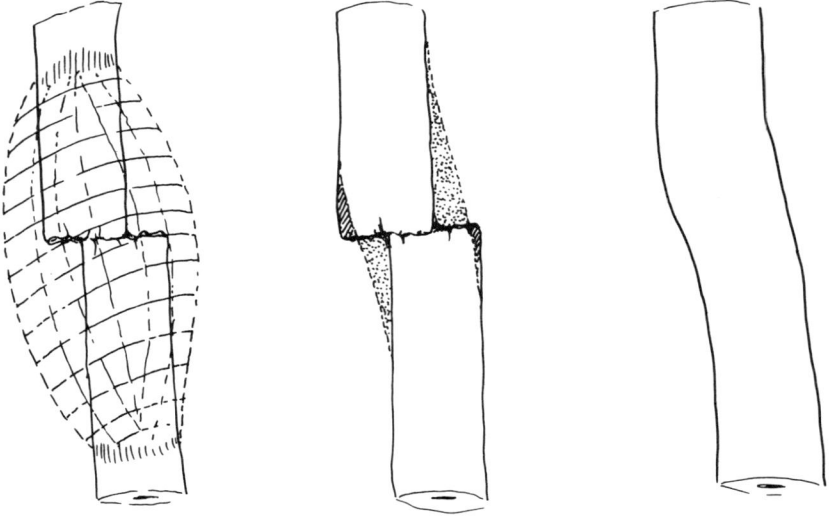

Fig. 4-2. Apposition. Lack of complete apposition can be justified as long as alignment is good and there is no shortening, as remodeling can be expected to take place as shown.

Angulation

Figure 4-3 demonstrates several principles that are important in evaluating the results of angulation. To start with, fractures that are near an epiphyseal center allow a considerably greater latitude of angulation since the almost invariable correction that occurs in the epiphyseal line will make up for a surprising degree of deformity. It is still better to obtain as good a position as possible even near the epiphysis. In a fracture that has lost position, a considerable amount of deformity can be accepted without remanipulation since it can be expected to remodel considerably because of its proximity to the epiphyseal plate. Other than this, remodeling occurs by the tendency of bone to adhere to Wolfe's Law. Wolfe's Law, simply stated, is that bone tends to be laid down along the lines of stress. If one considers a fracture that is angulated, such as Figure 4-3B the line of stress is across the concave side of the bone at the fracture level. Bone will naturally tend to be laid down along these lines of stress, which fall outside of the bone per se. These lines of stress will stimulate the laying down of bone in layers so that ultimate remodeling occurs both from this laying down of bone across the concave side and the gradual dissolution of bone across the unstressed convex side.

Finally, another point of considerable importance is the projection of angulation. Angulatory deformities near the distal end of a digit, for instance, are sometimes more acceptable than those that occur more distally in the ray. This is accounted for by the projection of angulation from the point of fracture distally to the tip of the digit. When the angulatory deformity occurs proximally the projection is much greater and a deformity of only 2 or 3 degrees is projected to a considerable distortion of the position of the tip when extended out over several centimeters.

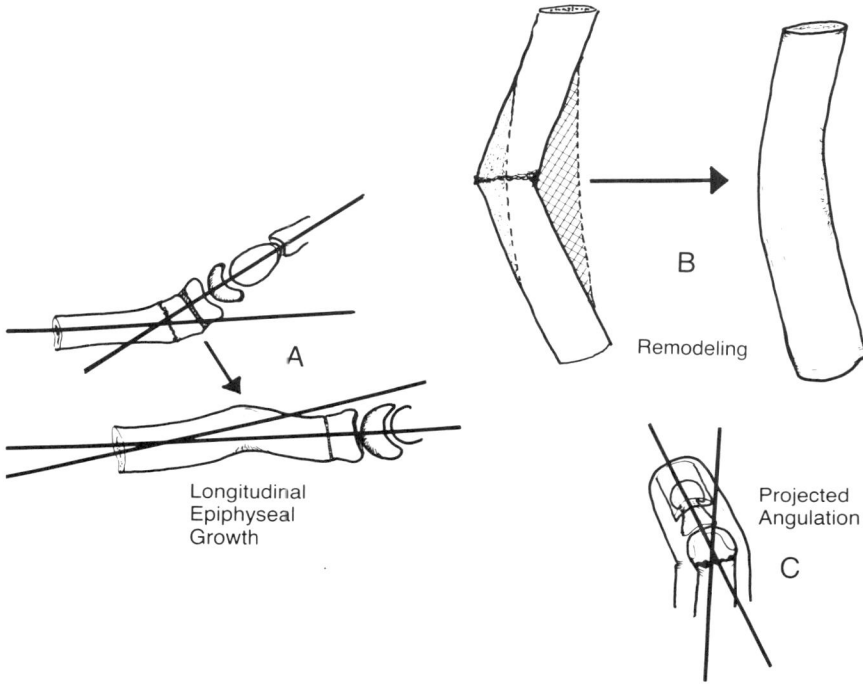

Fig. 4-3. Angulation is much more important than apposition, but **(A)** when it occurs in a child, particularly near the growth center, remodeling may occur by longitudinal epiphyseal growth. **(B)** In older individuals angulation may be somewhat improved by remodeling, though great amounts of angulation are unacceptable since they will not completely correct. **(C)** If angulation occurs in a digit it must be corrected more completely since projection of the small degree of angulation out to the tip of the digit will result in a considerable increase in the deformity and a poor cosmetic result.

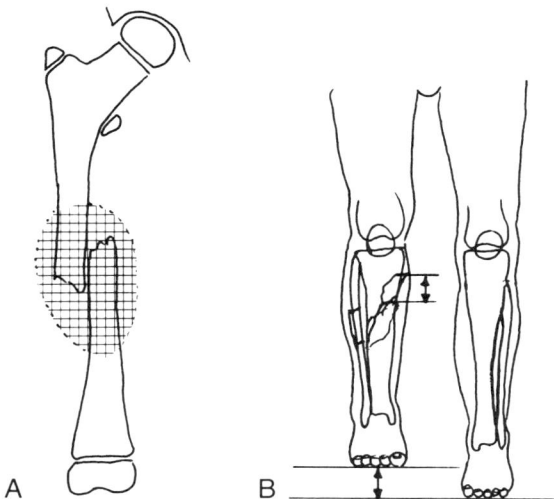

Fig. 4-4. (A) Shortening of an extremity may be allowable in the young child, since remodeling may occur as shown and stimulation of the epiphyseal plate will result in overgrowth to correct the shortening. **(B)** In the older individual, shortening of weight-bearing bones results in shortening of the extremities with the obvious gait abnormalities, which can be alleviated by building up the shoe.

Loss of Length

Loss of length is sometimes acceptable if the bone can be expected to make up the discrepancy as healing occurs (Fig. 4-4). This is particularly true in fractures of the femur in children in which a bayonet apposition is often acceptable. In fact some shortening may be desirable because of the expected stimulation of the epiphyseal center at the distal end of the femur which will make up some of the loss of length by overgrowth. Of course, great amounts of shortening cannot be accepted, but relatively small amounts of shortening are quite compatible with restoration of good function. On the other hand, loss of length in a weight-bearing bone, particularly in adults, is totally unacceptable. Fractures of the tibia, for instance, which result in a shortening greater than 1 cm considerably influence the function in the extremity by creating enough shortening that a lift under this foot will be necessary once healing has occurred. By the same token, loss of length in the upper extremity can be tolerated better than that in the lower extremity since the weight-bearing line is not disturbed. One must, however, be careful to refrain from allowing enough loss of length even in the upper extremity to cause cosmetic deformity.

Rotation

Rotation is probably the most often missed positional error in the treatment of fractures. This is particularly true in the hand, where rotatory deformities are often not discovered until after the fracture has healed. If one is careful to recognize the faulty level of the nail in comparison with those of the adjacent fingers when the finger is in flexion, one can often recognize rotatory deformity. By the same token, it is mandatory that fingers be examined in flexion after the fracture has been reduced, since rotation will show up much more dramatically if the joint is flexed because of the projection previously described. A final point is important, particularly in cases of fractures of the hand. The tip of each finger, when bent separately, normally points to a single point, namely, the tubercle of the scaphoid bone. Rotatory deformities, of course, will alter this congruency in the fingers (Figure 4-5).

Causes

Avoiding loss of position is often possible if one takes into the effect the importance of adequate immobilization. The old adage of including the joint above and below the level of fracture in the immobilization of fractures is still a good rule. Even though, on some occasions, this can be shortened somewhat, one can never make mistakes by following this dictum.

Fractures that tend to lose position are those inadequately immobilized, usually by too short a cast or splint. It is also important to remember the effect of position during immobilization: the position of the extremity often materially affects the stability of the reduction. Examples of this are seen in Figure 4-6 which demonstrates that fractures that are stable only in flexion are quite unstable in extension and often extension will result in loss of position. Simularly,

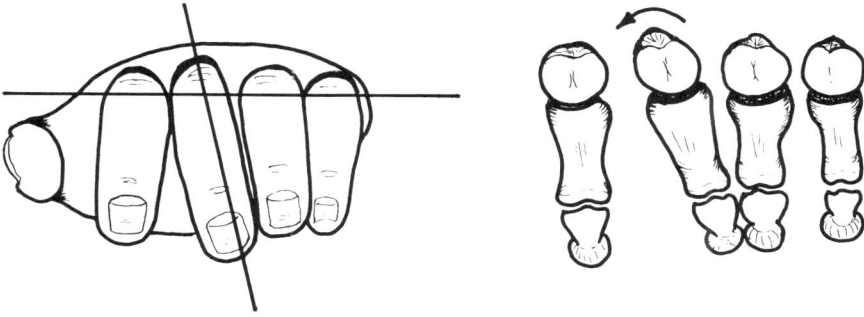

Fig. 4-5. The problem of rotation. Rotation resulting from a fracture of a proximal phalanx is quite noticeable when the fingers are flexed. Not only is this cosmetically poor, but it results in functional disabilities as wel .

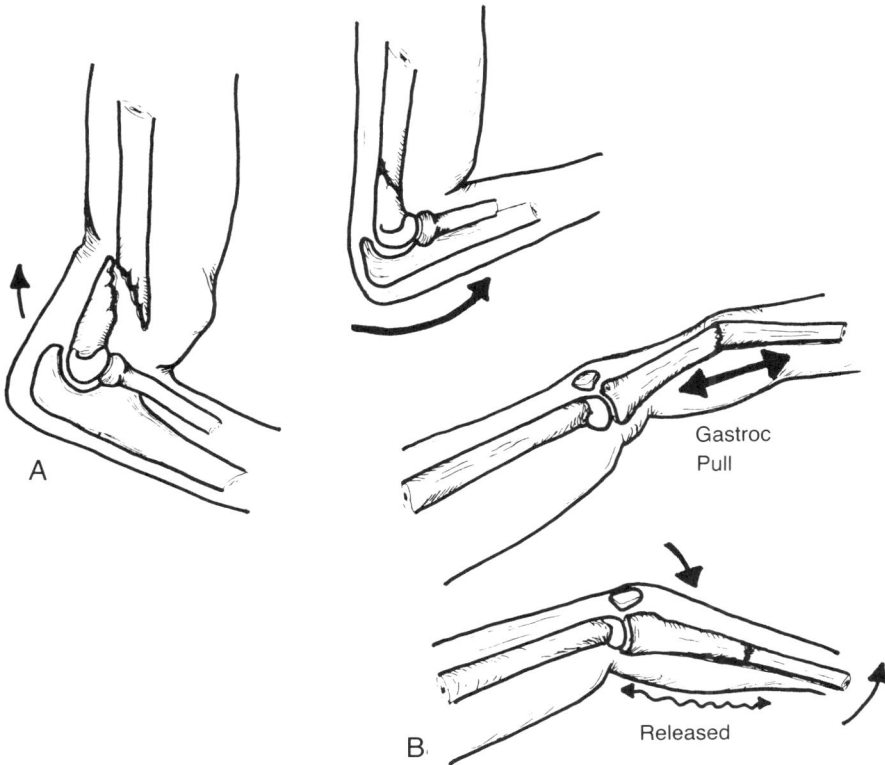

Fig. 4-6. Effect of position. **(A)** An example of the advantage of holding a fracture of the distal humerus in position. The over-pull of the triceps, which deforms the elbow posteriorly, is overcome with the elbow flexed. The fracture will be quite stable in the reduced position. **(B)** An example of angulation in the tibia caused by spasm and over-pull of the gastroc-soleus group which results in bolster ng an angulation of the fracture. Once the fracture has been reduced and the knee is flexed, the over-pull of the muscle is released and the fracture site will remain in the straight pos tion.

muscle pull in the lower extremity, will often result in loss of position of tibial fractures, from bowstringing of the gastrocnemius group. Simple flexion of the knee in the immobilization apparatus results in the relaxation of the gastrocnemius pull and obviates this abnormal deforming force.

Another example is seen in fractures of the wrist. These fractures are stable only in flexion and many instances of Colles-type fracture losing reduction can be directly related to failure to put the wrist up in flexion in the immobilizing splint or cast. Fractures must always be put up in the stable position if one is to maintain position (Fig. 10-3).

Loss of position can often be directly related to the application of too much or too little traction. When too much traction is applied, distraction occurs and nonunion will often result. An excellent example is seen in the treatment of a fracture of the midshaft of the humerus with a hanging cast. It is a common error to apply the cast with too much weight so that the fracture becomes distracted. By the time the physician has recognized this, fibrous union has already occurred between the bone ends. By the same token, too little traction is often just as bad. Not only does this allow for shortening at the fracture site but occasionally too little traction will also result in angular deformities and failure of reduction of the fractures due to pull of gravity, overpull of muscle groups, and similar forces.

VASCULAR COMPLICATIONS

Vascular complications are often seen in treatment of fractures of the extremity and are related to pressure on adjacent blood vessels either by the fragments themselves or by swelling and bleeding in the area, which results in compression. Direct damage to the vessels themselves must also be ruled out (Fig. 4-7). One should be aware of the triad of pain, power, and pulselessness (Figure 4-8), since these are the cardinal signs of arterial insufficiency in the extremity. Vascular complications occur as two types: immediate and delayed.

Immediate

Immediate vascular insufficiency usually results from disruption of the vessels, from impingement of the fragments against the vessel, or from acute torsional deformities in the vessel caused by loss of stability of the skeleton and faulty position of the extremity. These changes are seen immediately and the serious implications of immediate vascular insufficiency should be recognized by the physician so that appropriate treatment can be instituted.

Delayed

Delayed vascular complications usually occur more insidiously and are the result of late factors that cause occlusion of the arteries and veins by tamponade. This usually occurs as the result of the "compartment syndrome." Bleeding from

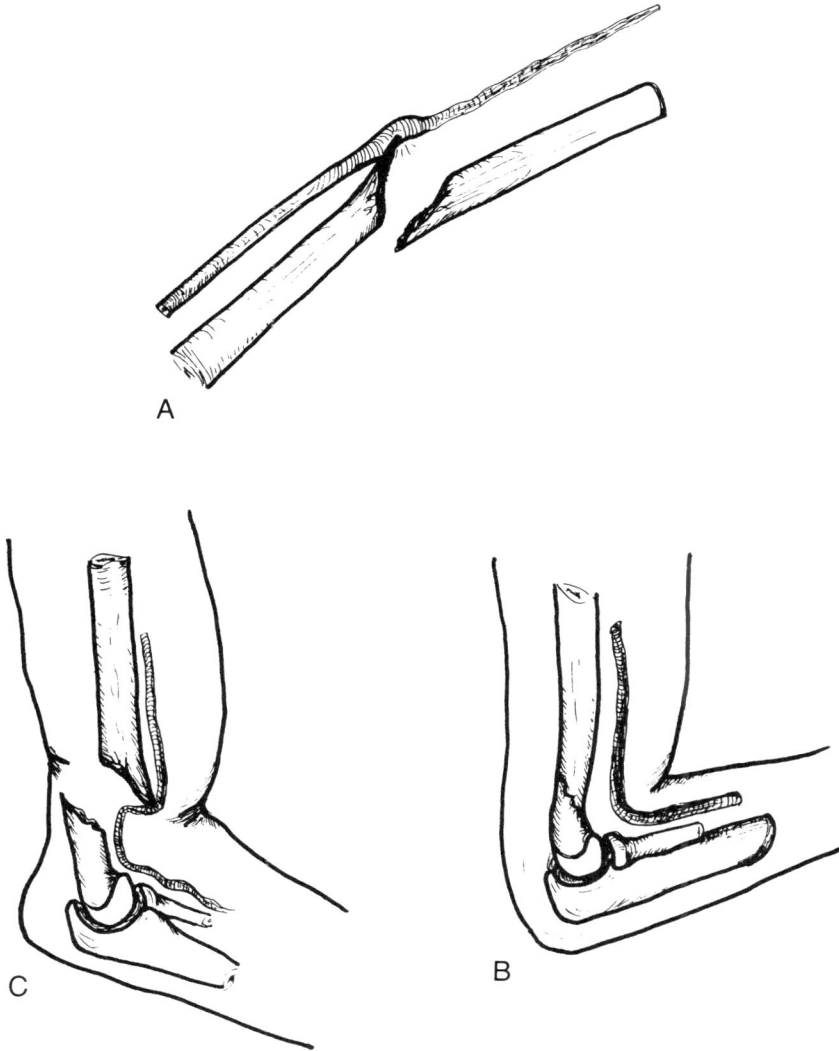

Fig. 4-7. (A) Impailment of fracture end into vessel wall with resulting arterial damage, spasm, and ultimate thrombosis. **(B)** The result of stretching or angulation of the artery by displacement at the fracture site. Impailment of the artery may occur over the end of the humerus, though most of the vascular loss is from crimping and stretching of the artery. **(C)** Reduction of the fracture returns the artery to its normal position and relieves the arterial insufficiency.

the fracture site itself along with the outpouring of inflammatory edema fluid all contained within a closed fascial space results in a tremendous increase of pressure. This occludes first the veins (which have a lower intrinsic pressure) and then the arterial supply. In the particularly traumatized closed fracture of the extremity, one should always be on guard for the signs of vascular insufficiency related to tamponade (Fig. 4-9).

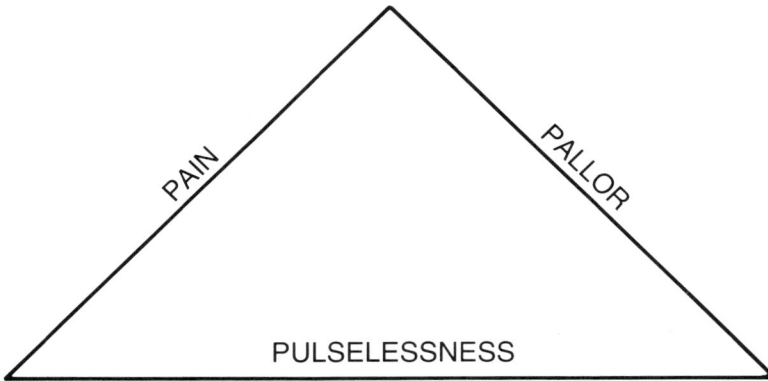

Fig. 4-8. The triad of acute vascular insufficiency showing the three "P's"—pain, pallor, and pulselessness.

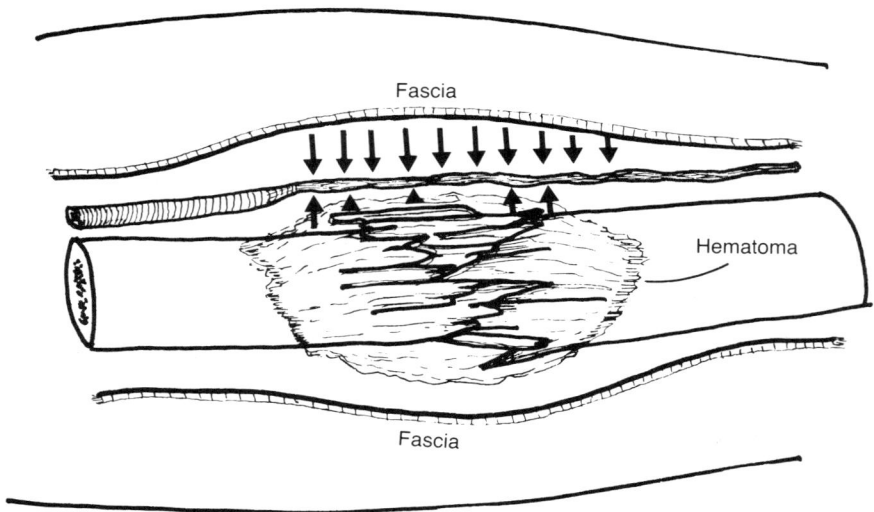

Fig. 4-9. Tamponade. A diagramatic example of a vascular complication taking place in a closed fascial compartment following a fracture. The hematoma around the fracture can be seen with the abutment of the margin of the hematoma against the arterial supply, which passes nearby. However, the increased pressure within the fascial compartment has resulted in a compression of the artery so that arterial circulation has been diminished or cut off distal to the swelling. Circulation can be reestablished by opening the fascial compartment surgically allowing the vessel to decompress by migrating away from the area of injury.

Treatment

Treatment consists of general supportive measures for the circulatory condition of the extremity distal to the fracture. The most important treatment of vascular complications is related to the reduction of fractures and the direct treatment of the vessels if severe injury to the vessel itself has occurred. Most of

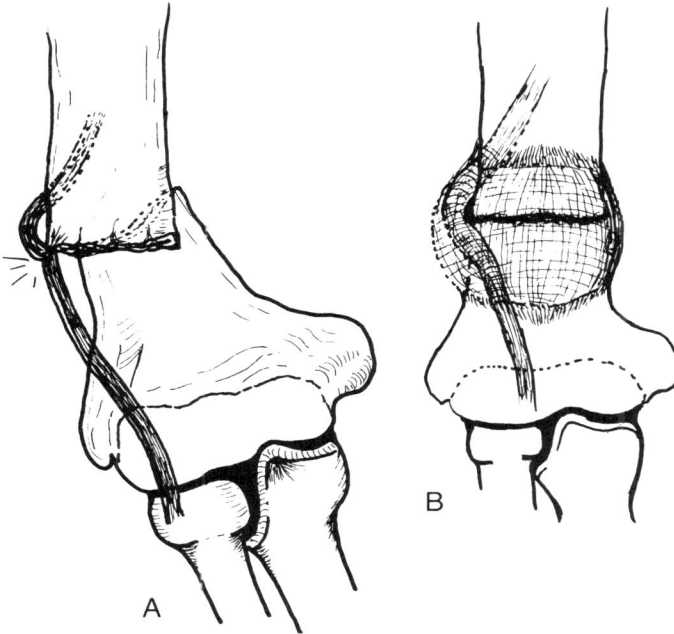

Fig. 4-10. An example of immediate neurologic deficit following a fracture of the humerus occurs when **(A)** the radial nerve becomes trapped and impailed by the margin of the proximal fragments as the nerve passes around the humerus through the musculospiral groove. This may result in a neuroplaxia, but often recovery will occur if reduction is established soon after the injury and the nerve has not been damaged. **(B)** Delayed nerve damage caused by incorporation of the nerve in the callus formation or in the area of scar tissue, is illustrated.

the time, the reduction of the fracture will result in the release of any bony impingement against the vessels and will at the same time relieve any torsional or kinking deformities that may have occurred at the fracture site. Finally, the restoration of skeletal stability results in a much better framework on which the vascular tree can work. Often merely reduction of the fracture with restoration of normal stability restores normal circulation to the extremity.

NEUROLOGIC COMPLICATIONS

Neurologic complications following fractures may be immediate or delayed (Fig. 4-10).

Immediate

Immediate deficit usually results from traction, impingement, or lacerations through the nerve involved. It is often not possible to render definitive treatment in the case of immediate neurologic deficit. It is extremely important, however, to examine and record the presence of neurologic deficit as soon as the patient is seen. Progression of the deficit is much more important, from the standpoint of urgency of treatment, than is the deficit present when first seen. Most nerve lesions can be very satisfactorily treated as a delayed primary repair. There is therefore not the urgency for treatment when the patient is first seen. Neurologic deficit with a fresh fracture may cause concern, but concern should be for restoration of stability to the skeleton and the stabilization of the vascular supply.

Delayed

Delayed neurologic complications occur from swelling, scarring around the nerve, and during the healing stages of the fracture by involvement of the nerve in callus formation. These delayed neurologic deficits can be identified as treatment progresses and depend basically upon the alertness of the treating physician in periodically evaluating the neurologic status of the extremity. It is important to recognize these deficits as they begin to occur so that the patient can be referred for evaluation and treatment.

REFLEX SYMPATHETIC DYSTROPHY

Reflex sympathetic dystrophy is a frequent complication following fracture treatment and is often not recognized until it has become quite severe. Too often the signs of reflex sympathetic dystrophy are misinterpreted as related to simple disuse caused by immobilization of the extremity. Not until the symptoms have become full-blown does one recognize the severity of the complication. The following symptoms *may* be present with simple disuse, but more often indicate the development of reflex dystrophy.

Persistent Swelling

Persistent swelling tends to occur in the extremity rather diffusely. It is not located directly at the injury site, but usually occurs in the entire extremity and is a rather woody hardness.

Joint Stiffness

Joint stiffness occurs as the result of swelling, with the organization of the inflammatory edema fluid in the joint capsule, and may be related to the pain that occurs and prevents the patient from moving the involved joint.

Contractural Phenomenon

Contractural phenomenon is a relatively late occurrence and is related, again, to the stiffness and to the pain that prevents stretching and motion.

Muscular Atrophy

Muscular atrophy may actually be related more to disuse than to reflex dystrophy. However, since disuse with reflex dystrophy is much more profound, the muscular atrophy is likely to be greater than one would expect from simple disuse alone.

Vasomotor Phenomena

Vasomotor phenomena such as hyperhydrosis, mottling of the skin, or perhaps a reddish color of the skin all indicate some abnormal response in the sympathetic nervous systems. The skin may develop a slick shiny appearance and be devoid of sweating or may be damp and clammy, with perspiration dripping from it. The latter is more characteristic.

Pain

The final and most characteristic symptom of reflex dystrophy is pain. Patients often develop a "touch me not" feeling; they will hardly allow the examiner even to touch the involved part. They often come into the office with the part wrapped in cotton or in a scarf to prevent even wind on the extremity since all of these stimuli tend to trigger the severe painful spasms characteristic of the phenomenon.

Treatment

Reflex sympathetic dystrophy requires early treatment once it has been recognized. It is much more common following injuries that result in involvement of major nerves though it may occur without this particular injury. It is likewise much more commonly seen in the upper extremity. Injuries to the hand far surpass the other types of injury in frequency of reflex dystrophy. Vigorous attempts to get the patient to move the extremity are imperative if one is to reverse the changes described. If the diagnosis is fairly well established, however, the patient should be referred to a specialist for possible sympathetic ganglion blocks, intravascular blocks using appropriate drugs, or other treatments.

PRESSURE PHENOMENA

Pressure phenomena are almost always due to the immobilization apparatus. This should be recognized as being the cause when pressure is seen in an extremity immobilized for treatment of fracture. Casts that have been too tightly applied and without padding over the bony prominences are the primary cause of these pressure phenomena.

Molding the casts over bony areas is particularly important. Often the cast that has been so greatly padded that it slips back and forth on the extremity results in the pressure phenomena. Pressure phenomena in the extremities may take the form of ulcerations, damage to the nerve (such as the damage to the common peroneal nerve seen in lower extremity casts with pressure over the fibular head area), and even vascular impairment if the cast is too tight or if constricting bands have been allowed to form while the cast is still wet. The basic factor to remember is the importance of early recognition. The physician should not ever fail to recognize and investigate a patient's complaint that the immobilization apparatus is causing pressure on the extremity. Many times these complaints are unfounded and examination will reveal that no harm is being done, but the physician should never fail to take the time to investigate these complaints to be certain that they are not valid and to be certain that these pressure phenomena do not occur.

5

MISCELLANEOUS AFFECTATIONS OF THE SPINE

Along with the problems that occur in the cervical spine and the low back area (see Chs. 6 and 7) a number of conditions involve the spine as a whole and, because of their unique characteristics, deserve special consideration.

SCOLIOSIS

Scoliosis describes a lateral curvature of the spine. This may be in either direction from the midline and the configuration may be a single C-curve, an S-curve, or the SS-curve. There are, of course, many variations along with these more common configurations, but certain types of curves are more characteristic of certain causes. Along with the lateral curvature, scoliosis, if it is of any magnitude, is ordinarily associated with a certain amount of rotation. The architecture of the spine is such that when a considerable amount of lateral stress is placed on a vertebrae the relationship between the body anteriorly and the two facet joints posteriorly is such that rotation is necessary to accommodate the lateral curvature. The more severe scoliotic curves, therefore, are often associated with enough rotation that the rotatory deformity overshadows the curve. This is particularly true in thoracic curves, where rotation results in a considerable amount of rib deformity. This deformity of the thorax is cosmetically unacceptable and physiologically damaging, since the vital capacity is often compromised in severe cases.

Scoliosis is related to various causes. No matter what the cause, the condition is likely to be much more progressive during the growth years and to become much more static after the spine has stopped growing. The three basic kinds of scoliosis, from the standpoint of cause, are (1) congenital, (2) neurogenic, and (3) idiopathic scoliosis. Many types of much less common forms are also seen by the orthopedic surgeon, but most all will fall into one of these three categories.

Congenital

Congenital scoliosis is present to a certain degree at birth and is related to a specific congenital abnormality of the spine. In its true form, congenital scoliosis usually is related to a hemivertebra. In this condition, the vertebral bodies of one or more vertebrae are wedge-shaped due to failure of complete formation of one side. Instead of the square vertebral bodies being stacked on one another in a straight line, the wedge-shaped vertebra in the center of a group of vertebrae will result in an apex about which a scoliotic curve may develop. These hemivertebrae are usually associated with other abnormalities of the spine and are usually multiple, with abnormal fusions between various of the vertebral bodies often seen.

The congenital scoliosis may or may not be compensated. The patient will often present with a decompensated condition in which the head and shoulders are not positioned directly over the pelvis. On the other hand, many cases of congenital scoliosis have enough counterdeformity that an automatic compensation has occurred and the process is quite stable.

While congenital scoliosis is subject to exaggeration with growth, these curves are not apt to show the rapid progression seen in other types of scoliotic curves. For the most part, they tend to be somewhat more stable than the other two types. Occasionally at the center of the apex there will be a group of vertebrae fused together without much differentiation and with such loss of anatomical identity that they can be considered a single vertebra. As indicated, these tend to be relatively stable. Unless there is a great amount of decompensation that promotes progression of the deformity, they usually are not prone to rapid progression.

Congenital scoliosis is frequently associated with rib deformities since many of these are seen in the thoracic and cervical spine. Rib deformities may take the same form as the vertebral deformities; there may be a fusion of multiple ribs so that each rib has lost its identity. This may be extremely difficult to treat because it constitutes such a severe deformity. However, if this fusion is not progressive, it may be cosmetically and functionally acceptable. These cases, however, should be evaluated by an orthopedic surgeon who is more experienced in determining the possibilities of progression and the level at which further progression is unacceptable.

Congenital scoliosis is occasionally associated with other congenital abnormalities such as abnormalities of the kidney, gastrointestinal tract, or heart. One should watch out for these other associated abnormalities, particularly if the patient is to undergo surgical correction.

Neurogenic

Neurogenic scoliosis is a form of lateral curvature of the spine seen much less frequently today, because many of the paralytic curves seen in postpoliomyelitis patients are not seen in this age of proper immunization against this disease. Occasional cases are still seen in older individuals or in those coming into this country who have not been immunized.

When a scoliotic curve is related to motor paralysis of the supporting musculature of the spine, it tends more commonly to be a long C-curve and, of course, is related to the inequal pull of the supporting musculature on the two sides. Likewise, the loss of abdominal musculature strength leads to a progression of the scoliosis. Many of these cases of severe lateral curvature are also accompanied by a severe lumbar lordosis.

One type of neurogenic scoliosis is caused by a neurofibroma in the spine. The neurofibroma occurs within the vertebral body, usually as a radiolucent area. For some unknown reason it results in a rapidly progressive scoliosis that can be severe in a matter of months. It usually occurs in slightly younger patients. Because of this condition's tendency to rapid progression, the child suspected of having this type of scoliosis should be referred to an orthopedic surgeon so that the spine can be watched very closely with serial radiographs taken quite often and a brace or surgical stabilization can be used as needed.

The patient with a paralytic curve usually will show a long C-type curve, which may extend all the way from the upper dorsal to the lower lumbar area. An S-type curve may develop due to collapse of the vertebrae, but this is more often the case when there is loss of muscular tone on both sides of the spine.

Patients with severe muscular paralysis in the torso usually have severely deformed spines and treatment is particularly difficult because they present a high operative risk.

Idiopathic

The term idiopathic actually means "caused by itself," which is another way of saying that the cause is unknown to the physician. Idiopathic scoliosis occurs almost always in adolescence; however, it may sometimes begin earlier and merely show progression during the adolescent growth years. As a general rule idiopathic scoliosis occurs in late childhood and early adolescence and ordinarily girls are more often affected than boys. In some series the ratio is as high as 9 : 1. The reason for this sexual predisposition is not known.

Idiopathic scoliosis may occur all the way from C7 to S1 but it is seldom seen in the cervical spine unless compensating for a curve lower down. There may be many types of configurations with idiopathic scoliosis: an S-type curve is somewhat more prominent because of its tendency to compensation. Long C-curves almost invariably have compensatory curves at the top and bottom of the longer curve, if compensation has occurred. A curve that is not compensated results in a severe functional disability and cosmetic deformity since the head and shoulders are not aligned with the pelvis.

The idiopathic curve is characteristically seen during the period of the greatest growth of the skeleton. Progression of these curves is often related to the growth factor itself. The apex of the curve can be ascertained by finding the point of greatest lateral deviation of the spine. On the convex side of the curve the disc space is wider than on the concave side. On reaching the end of the curve, the wide part of the disc space will occur on the concave side. Therefore, you may know that you have reached the end of the curve by this change of the disc space appearance. Even with an S-shaped curve the same principle applies. Rotation is quite noticeable in idiopathic curves; when this occurs in the thoracic spine the chest deformity may be quite severe.

The important issue with idiopathic scoliosis is whether or not the curve will progress.

A curve of less than 30 degrees is usually considered the upper limit of acceptability from a cosmetic and functional standpoint. Therefore, a 30 degree curve in a 25- or 30-year-old patient is not likely to progress and probably requires little or no treatment. On the other hand, a 30 degree curve in a 12-year-old will very likely progress and, because of this, must be carefully watched by the orthopedic surgeon. It is often possible to predict the patient's ultimate height at maturity by calculations made from the appearance of the bones of the hand and wrist. Charts are available to plot out the chronologic and skeletal age of children and their anticipated maximum height at maturation. These charts can be valuable in predicting the amount of growth that will occur in a given individual.

Treatment of scoliosis should be relegated to the orthopedic surgeon familiar with this condition and the patient should be referred as soon as the condition is diagnosed. It is proper for the family physician to help in the follow-up of these patients, but the final decision as to the type and extent of treatment should be made by the specialist to whom the patient is referred.

RHEUMATOID SPONDYLITIS

Incidence and Findings

Rheumatoid spondylitis is a collagen disease involving primarily the spine. It occurs 90 percent of the time in males. The condition is one of gradual involvement of the perispinous ligaments and capsules with an acute inflammatory reaction that often ultimately causes fusion of the entire vertebral column. It usually begins in younger men, aged 25 to 35 years, and is slowly progressive over the remainder of their life span. Since the major involvement is of the spine, this condition is largely unlike its counterpart rheumatoid disease in general, in which the involvement is systemic with multiple joint involvement. Peripheral joint involvement with rheumatoid spondylitis occurs in about 10 percent of the cases. In each instance the majority of the involvement is of the hip joints and, in very rare instances, other peripheral joints of the extremities are involved. For the most part, however, it should be considered to be basically a disease of the spine with occasional hip joint involvement.

The symptoms are usually insidious, with a first complaint of morning stiffness in the spine and gradual increase in the severity of the symptoms over time. There is a generalized feeling of malaise and an aching of the entire spinal area that gradually begins to occur all of the time, with exacerbations during periods of increased stress to the back or during other systemic disease such as throat infections, influenza, and the like.

The patient is usually thin and asthenic, and very early in the course of the disease will be noted to have marked diminution in movement through the spine. While the neck is often spared during the early part of the disease, involvement of the cervical spine is most incapacitating during the later stages of the disease since it completely precludes movement of the head and neck. In some instances in which the patient is more or less bedridden, the neck becomes fused in relatively grotesque positions such as looking to the side or, more often, tilted to one side looking at the other. Relatively soon after the onset of the severe symptoms the patient begins to have recurring episodes of acute pain in the back with muscle spasm and occasionally radicular type pain. Between these acute exacerbations, however, the patient basically has the dull aching type of pain throughout the spine. One of the characteristic findings even early on the natural course of the disease is a marked diminution of chest expansion. The usual patient with widespread involvement will have virtually no chest expansion, whereas the normal individual should have at least 2 inches of change in circumference of the chest from the completely exhaled to the completely inhaled position.

Laboratory studies early on reveal an anemia that seems to be out of proportion to the state of the disease. The anemia is often unnoticed but the patient complains usually of a feeling of lassitude and depression. The anemia is only moderately responsive to treatment with various hematinic preparations. The other test that is routinely strongly positive in the later course of the disease is the rheumatoid fixation test. Early, the findings of the rheumatoid fixation test may be negative or equivocal but invariably after the patient has begun to have symptoms of any severity the results become strongly positive. Other laboratory studies are usually within normal limits, with the exception of the erythrocyte sedimentation rate, which may be quite high. X-ray examination begins relatively early to show calcification and ossification of the periarticular ligaments, with a gradual filling in of the longitudinal ligaments of the spine with bone. These changes relatively early have a characteristic appearance and will often advance to the complete ''bamboo spine,'' the picturesque name given to the complete fusion of the longitudinal spinal ligaments that on AP radiographs appears not unlike a bamboo pole.

One of the unusual predilections for rheumatoid spondylitis is into the sacroiliac joint. Symptoms there may be the first recognizable symptoms of the disease. It is not certain why spondylitis involves the sacroiliac joints, but it is a well known phenomenon and a high percentage of patients will at some time or another show radiographic changes in their sacroiliac joint. These may be some of the earliest findings and may first establish the diagnosis before the patient has begun to have significant signs or findings in the spine.

Treatment

General Supportive Measures

General supportive measures, such as the maintenance of normal resistance and good nutrition, are very important since these patients tend to become debilitated quite readily. Adequate rest, avoidance of stress, and other things that are likely to cause the acute flares are to be avoided. Particular attention should be paid to maintaining as much motion as possible in the areas that are becoming stiff and maintaining functional position in areas becoming totally ankylosed. For instance, the cervical spine may become completely fused. However, as long as the head is completely straight with the chin down and the eyes looking straight ahead one can tolerate the ankylosis better than with the head turned to the side and tilted or with the chin pointed upward, as is sometimes characteristic, particularly of bedridden patients. A good firm mattress is necessary and will quite often considerably improve the symptoms. A soft sponge rubber mattress can be used as long as it is placed over bedboards that do not allow sag in the back nor unusual repetitious motion through the spine each time the patient moves. To be avoided, for the most part, are the very relaxed bed springs that allow the mattress to sag and cause unusual strain on the back even with the slightest amount of motion. Of course, the usual applications of heat and rest during the acute episodes considerably improve the symptoms, as does the placing of the spine at rest using various extrinsic supports. Exercise to maintain as much motion as possible is excellent and the patient should be referred to a physical therapist for instructions in a home program that can be done twice daily.

Splinting

Splinting is often effective during the acute episodes and will even improve the deep aching type of pain that the average patient has during the progressive stages. Be certain that splinting maintains the position ultimately desired when ankylosis occurs, since this will most certainly happen with the passage of time. The splints range from the full spinal brace, as described by Taylor many years ago to canvas corsets for support in milder cases. These this may be altered with various outriggers or extensions to include other parts of the spine, such as the cervical area. Splints will hasten the occurrence of ankylosis, however, and if bracing is used it should be accompanied by an even more rigorous exercise program to maintain as much motion as possible. Canvas corsets with a high back, such as the "Hoke" corset, are excellent for giving support without maximum immobilization. Until the disease becomes severe the patient may well get by with periodic use of a canvas corset of this type. Later on, or during the acute episodes, he may be more comfortable in a Taylor-type brace that does afford relatively rigid fixation of the spine.

Medication

Medications are of considerable value in most cases and should be begun by using the least toxic dosage and gradually increasing as necessary based on clinical response. Salicylates have been shown to have excellent therapeutic effect by their anti-inflammatory action and represent a primary treatment of choice soon as the diagnosis has been made. Many people can be treated over long periods of time with salicylates alone and remain relatively comfortable as well as demonstrating decreased progress of the inflammatory disease. Many of the nonsteroidal anti-inflammatory medications other than salicylates may be of value and their dosage can be adjusted by clinical trial. It is interesting that the nonsteroidal anti-inflammatory drugs all have certain predilection. While some work better in a given patient, others will work better in other patients; many times it is a matter of trial and response to a given medication.

Cortisone and its derivatives, of course, have a very dramatic effect on rheumatoid spondylitis but because of their inherent dangers from metabolic and other responses, they should be used only sparingly.

There is probably no harm in giving occasional episodic doses of prednisone orally during the acute episodes of pain. A good plan is to give a gradually diminishing dosage schedule over a 3-week period. This may be quite effective and will not result in a rebound of symptoms once the steroids have been discontinued. My preferred routine has been to give prednisone in 5 mg doses, four times daily for 5 days, three times daily for 5 days, two times daily for 5 days, and then 2.5 mg twice daily for 5 days. This should give a maximum clinical response during the first 5 days with a maintenance of this response as the dosage is gradually diminished. We have not seen any untoward effects of this 20 day schedule, which delivers only a total of 250 mg. During the last few days of this regimen the patient should be started back on one of the nonsteroidal anti-inflammatory medications so that he will have good blood levels as the prednisone level drops to zero.

Low-Voltage X-Ray Therapy

Finally, a very effective treatment regimen that has been used is low-voltage x-ray therapy over the spine. The serious side effects of the administration of great quantities of x-rays over the spine are well known. However, the dosage regimen used in rheumatoid spondylitis can be quite low since the inflammatory reaction tends to respond to this. The response to these small doses is often quite prolonged, so the patient may remain comfortable and show no evidence of progression of disease for many months following cessation of therapy. Therapy is likewise particularly useful in patients with symptoms referable to the sacroiliac joint area, since the inflammatory disease here tends to respond quite readily to small doses of x-ray. Often a single treatment will be followed by permanent relief of symptoms in these joints.

EPIPHYSITIS JUVENILIS

Incidence and Findings

Epiphysitis juvenilis (Scheuermann's disease) has been long recognized as occurring primarily in the thoracic spine in adolescent boys. Girls may be affected but the instance in boys is much higher. The usual age of onset is during the adolescent growth spurt, though it may occur at any time between the ages of 12 or 13 on up to 16 or 17.

The symptoms are usually pain and aching in the thoracic spine or upper lumbar area. These are not related to trauma except that they occur in a patient who is quite active and often participates in sports. The original symptoms are often related to an episode of trauma even though this may not be the etiologic factor. These symptoms become gradually more severe. The patient complains of nocturnal pain and will occasionally have fairly acute episodes of pain in the back, particularly following episodes of trauma, such as playing football.

The confirming evidence of epiphysitis of the spine in the adolescent is the x-ray appearance. The changes occur in the ring epiphysis, which surrounds the superior and inferior margins of the vertebral body, and are best seen on the lateral views of the spine. A moth-eaten appearance of the upper or lower margin of the vertebral body signifies the inflammatory reaction in the ring epiphysis that has extended out into the adjacent bone of the vertebral body. These changes may be quite marked on occasion. In instances in which the upper and lower plates are involved in a single vertebra there may be considerable wedging of a vertebra. This is due to the softness of the involved bone and weight-bearing with repeated small episodes of trauma, which result in wedging of the vertebral body as seen on the lateral films. Changes may become marked enough on occasion to be frightening when viewed on the radiograph, but the clinical history as well as the location of the moth-eaten area should give unmistakable evidence of the diagnosis.

Treatment

As with other instances of epiphysitis in the adolescence, the treatment of choice is rest without weight-bearing. In the more advanced cases, or with marked changes, this can be accomplished only by the wearing of a steel brace while in the vertical position. The patient is usually more comfortable in a Taylor-type brace though the Jewett brace with three-point pressure (over the sternum, pubis, and spine) will give considerable relief of symptoms and allow healing without distorting the vertebral body by avoiding weight-bearing on these bones. Bracing should be started as soon as it is evident that the condition is progressive and the changes are likely to become marked. The patient should be maintained in the brace at all times except while in bed at night. This is often very difficult to persuade a youngster to do but it is mandatory if one is to avoid the compression of the softened bone, with resulting mechanical changes and symptoms at a later date. Wearing the brace, of course, also precludes participation in most types of contact sports.

The brace is maintained in position until definite x-ray evidence of healing can be seen in the areas of involvement of the spine. The patient and his parents should be warned early that this process requires many months; the brace usually should be worn for at least 2 years and perhaps more. The brace cannot be safely removed until x-ray evidence of healing of the lesions is demonstrated. Allowing the patient to resume full weight-bearing on the spine will result in a progression of the compressive lesion, even after some healing has been accomplished. For this reason it is much better to wait until the radiographs shows good evidence of healing before allowing the patient to remove the brace, even for short periods of time other than when lying completely horizontal.

During immobilization, the patient should be encouraged to do extension exercises for the thoracic spine twice daily. These exercises are easily done and do not take a great amount of time. They involve lying prone on the floor or table with the arms to the side. While keeping the abdomen on the table, the chest is gently elevated, using the erector spinae muscles on either side. The thorax is usually raised up with these muscles, held for a count of five, and then allowed to return to the resting position. This exercise is repeated ten times before a short rest. Six sets of ten repetitions are done twice daily. It is often better to place a small pillow under the abdomen to prevent hyperextension of the lumbar or lumbosacral spine during these exercises. Otherwise this will cause the patient to complain of low back pain due to the stress placed on these lower spinal joints by hyperextension. The exercises can be done twice daily even when the patient is wearing the brace but should be continued for a period of a good many months after the brace has been removed. Likewise, when the changes are very early and not severe enough to warrant use of a brace, the exercise routine done twice daily as directed will usually result in control of symptoms and perhaps abort the progression of the disease.

Once healing can be shown on the radiographs, with filling in of the defects, the patient is considered to be over the disease and can be allowed to stop the regimen.

COMPRESSION FRACTURES

Traumatic

Compression fractures in the spine are the usual type of fracture seen in the vertebral body. There can, of course, be more disruptive fractures of the vertebral body with separation of the dorsal elements and an "exploding" of the body itself but these are always due to more violent trauma. Actually, the compression fracture is often due to very minor trauma in a bone weakened by demineralization.

The typical compression fracture that results in wedging of the vertebrae will ordinarily involve the compression of the body anteriorly, since the dorsal elements give a stronger support posteriorly and most of the time will maintain the integrity of the posterior wall of the vertebral body. Thus, the average compression fracture, whether due to trauma or to osteoporosis alone, results in a pie-shaped deformity with the compression occurring anterior, either with a depression of the superior inplate and an elevation of the inferior inplate, or a combination of the two. In some cases of trauma there may be enough force to compress the anterior aspect only. If, however, the trauma is of great enough magnitude, after simple compression has occurred there may be continued force on the posterior elements so that they may become detached or broken. The compression fracture may therefore be associated with subluxation or even dislocation. Except for these relatively severe cases, however, the usual compression fracture of the vertebral body with intact dorsal elements is treated in much the same way, whether caused by severe trauma in a normal bone or minimal trauma in a demineralized bone.

Demineralized

Our increasing life expectancy has made osteoporosis and similar metabolic demineralization of bone much more common. Demineralization, which ordinarily is associated with advancing age, is seen much more frequently in women than men because of the lack of osteoid formation occasioned by the cessation of hormone production in postmenopausal women. While the treatment of osteoporosis is not within our scope, most primary compression fractures in older women with osteoporosis occur in those who have not had treatment for osteoporosis or despite treatment of the osteoporosis. Estrogen and calcium metabolism as well as high-protein diets all have a part in the treatment of osteoporosis, but in many instances none of these will provide the extra strength to the vertebral body to prevent compression fractures.

These fractures should therefore be expected in most women past the age of 50 in whom sudden back pain in the dorsal or lumbodorsal spine occurred with minimal trauma of "sitting down too hard" or of coughing, or sneezing, or other sudden flexion of the upper part of the torso on the fixed pelvis. The patient will have usually rather sudden severe pain associated with muscle spasm and often time requires sedation for this pain. A gibbus can sometimes be felt by the prominence of the spinous process at the apex of the triangle created by the fracture. Often this is visible later after some settling has occurred. These fractures will usually result in almost complete loss of height of the anterior aspect of the vertebral body but, as mentioned previously, the posterior wall will usually remain intact along with the dorsal element.

As soon as the patient can tolerate it she should be fitted with a supporting brace to immobilize this portion of the spine as much as possible. The Taylor brace, which is a chair type with double posterior uprights and a pelvic band with shoulder straps to hold the upper torso, is the standby and probably the immobilization of choice since it is well tolerated and effective. The so-called Jewett brace is composed of three pads that maintain the extended position of the spine. One of these pads is placed in the upper sternal area and one in the pubic area, and these are attached to a belt in the central portion that constitutes a fulcrum by which the two anterior pads keep the two ends of the spine straight against the central portion, which pushes forward. These braces are much more effective than the Taylor brace but are very poorly tolerated since they make sitting difficult because they punch down in the groin and up into the neck when the patient sits.

Since the primary purpose of the support in compression fractures associated with osteoporosis is to stabilize the spine and hold it in its present position without any thought of correction, the Taylor brace is adequate and probably the method of choice. The brace should be worn for approximately 12 weeks so that adequate healing of the spine may occur. After 6 weeks, however, the patient can begin to take the brace off for short periods of time but still should wear it while up for extended periods or for such things as riding in an automobile or other activities that put pressure on the spine.

During this time, if possible, the patient should exercise to strengthen the erector spinae musculature and provide muscular support for extension of the spine once the brace has been removed. Since exercises of this type are poorly tolerated in many older people this is often not possible. However, attempts should be made in instances in which the patient is capable of doing extension exercises; these should be done twice daily much as described in the section on epiphysitis juvenilis.

Traumatic compression fractures tend to have similar characteristics except for those caused by severe trauma, as mentioned above. In patients in whom the posterior elements are intact, they can be treated in much the same way as previously described in the older individual. In the younger patient, however, who can expect to want to be much more active after healing, there is a considerable stimulus to consider surgical stabilization of the spine at the injured level. Angulation of the spine at a point of compression of the vertebral body changes the mechanics of the spine at that level considerably. This is caused by the alteration of the positions of the posterior elements, with a considerable increase in the amount of strain on the supporting ligaments caused by this unusual position.

Because of this, a patient who expects to be quite active will probably continue to have a considerable amount of discomfort because of these altered mechanics. If this occurs, consideration may be given to surgical stabilization of this level to stabilize these painful mechanical deficiencies. The average individual, however, if older and more sedentary, will probably gain enough stabilization to be comfortable and should be allowed to heal in this position, with the prospects of being able to return to normal desired activities without much difficulty.

In the younger individuals with compression fractures related to trauma, healing time is somewhat longer and more rigid support will be required. The Jewett brace is probably more satisfactory since the patient can tolerate the brace somewhat better and it does afford more reliable immobilization in extension.

Depending upon the level of the fracture, after 6 or 8 weeks patients can sometimes use a lighter, less constraining type of brace. For the most part, a full 12 weeks is required for good stability to develop and these patients should be immobilized in an acceptable manner for that period of time. It is also imperative that the extension exercises previously described be done.

These individuals usually are more agile and have a musculature that is more responsive to exercise hypertrophy. They should therefore expect to gain considerable improvement of stability in the spine by doing these exercises faithfully twice a day, beginning as soon as the symptoms will allow.

Neoplastic

The third type of compression fracture is related to bone destruction by a neoplasm. Since the spine is a relatively common place for metastasis, it can be expected to be involved frequently in patients with proven diagnosis of malignancy in other organs. The appearance of the fracture on the radiograph will be somewhat different, however, because there is not only a loss of stability of the vertebral body with collapse but usually also an involvement of the dorsal elements, particularly the pedicles on either side with the tumor. Collapse is not likely to be uniform and may involve a considerably greater loss of structural sufficiency than the simple compression fractures described previously. Along with this, the patient may have radiographic changes more indicative of a bone destructive lesion occurring at the margins of the fracture; this should lead one to suspect a metastatic lesion. While many of these compression fractures due to bone destruction from metatastic disease do occur with very minimal trauma, the patient usually has a known disease to start with, which should increase the index of suspicion rather markedly. Treatment of metatastic lesions, of course, depends upon treatment of the tumor itself and support of the spine is basically done with braces as indicated previously. Certainly, these patients should be referred to one specialized in treatment of malignant diseases so that the primary lesion can be treated. In most instances x-ray therapy is given over the pathologic fracture of the spine to diminish pain and promote bony healing of the compressed vertebrae.

6

THE CERVICAL SPINE

ANATOMY

The cervical spine has a unique function because of its location between the torso and the head (Fig. 6-1). In a distance of a relatively few centimeters this portion of the spine has become adapted to its unique function by developing a compromise between stability and mobility. The upper part of the cervical spine, along with its attachment to the occiput, is functionally adapted to allow for the extremes of rotation. The unique arrangement between C1 and C2 allows for enough rotation that in the normal individual the chin can be placed at approximately 90 degrees to the midline in either direction. This portion of the spine, however, has only limited ability in flexion and extension, this function being the priority of the lower portions of the spine from C3 down to T1. While this lower segment of spine participates to a certain extent in rotation, its primary function is that of flexion, both forward and backward as well as lateral. Because of this unique functional adaptation, the cervical spine has a unique set of articulations between the adjacent vertebrae which allows for more of a gliding type of motion, particularly in rotatory movement, compared to the lower segments of the spine.

The central articulation between the vertebral bodies is, as in the remainder of the spine, through connecting fibrous tissue structures known as intervertebral discs. In the cervical spine, however, these discs spaces are relatively narrow and the disc, therefore, has much less of a functioning hydraulic system. Cervical discs contain very little material in the nucleus pulposus but instead represent relatively firm and rigid fibrous tissue elements connecting the vertebral bodies. The facet joints are likewise altered in their structure from those of the lower part

57

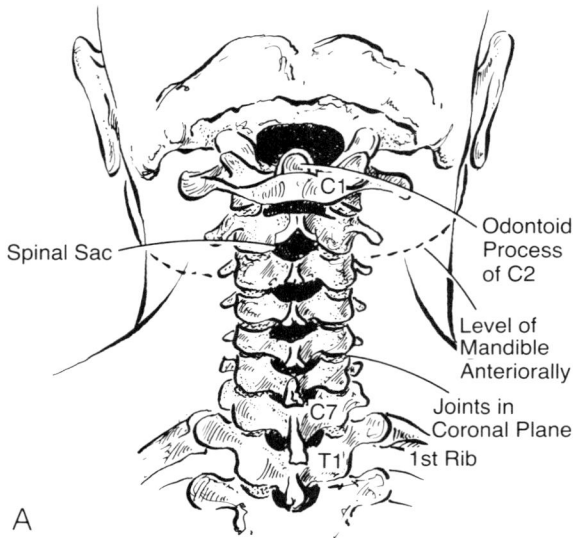

A

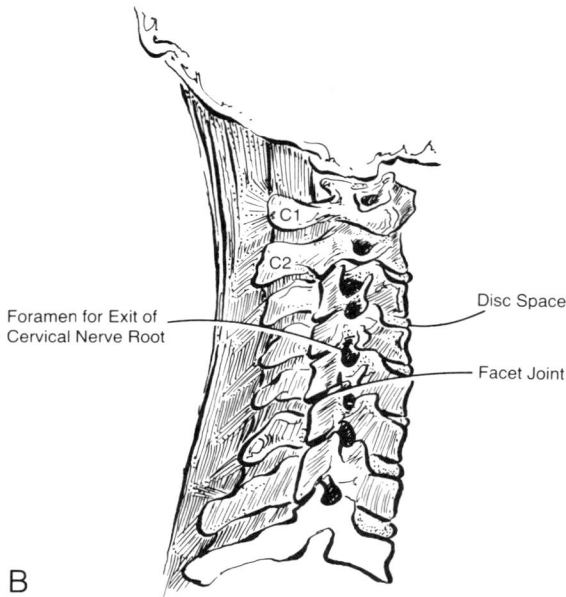

B

Fig. 6-1. (A) Posterior view of the cervical spine shows the close relationship between the vertebral bodies with the facets being located, for the most part, in the coronal plane. Dotted line indicates the line of the mandible: the first two cervical vertebrae lie superior to this. **(B)** Lateral view of the cervical spine. Note the close relationship between the vertebral bodies, with the spinal cord being almost completely encased in a bony canal. Notice the interwoven effect of the ligamentum nuchae extending posteriorly past the tips of the spinous processes to create additional strength in stability of the various articular bodies in flexion.

of the spine: they are elongated and relatively slanted in their position to allow a gliding type of motion in the forward flexion and extension while remaining relatively stable as the rotatory component of cervical spine motion comes into play.

The unusual structure of C1 and C2 has already been mentioned as being modified by their primary function in rotation. The first cervical vertebra is actually a large ring containing a lateral mass on either side representing, for the most part, the articular facets for the skull above and the second cervical vertebra below. The anterior part of the ring is sectioned off by a stout transverse ligament that creates a cylindrical compartment for articulating with a pinion-type projection from the second lumbar vertebra, known as the odontoid process. This "pinion and ring" structure allows the great amount of stability this articulation exhibits while still allowing maximal rotatory motion. The upper facets of C1 articulate directly with opposing facets on either side of the foramen magnum of the skull. These articulations are likewise created to allow maximum mobility in both flexion and extension as well as rotation. From the second cervical vertebra down, the laminae create a series of overlapping shelves, so that the cervical spine is covered by an armored plate made up of the successive layers of cervical laminae that overhang one another, much like an armadillo shell.

Since the torso acts as a relatively immobile foundation for the cervical spine and the head represents a 5 to 7 lb weight attached to the other end of this short segment of spine, these seven cervical vertebrae must have a great amount of additional supporting mechanism despite their architecture. The ligaments connecting the vertebrae are very strong and sturdy in the cervical spine but have enough elasticity to allow for the great range of motion previously described. In the normal individual these ligamentous structures almost completely encompass the cervical spine so that the stability of the relationships between adjacent vertebraes is ensured, unless a great amount of trauma disrupts these ligments and allows for alterations in the normal relationships between these vertebrae. Only when the trauma is severe enough to result in tear of these ligaments is it possible for the vertebrae to become separated or dislocated from their normal attachment.

Add to this already unique system a group of short, thick, heavy, muscles that not only serve as the motors for activating motion of the head on the body but also act as stabilizing mechanism to give additional support to the cervical spine. By their integrated pattern of resistance against each other, they maintain the head in a spectacular balancing act through its many different positions relative to the body. When this musculature becomes irritated with injury it usually goes into severe spasm that limits the motion of the head and causes severe pain. At the other end of the spectrum, however, when some abnormality results in paralysis of the supporting musculature not only is the control of head movement lost, but also the ability to maintain the upright position of the head over the torso in the erect position.

Add to these other anatomical features the fact that the neural control of the entire body from the brain passes through the neural canal of the cervical region and the blood supply to the brain from the heart likewise courses through the anterior aspect of this relatively small passageway. Finally, the two tubes that carry oxygen to the body for metabolic purposes and nutrition as well as fluids to the body for absorption through the gastrointestinal tract course through here. One can see the great importance of this relatively small segment of the body.

PHYSICAL EXAMINATION

Since the innervation of the upper extremities is derived from nerve roots that arise in the cervical spine area of the cord, examination of the neck must include specifically an examination of the upper extremities. Since the neurologic communication to the entire body from the brain courses through the cervical spine canal, a neurologic examination of the lower extremity is necessary when evaluating the cervical spine. The patient must, therefore, be disrobed for an adequate examination of the neck. The examination should be done with the patient sitting on an examining table at a comfortable height in an examining gown that exposes the neck as well as the upper extremity.

Attitude

The examination is begun by first noticing the attitude of the head and cervical spine, noting whether abnormal positions occur and whether the patient moves the neck well during conversation. Muscle spasm in the cervical spine can usually be identified from merely observing the patient, who often presents with a complaint of a "crick in the neck." The crick in the neck is, of course, due to muscle spasm in the supporting musculature of the spine. The head is usually drawn into a position indicating an overactivity of the muscles that happen to be in spasm. The cervical spine is next palpated in an effort to determine the location, extent, and severity of the muscular spasm, if present. Likewise, tender areas may be identified either overlying the spastic musculature in acute cases or overlying the points of muscular attachment in more chronic cases. This is particularly true in patients with long-standing tightness of the posterior cervical musculature in whom point tenderness can be elicited over the occipital attachment of the musculature on either side. This pain may sometimes be quite exquisite and even result in a radiating pain over the course of the occipital nerve on that side into the occipital and frontal areas of the skull. As a matter of fact, many people who complain of severe headaches with cervical spine problems have this continuous irritation of the attachment of the musculature to the occiput and the corollary of neuritis of the occipital nerve that passes through that area of muscular attachment. This so-called occipital neuritis is a very common cause of chronic headache in these patients.

Other points of tenderness may be over the ligamentous attachment to bone, such as at the tips of the spinous processes, and out over the shoulder girdle area where the associated musculature attaches. A favorite spot for tenderness in these patients is over the medial scapular angle, where an area scarcely larger than 1 cm in diameter often is exquisitely tender and thought to be related to the point of attachment of the levator scapulae muscle to this medial scapular angle. It is usually related to chronic cervical stiffness and/or muscle spasm.

Motion

The motions in the cervical spine are evaluated next. The patient is asked to touch his chin down to his sternum or come as closely as he can to this maneuver without assistance. While he is doing this, notice whether this flexion is possible and then whether the flexion is accomplished by a rounded, well-diversified flexion of the entire neck in a gentle curve or by an angular flexion with motion mainly at the base of the cervical spine or in a single level of the midcervical spine area. It will be quite often seen that the entire neck remains relatively straight and one can observe motion only at this limited level. It should be noted whether the patient has pain on this maneuver. The patient is next asked to extend the head as far as he can backwards and again the amount of motion is noted as well as the apparent degree of participation of all the vertebrae in the movement. The posterior curve of the spine in extension tends to be more nearly a smooth uniform curve, with participation of all vertebrae equally, rather than the angular curve seen in forward flexion. Finally, the patient is asked to demonstrate lateral flexion to either side, by attempting to place each ear to the shoulder on that side without elevating the shoulder and then to place the chin on either shoulder to demonstrate rotation. All of these motions should be evaluated to the limitation of motion and the absence or presence and degree of pain.

Sensory Function

The neurologic examination, as mentioned previously, should include the upper extremities primarily, though attention should be given to the lower extremities regarding the motor and sensory function and the presence or absence of Babinski's sign. The upper extremities are tested against the other. Inspection is made for muscular atrophy and then the muscles are tested for strength. Elbow flexion and extension, wrist flexion and extension, and finally intrinsic power in the hands are all evaluated. The thenar muscular strength is evaluated as is the function of the interossei and the adductor of the thumb. Sensation is then evaluated. While one commonly evaluates the hand with respect to the median, ulnar, and radial nerve functions, when testing in relation to the cervical spine function the sensation and motor power must be evaluated with respect to their cervical root origin rather than the actual peripheral nerve distribution, since the two may not completely coincide. Finally, reflexes are tested at the biceps, triceps and brachioradialis levels. Any obvious gross neurologic deficit will require a more thorough neurologic investigation by a neurologist or neurosurgeon.

X-RAY EXAMINATION

X-ray examination of the cervical spine should be done with multiple projections. The anteroposterior (AP) projection must be done with a single AP view of the cervical spine and then an additional odontoid view. In a straight AP view of the cervical spine the odontoid and the C1-C2 articulation are obscured by the jaw. The odontoid view is taken with the mouth open so that the jaw is displaced inferiorly and the AP picture taken through the open mouth. This will ordinarily give an excellent projection of the odontoid process of the second cervical vertebra along with its surrounding anatomical structures. Three lateral views should be taken. On the straight lateral view with the head in neutral position one can evaluate the relationship between the cervical spine bodies. Take care to determine that there is no evidence of displacement of the posterior line passing through the margins of the vertebral bodies. A normal cervical spine in the resting position will have a gentle forward curve indicative of the normal stance of the cervical vertebrae. With a neck that is injured or causing severe pain, this cervical lordosis is ordinarily absent due to muscle spasm and this can be easily ascertained on the lateral radiograph. A second lateral film should be taken with the neck in maximum extension and the head tilted as far backward as possible. The forward flexion film should be taken with the head tilted forward and the neck bent as much as possible. These views are mandatory if one is to evaluate the changes in position of the vertebrae relative to motion in the cervical spine. Extension of the spine is almost always associated with an increase of the gentle lordotic curve and seldom is any serious abnormality seen in the extension film.

Instabilities of the interveterbral relationships may be manifested in the hyperextension films but changes in alignment are much more likely to be noticed on the flexion films. The flexion film will, in a normal neck, reveal a gentle forward curve if all vertebrae are freely moving. However, in the usual instance, particularly if there is some straightening of the normal curve in the resting stance, there will be a continued straightening of the spine even in forward flexion. Occasionally, the normal lordotic curve of the cervical spine will be maintained even in flexion. This maintenance of the cervical lordosis in flexion is usually segmental and is ordinarily associated with some flexion occurring at various single levels, more commonly the C5-C6 interspace. This finding is more likely in the chronically painful stiff neck. The fact that this may go on unnoticed for great lengths of time probably accounts for the tendency for the greatest amount of wear and tear changes in the cervical spine to occur at the C5-C6 or other midcervical levels. Aside from these more subtle changes indicative of cervical musculature spasm or long-standing stiffness in the neck, other changes are more visible in the forward flexion film. Any gross instability in the cervical spine is usually much more noticeable and is accentuated in the forward flexion films. The tendency of one vertebral body to slide forward with respect to the adjacent vertebra will usually be accentuated in forward flexion and can be readily appreciated.

A word of warning seems pertinent in the examination of the patient who has been severely injured, such as in a motor vehicle accident, and who is brought into the emergency room on a stretcher, either with or without loss of consciousness. Scout AP and lateral films of the cervical spine should be taken before he is moved, to ascertain the general relationship between the vertebral bodies in the neck. Any serious injuries to the neck will be manifested by gross alterations in the normal alignment of the vertebrae. If this occurs, recognition prior to movement of the patient will many times prevent serious injuries to the spinal cord. A single AP and lateral film is all that is necessary to determine these gross relationships and these can be done quickly before the patient is moved. After these have been found to be essentially normal, somewhat more liberties can be taken in the changes of position necessary to obtain a more adequate cervical spine series for better visualization of the cervical vertebrae.

CONGENITAL MALFORMATIONS IN CHILDREN

Congenital skeletal malformations in the cervical spine are seen occasionally and are usually recognized relatively early. There is usually obvious deformity in the neck and many of these cervical spine abnormalities create angular deformities that result in some alterations in position of the head with relationship to the body. Changes such as seen in the Klippel-Feil syndrome are usually manifested by short thick necks with obvious loss of motion and abnormalities in the spine. These can be evaluated by x-ray examination and most cases should be referred to the orthopedist for evaluation of treatment. For the most part, nothing can be done in the majority of these instances. As with any congenital abnormality of the spine, the patient must be evaluated over time to be certain that progressive changes in alignment do not occur.

Congenital hemivertebrae and other abnormalities causing angular deformities will often be progressive, since the angular deformity, which may not be noticeable to any great extent at first, will become magnified by growth and may become unacceptable from a cosmetic and functional standpoint. These cases should, therefore, be monitored in most instances by an orthopedic surgeon.

The most significant condition seen in the early neonate is torticollis. In many instances the newborn will tilt his head slightly to one side or the other; this should be the signal for a very careful evaluation by the examining physician. In instances in which a torticollis is developing, a hard small nodule will be palpated in the sternocleidomastoid muscle soon after birth. This nodule is usually present in the muscular belly of the sternomastoid and is usually easily palpated. Its cause is unknown but it is recognized as the precursor to severe torticollis if left untreated.

This nodule should indicate that the parents start a vigorous stretching program, even with the very young infant. If this is done and done expertly and faithfully, ensuing deformities can often be prevented. The youngster with a typical torticollis has an extremely tight sternomastoid muscle. The sternomastoid muscle attaches from the mastoid process of the skull to the manubrium of the sternum in the region of the sternoclavicular joint. Tightness in this muscle will cause a characteristic deformity in which the head is tilted towards the side of the tightness but the face is tilted towards the opposite side. The examiner will visualize that by bringing these two points as close together as possible to reproduce the characteristic deformity. Stretching, then, will depend upon manipulation in precisely the opposite direction. The mastoid process and the sternum must be identified as two points and then separated as widely as possible. The head must be tilted to the opposite direction from the tight muscle and the face tilted or pointed toward the side of the muscular tightness.

The stretching procedures should be done by both parents: one holds the infant and stabilizes its shoulders while the other is charged with manipulating the head. With one parent sitting down, holding the infant on its back in his or her lap, and stabilizing the shoulders, the other parent can then stretch the tight muscle. The second parent should hold the infant's head in both hands and the infant's body should be moved out so that the shoulders lie at the level of the knees of the other parent. The infant's head can then be gently tilted backward and laterally away from the tight muscle and the head rotated so that the face is pointing toward the tight muscle. This should be done gently and without any real force being applied, merely carrying the infant's head through what is considered a relatively complete normal range of motion.

The stretching procedure should be done six or eight times at a session for two sessions daily. The infant can be checked periodically in the office. If the deformity appears to be improving, treatment can be continued on this basis. If, however, no improvement is seen or if the deformity appears to be getting worse, the child should be referred to the orthopedic surgeon for further evaluation. The nodule in the muscle occasionally will become quite large but in no circumstance should removal ever be recommended. As the child grows, the mass will gradually diminish and by the time the infant is several months of age it will have completely disappeared. If stretching has been carried out effectively the tightness of the muscle will be minimal. If, however, the mass has not been identified or if stretching has not been started, a considerable tightness of the muscle will be found and other marked deformities will be seen.

When the child has not been treated from infancy, the typical wryneck deformity will be seen to form and progress. Even in babies around 1 year of age in whom the deformity has become evident, stretching will often still be effective and the muscle tightness can be relieved. However, if the child is much older or if the deformity has become more definitely established, surgical release of the tight musculature will most likely be necessary and the child should be referred to the orthopedic surgeon. In the older child in whom the torticollis has been untreated, marked facial deformity will result from the prolonged pull on the attachment of the muscle to the skull. These children will often have a very noticeable flattening of the face on this side. Ultimately the deformity becomes severe enough that diplopia will occur. In the untreated child who reaches the age of 8 or 9 years, diplopia will often be the complaint that brings the child to the physician for care.

CONDITIONS IN THE ADULT

Acute Trauma With Fractures and/or Dislocations

Cases of acute trauma with fractures of the cervical spine should be identified and quickly transferred to the orthopedic surgeon for care. As mentioned earlier, extreme caution should be exercised in injuries in which bony damage to the cervical spine might possibly have occurred so as not to aggravate the situation. The patient should be handled very cautiously at the site of the accident and the neck immobilized with a cervical collar prior to transport. If there is evidence of a cervical spine injury the patient should be gently placed on a stretcher and sandbags applied to either side of the head to prevent motion. The scout films previously described can be taken as long as they can be done without moving the patient. If these can be found to be unquestionably negative for fracture or dislocation, treatment can be done by the primary care physician. If obvious deformity of the cervical spine exists or if the symptoms create a question of cervical spine injury, the patient should be transferred immediately to the care of an orthopedic surgeon. Even when no abnormalities can be demonstrated on radiograph, if serious symptoms are present the patient should be admitted to the hospital for observation and treatment.

Acute Trauma Without Fractures or Dislocation

Acute injuries to the neck in which no fractures or dislocations exist and in which stability of the cervical spine can be demonstrated to be intact must be assumed to be acute cervical sprains. This implies overstretching and possibly incomplete tears of the ligamentous structures and overstretching of the supporting musculature. These patients will often have severe, acute, symptoms. As mentioned earlier, if these symptoms are severe enough hospitalization is indicated. The patient should be placed in a halter traction in the hospital bed with the head of the bed inclined to about 30 degrees and the hips and knees flexed so that the leg from the knee to ankle is horizontal but the hips and knees flexed to around 45 degrees. Cervical spine traction should be in the line of pull so that a completely straight line can be drawn from the base of the neck to the pulley at the top of the bed. This will yield a completely straight line of traction as a starting point. If the patient seems somewhat more comfortable in flexion, the head of the bed can be lowered slightly. If the patient seems to be somewhat more comfortable in extension, the head of the bed can be elevated slightly past 30 degrees. The chin and occiput must be well padded and the halter should be removed periodically so that the pressure on the chin particularly can be relieved, the skin massaged, and pressure sores prevented. Heat and medication will usually be beneficial for the muscular spasm and sedation will be required for the relief of pain and spasm. After a few days physical therapy can be started in the forms of heat, massage, and gentle exercises and the patient allowed to begin ambulation in a soft cervical collar.

A word of caution should be given concerning the tendency to dependence on cervical support. A soft cervical collar has a very important place in the treatment of these acute cervical sprains since it does help to support the head and gives the cervical spine and the associated muscles a degree of immobilization and rest. However, in no instance should this be used for longer than 6 weeks without the advice of the orthopedic surgeon. Dependency upon this support can very readily develop and become difficult to treat.

Acute sprains of the cervical spine should respond to these relatively simple measures so that the patient gradually improves over a relatively short period of time. If the patient fails to respond to treatment, if response is slower than is considered normal, or if there is obvious litigation pending in the case, the patient should be referred to the orthopedic surgeon for consultation and probable treatment.

Mention should be made about the so-called "whiplash" injury. This usually describes acute flexion and extension classically caused by a rear-end collision. If the patient is sitting still in an automobile that is struck from behind, there is a tendency for the head to remain in its original position while the thorax, which is supported by the seat, is suddenly propelled forward with great force. This results in acute hyperextension of the neck and a sudden axial loading or compression of the cervical spine caused by the spine being forced between the relatively immobile head and torso. As the body continues to move forward the head reaches the end of its connection to the neck and is then propelled forward. The original hyperextension is followed by acute flexion of the neck as the head goes forward relative to the torso.

There are, of course, different degrees of severity, depending upon the force and myriad other circumstances. These patients generally do not have any great amount of bony damage but they can be considered to have an extremely acute cervical spine sprain. The symptoms are usually acute and the most severe are often present in the musculature of the anterior neck, caused by the original sudden acute hyperextension of the neck. The more acute joint sprains occur following acute flexion of the neck. If the force is severe, there may be areas of partial tears of the ligamentous structures with intrinsic bleeding and swelling followed by acute muscle spasm and ultimately by considerable loss of neck motion due to scarring.

Damage to the bony attachments of these ligamentous structures can be seen after the passage of many months by the formation of marginal osteophytes along the rims of the vertebral bodies. These osteophytes occur as a bony proliferative reaction to the bleeding and inflammation that results from the partial tear. Patients with relatively severe flexion and extension injury should be referred early to an orthopedic surgeon. Treatment is often complicated and continuation of symptoms prolonged; the possibility of some permanent impairment is great. These injuries also occur for the most part in motor vehicle accidents. Litigation is often pending that will probably require an expert opinion subsequently. For all of these reasons, cases of this type should be best referred to the orthopedic surgeon who is better equipped to accept responsibility for their care.

Chronic Conditions

Chronic conditions involving the adult cervical spine involve two specific clinical pictures: a stiff painful neck with or without degenerative joint and a protruded cervical disc.

Stiff Neck

The patient with cervical spondylopathy or a stiff painful neck generally has more or less chronic neck pain almost daily, but characterized by acute episodes at periodic intervals. These acute episodes may either be precipitated by some injury, even though trivial, or they may occur without any known reason. The common denominator in these individuals is a marked loss of motion in their cervical spine. This can be seen on examination particularly on the radiograph, with loss of motion seen on flexion and extension films in the lateral view. In most instances there is marked loss of motion throughout the cervical spine with most of the flexion present being through a single interspace, usually in the midcervical area.

Some of these patients have very little evidence of degenerative changes in the cervical spine, but they nevertheless have markedly limited motion with chronic neck pain. Others have marked degenerative disc disease manifested by narrowing of the disc space and marginal osteophyte formation. These patients, however, also have a stiff painful neck. The implications are virtually the same except that the patient with marked degenerative changes has less chance of regaining motion in the cervical spine than does the patient with normal x-ray findings whose loss of motion is based on ligamentous tightness. By the same token, the individual with cervical spondylopathy without serious degenerative changes usually has virtually no radicular pain. The patient with marked osteophyte formation will often have encroachment on the cervical roots as they pass through the neural foramina. These patients may have radicular pain that is indistinguishable from an acute cervical disc protrusion. Patients with ligamentous tightness in the neck may have a small amount of motion, particularly in rotation but be markedly in flexion. During the acute episode, however, there will be marked muscle spasm added to the clinical picture as nature's attempt to immobilize the painful spine.

In most of these individuals the pain occurs from the stiff joints present at each level, in much the same way that any joint in the body that loses motion causes pain on attempts to regain that motion. This same phenomenon is true in the cervical spine but is magnified by the fact that there are four separate joints at each articular level.

Early degenerative changes may occur as marginal osteophyte formations and, as was discussed under flexion and extension injury, osteophyte formation along the marginal attachments of the ligamentous structure may result from acute injury with partial disruption of the ligamentous attachments and subsequent reactive bone formation. Most degenerative changes, however, result from long-standing changes from wear and tear in the cervical spine or perhaps from repeated episodes of trauma to the neck. When radicular pain occurs the clinical picture is still essentially the same except for the extension of pain out into the upper extremities, which markedly increases the severity of symptoms. Most of the time, however, people with radiculitis coming from degenerative changes in the cervical spine have only slight pain in the extremities most of the time but develop acute episodes, in which radicular pain may extend down into the nerve root distribution in the hand on the affected side.

Treatment.   Treatment of the cervical spondylopathies consists of the following features.

Heat and massage to the neck often result in relief of muscle spasm and tightness and generally give considerable symptomatic relief. The heat is usually best applied as moist heat either with compresses or with hot packs.

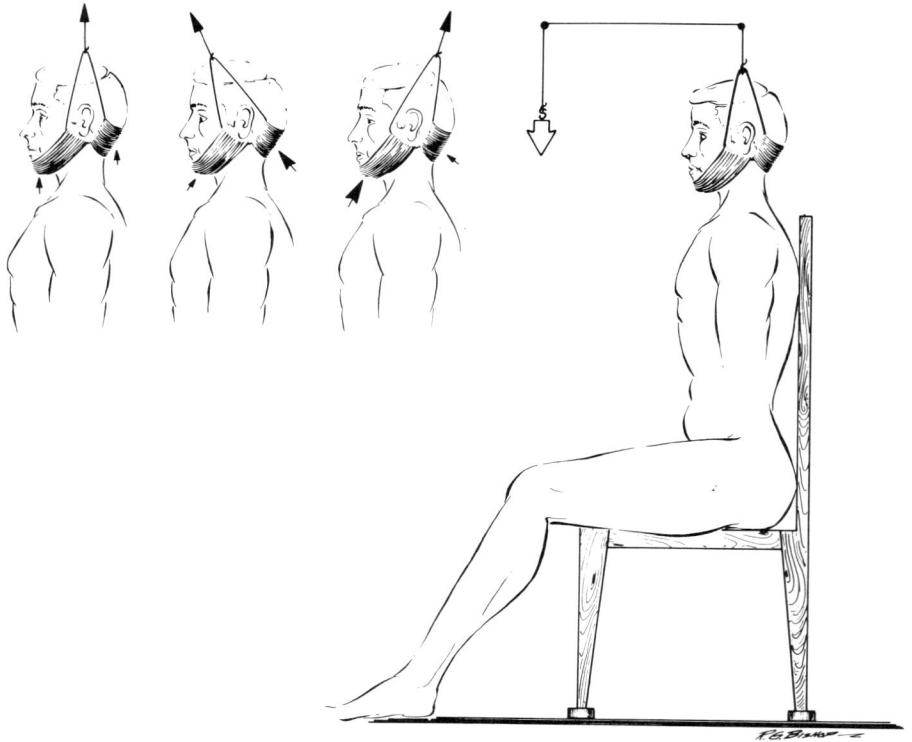

Fig. 6-2. Pull applied with the patient in the erect position is accomplished by using the same type of halter, but with two pulleys that are attached to a doorjamb by eye screws. The traction is applied as shown (right), with the amount and duration of traction prescribed by the physician. Ordinarily, 10 minutes of traction with 15 lb of weight, twice daily, is suitable. The amount of pressure on the occiput or the chin may be varied by moving the chair forward or backward to cause the line of pull to be somewhat posterior or anterior, respectively. (Lewis RC, Jr: Handbook of Traction, Casting and Splinting Techniques. JB Lippincott, Philadelphia, 1977.)

Cervical spine exercises should be instituted and instructions probably should be given by a professional physical therapist. For the most part the exercises aim to restore motion in these cervical levels and the exercises, particularly in flexion, must be done with the aim of stretching the ligamentous structures in the cervical spine without accentuating the changes present at the level where most of the flexion and extension occurs. This type of exercise, done after the application of heat to relax the muscle spasm, should be done by tucking the chin in toward the chest as the neck is flexed, thereby causing a generalized stretching of the cervical musculature and ligamentous structures rather than merely a bending at the midcervical level. The exercises done as instructed by the physical therapist twice daily basis will usually result in gradual improvement in motion in cases without severe degenerative disease. Even patients with marked degenerative changes will exhibit some improvement of motion with appropriately administered cervical spine exercises.

Cervical traction is probably the most important physical therapy for neck pain, even radicular pain. Traction is best applied with a halter and can usually be applied twice daily with the patient in a sitting position. Figure 6-2 demonstrates the proper method for the application of cervical spine traction using a relatively simple apparatus created from two pulleys attached to "eye" hooks in a door jam. A 10 lb weight is attached to one end and the opposite end is attached to the spreader bar, which in turn attaches to the cervical halter. Slightly more weight can be used if desired but, as a general rule, very heavy weights cannot be tolerated for long periods of time because of the pressure caused on the inferior manibular ridge of the chin. If the pressure on the chin is great, the chair can be moved back slightly to decrease the pull anteriorly and increase it posteriorly. If, on the other hand, the traction causes the patient to have headaches from posterior muscle attachment stretching, the patient's chair can be moved slightly forward to increase the chin pressure but decrease occipital pressure. Alterations can be made for comfort. Traction is usually continued for 10 or 15 minutes and the patient usually rotates the neck slowly from side to side, pointing the chin towards each shoulder alternately during traction. It is usually better to precede the traction with the application of heat.

Various medications have been devised for the relief of cervical spine pain, particularly muscle spasms. These preparations all have merit and can be used with some degree of success in most cases, particularly when muscle spasm is a factor. Most of these preparations cause considerable drowsiness and the patient should be warned of this. Medications such as the nonsteroidal anti-inflammatory agents may be of value. particularly in cases with considerable degenerative disease, since this pain is often magnified by the degenerative changes present in the joints, much as it is in other joints of the body. In these instances, nonsteroidal anti-inflammatory agents may give considerable relief of pain and improvement in motion.

Protruded Disc

Manifested primarily by radicular pain, protrusion of some of the disc material out into the neural foramen puts pressure on the corresponding nerve root. Because the cervical disc is composed of much more fibrous tissue and has a less demonstrable nucleus pulposus, protrusions of cervical discs are much less common than those in the lumbar spine. However, a patient who has persistent arm pain or pain suggesting radicular involvement should be referred to the orthopedic surgeon for a more thorough evaluation and treatment as indicated. Conservative measures for the treatment of disc protrusion are the same as those described for the cervical spondylopathies and may be used for a short time to determine whether improvement might occur. However, the treating physician should be ready to refer the patient for more expert care as soon as it becomes obvious that he is not responding to conservative management or that neurologic deficit, either motor or sensory, is developing.

7

THE LOW BACK

LOW BACK PAIN

When one begins an examination of the low back it is important to realize that all the causes of low back pain are not related to the musculoskeletal system. Before one pinpoints the examination to the musculoskeletal system one must ascertain whether other of these etiologic factors are present.

Viscerogenic

A variety of visceral organs can cause pain in the low back that sometimes is very difficult to differentiate from musculoskeletal pain. For instance, gynecologic causes of low back pain include malpositions of the uterus, endometriosis, fibroids or other tumors, pelvic infections, or even chronic cervicitis. These are usually easy to differentiate by careful history and examination. Prostatic difficulties may occasionally be very difficult to differentiate. Chronic prostatitis is a relatively common cause of low back pain but infection, malignancy, and benign hypertrophy of the prostate all may cause symptoms referable to the low back. Various renal causes such as calculi, infections, and neoplasms all may result in pain in the low back but the symptoms referable to renal difficulties are usually more in the flank region and should be easier to differentiate.

Vascular

Vascular causes of low back pain include such relatively rare but catastrophic conditions as aortic aneurysm. Much more common, however, is Leriche's syndrome, in which vascular insufficiency in the lower extremities relative to occlusion in the iliac or upper femoral vessels results in pain in the lower extremities, particularly with some pain in the low back. It is sometimes difficult to differentiate a vascular insufficiency type of pain from that occurring with a protruding lumbar disc, but with the absence of pulsations in the arteries of extremities one should at least be suspicious and include this in the differential diagnosis.

Neurogenic

Neurogenic causes of low back pain resulting from conditions other than herniated intervertebral disc are usually in the form of tumors of the spinal cord or adjacent structures. Extradural tumors such as hemangiomas and fibroblastomas may cause pain by compressing the nerve root. Much more commonly, pain in the low back and lower extremity is related to intradural tumors that may occur either alongside the cord with compression of the nerve roots or even as an intramedullary tumor such as an ependymoma. Most of the neurogenic cause of pain related to trauma, of course, should be self-evident.

Psychogenic

Psychogenic pain in the low back is common and is probably the most difficult to identify and differentiate from organic pain. The hysterical patient who complains of severe pain in the low back, but has completely normal findings, is usually relatively easy to identify. This patient, however, should have the benefits of a complete work-up to be certain that no organic cause of the pain persists. The patient will usually have a picture of pain out of proportion to what one might expect, particularly in the absence of true muscle spasm or any other organic findings.

More difficult than this is the malingerer. Since many of the instances of low back and lower extremity pain are work-related, the presence of secondary gain as a causative or exaggerating factor must be considered. Similarly, cases in the patient who has a liability claim from an injury in an automobile accident, a slip on a slick floor in a business establishment, or other instances in which secondary gain possibilities exist are often hard to prove. One of the primary proofs that the patient is malingering is that usually there is some underlying basis for his pain and the pain merely exaggerates this or fails entirely to respond to appropriate therapy. In these instances it is extremely hard to differentiate the true organic pain from that which is purely subjective. For the most part, this requires the experience and expertise of an orthopedic surgeon. These patients should be referred for consultation.

Spondylogenic

Spondlylogenic pain, or pain related to musculoskeletal structures of the low back, represents the fifth category of causes of low back pain but includes the vast majority of patients seen by the family practitioner. The pain related to the spine may arise either from bone and associated structures or soft tissue. Osseous lesions may be due to the following etiologic factors: trauma, infection, neoplasms, metabolism, degeneration, arthritis, spondylolisthesis or congenital instability syndrome, and spinal stenosis. Before these are discussed, the anatomy of the low back and method of clinical examination should be discussed.

ANATOMY

The low back is ordinarily thought of as consisting of the lumbar vertebrae and the sacrum (Fig. 7-1). While there are ordinarily five lumbar vertebrae, occasionally a sixth vertebra is present in a normal individual and represents a normal anatomical variation. However, when six lumbar vertebrae exist the sixth may represent a lumbarization of the first sacral segment and, as such, will probably have abnormal articulation with the underlying sacrum or with the L5 vertebra above it. These vertebrae are suspended on one another by three points of contact. Anteriorly, the vertebral bodies are separated by the intervertebral disc. The disc per se is made up of a heavy fibrous casing called the annulus fibrosis, which contains a small nucleus of gelanous or mucoid material known as the nucleus pulposus. When the disc is intact this material is contained within the central portion of the disc and acts as a more or less "hydraulic" shock absorber. Just behind the intervertebral disc the spinal sac runs through the neural canal (Fig. 7-2). The canal is formed by the vertebral bodies and the discs anteriorly and the pedicles and laminae of the vertebra posteriorly. The two other points of suspension of the spine are the facet joints posteriorly. The inferior articular facets point outward from the midline and occur on either side of the vertebrae, extending downward from the pedicles. The superior articular facets extend upward from the pedicles and have small articular areas that face toward the midline and articulate with the inferior facets of the vertebrae above. These articulations on either side create the so-called facet joints and represent the only true synovial joints in the vertebral articulations. In the architecture of the posterior elements of the vertebrae, the pedicles are depressed to create a small passage way through which the nerve roots exit from the spinal sac. These are known as the neural foramina and pass between the posterior aspect of the intervertebral discs and the anterior aspect of the articulation of the facet joint.

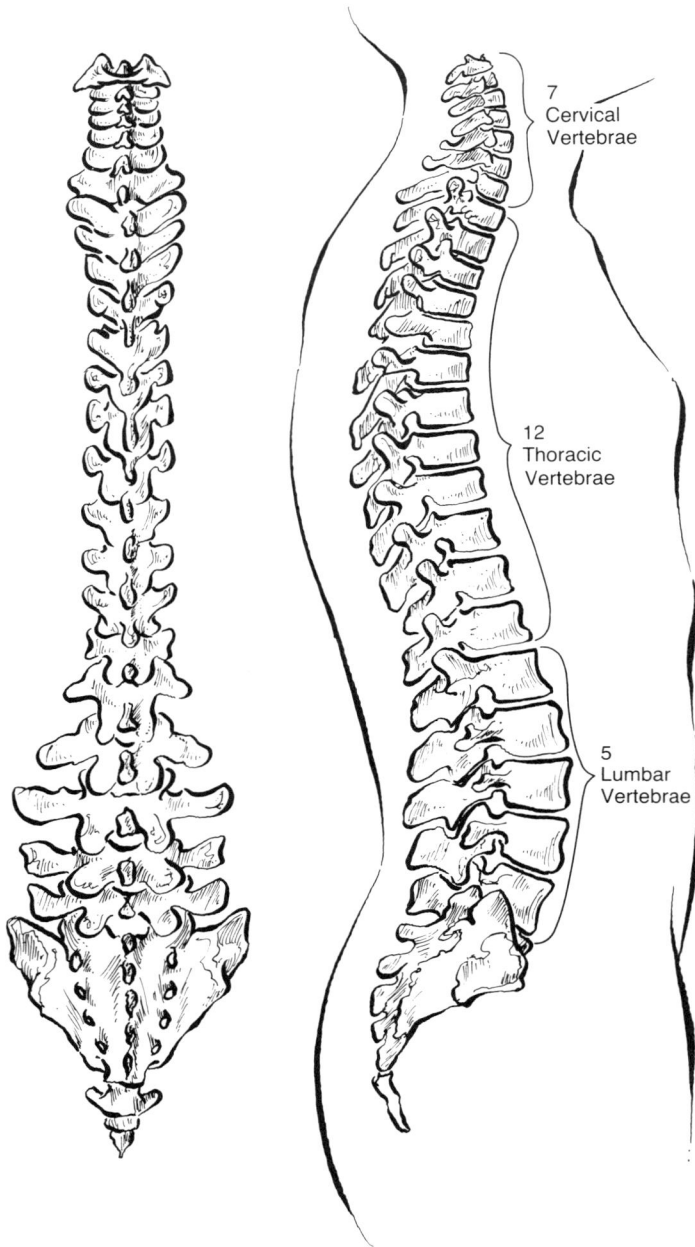

Fig. 7-1. Comparison views of the posterior and lateral projections of the entire spine. Note the difference in the shape and appearance of the vertebrae in various regions. The 5 lumbar vertebrae are much heavier and have much larger dorsal elements than the others and extend up to the thoracic cage. The 12 thoracic type vertebrae have a somewhat different configuration: much smaller slanted dorsal elements and spinous processes that point downward allow for overlap of the laminae posteriorly. Note the cervical vertebrae that extend from the articulation with the occiput down to the superior aspect of the thoracic cage. Note that the cervical and lumbar areas have a normal lordotic curve, whereas the thoracic area has a kyphotic curve.

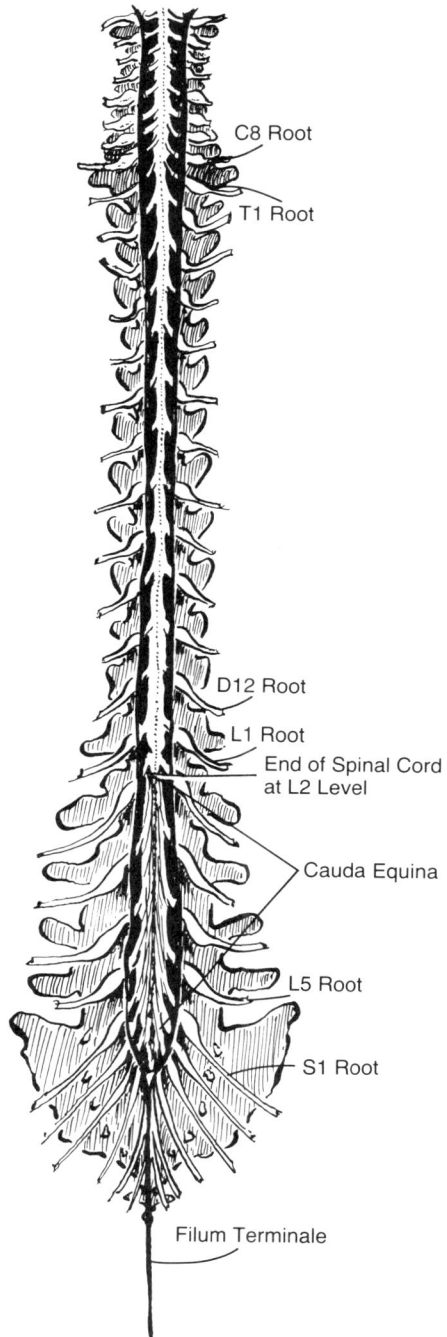

Fig. 7-2. Cutaway view shows the relationship of the spinal cord, the spinal roots, and the vertebral levels. Note that the eighth cervical root arises just inferior to the C7 vertebra and from the interspace between C7 and T1, the T1 root arises from underneath the body of T1 at the T1-T2 level. The spinal cord, as an identifiable structure, ends at about L2 and the nerve roots that extend distal to that lie in the spinal canal as individual roots passing together and are known as the cauda equina. Note that the L5 root rises at the interspace between L4 and L5 and that the S1 root rises at the lumbosacral level between L5 and S1.

Because the canal is relatively small and the fit of the nerve root going through it is relatively close, any impingement upon this space by a herniation of the nucleus pulposus of the intervertebral disc anteriorly or any encroachment by the creation of marginal osteophytes from the facet joint surfaces posteriorly results in a compromise of the space with compression of the nerve root. When the compression occurs from a herniated nucleus pulposus this is the so-called protruded disc syndrome. When the compression occurs from marginal osteophytes occurring along the vertebral margin, this is usually described as degenerative disc disease with nerve root compression. When the compromise of the neural foramen occurs from osteophyte formation along the margins of the facet joints, the compression is usually related to degenerative changes within these small joints themselves.

The ligamentous structures supporting the vertebral column consist of those surrounding vertebral bodies both anterior and posterior. The communications between the laminae or the so-called ligamentum flavium and the ligamentous structures occur as joint capsules around the facet joints. These ligamentous structures are all quite strong and destruction of the anterior or posterior longitudinal ligaments attached to the vertebral bodies is rare because of their strength. However, disruption of the facet joints does occur with some frequency in severe injuries but the majority of the injuries to the facets represent sprains of these supporting ligaments. The final ligamentous structure occurs between the spinous processes and is known as the interspinous ligament. This can quite often be sprained, with acute stretching or with compression between the spinous processes over a long period of time. Symptoms are usually prolonged and require specific treatment such as injections with hydrocortisone, x-ray therapy, or occasionally even excision of the ligament itself. Since the majority of disc protrusions occur at the L3-L4 level with compression of the L4 root, and the L4-L5 level with compression of the L5 root, or the lumbosacral level with compression of the S1 root, these three roots will be described in some detail as far as their clinical manifestations are concerned (Fig. 7-3).

L4 Root

The L4 root arises from the L3-L4 disc level. The L4 root has a motor component in innervation of the quadriceps muscle and, of course, a neurologic deficit here results in the diminution of the strength of the knee jerk reflex. The sensory level of L4 is the very medial aspect of the foot including the very medial side of the great toe and the balance of the foot back to the heel.

L5 Root

The L5 nerve root arises from the L4-L5 disc level and is probably the most common of the levels for disc protrusions. The L5 root innervates the extensor digitorum longus; motor deficit at this level renders the patient unable to extend his toes, particularly the great toe. There is no reflex loss with an L5 deficit since the knee jerk and the ankle jerk are both supplied by different levels. The sensory level of the L5 root is that of the medial side of the dorsum of the foot, extending

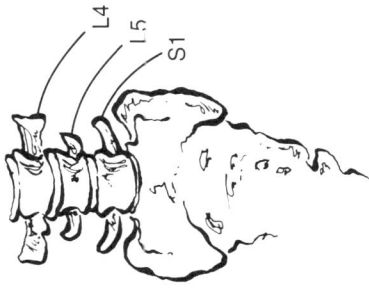

Fig. 7-3. Motor, reflex, and sensory components of each of the three lower lumbar roots. The L3-L4 interspace provides the L4 root and the changes are as shown. The L4-L5 interspace contributes the L5 root: there is no reflex component of the L5 root. The lumbosacral interspace provides the S1 root. Pressure on any one of these roots by herniated disc will result in disruption of motor power, loss of sensation, or alteration of the reflex component provided by the nerve root at that level.

across the great toe and the dorsum of the smaller toes to the little toe and lateral side of the foot, which comes from S1.

S1 Root

The S1 neurologic level arises from the L5-S1 disc level (lumbosacral level). The motor innervation of the S1 root can be tested by the function of the peroneus longus muscle and also by the calf musculature, particularly the gastrocnemius soleus group. Neurologic deficit of this level renders the patient unable to contract his muscles in pulling the foot to the lateral side and in pointing the toes in equinus. The reflex component of the S1 root is that of the Achilles tendon reflex, or ankle jerk; neurologic deficit of this root renders this reflex markedly diminished to absent. The sensory level of the S1 root is present over the lateral aspect of the foot and ankle and ordinarily includes the little toe.

Summary

There are, of course, variations in the degree of nerve root compressions and, therefore, in the degree of deficits responsible for varying clinical pictures, but the aforementioned comprise the absolute anatomical distribution of these three nerve roots and should serve as guidelines during the clinical examination. The spinal cord ends at the L2 level. Distal to that the spinal roots are contained within the dural sac and are known as the cauda equina. Each of the paired roots exits at each level for its transverse into the lower extremity. A discussion of the innervation of these roots is given in greater detail in the section on examination of the low back. The normal lumbar spine exhibits a mild lordosis with a lumbosacral angle created by the somewhat less than completely parallel position of the inferior surface of the vertebral body of L5 and the superior surface of sacrum. Ordinarily this interspace is more narrow posteriorly than it is anteriorly, resulting in the tendency for closure of the neural foramen and nerve root irritation with acute leg pain.

PHYSICAL EXAMINATION

Examination of the low back is done first with the patient standing, then with the patient lying down, and then the patient sitting up. The routines shown in Figure 7-4 A and B may be reproduced in condensed form as a rubber stamp (Fig. 7-4C) and can be used to document findings at the examination of the low back, so that the same information can be obtained each time the patient is examined and recorded appropriately. Thus nothing will be left out and comparable results can be obtained to demonstrate either improvement or deterioration of the patient's condition with treatment.

Standing

Inspection (Fig. 7-5)

1. The habitus of the patient should be noted. If he is unusually obese or has any unusual configuration of body type, this should be noted.

Mark tender areas as to location and amount (0 to +4)

Mark spasm

Mark sciatic notch and trochanteric bursa tenderness here (0 to +4) and, if none, write "No" in area

$$\frac{-2}{+2}$$

$$\frac{-1}{0} \leftarrow \bigcirc \rightarrow \frac{-1}{0}$$

$$\frac{-3}{+3}$$

Denote loss of motion, if any, as 0 to −4 and any pain as 0 to +4

SLR

(R) *range* n degrees from 0 to 90 and show *amount* and location of pain

(L)

HIPS: R/L range, pain, etc.

PULSES: R/L adequate pedal pulses?

LEG LENGTHS: (= or not)

Neurologic   (R) (L)

	R	L
Motor		
Sensory		
Reflexes		
Knee		
Ankle		
Babinski		
Circumference of the calf		

REMEMBER
L3-L4—Ant. thigh—Quad.—knee jerk
L4-L5—Great toe—Foot and toe dorsiflexion—no reflex
L5-S1 (L-S)—Lat. foot—Gastroc. soleus—ankle jerk

A

Fig. 7-4. (A) Form for evaluation of the low back. (*Figure continues.*)

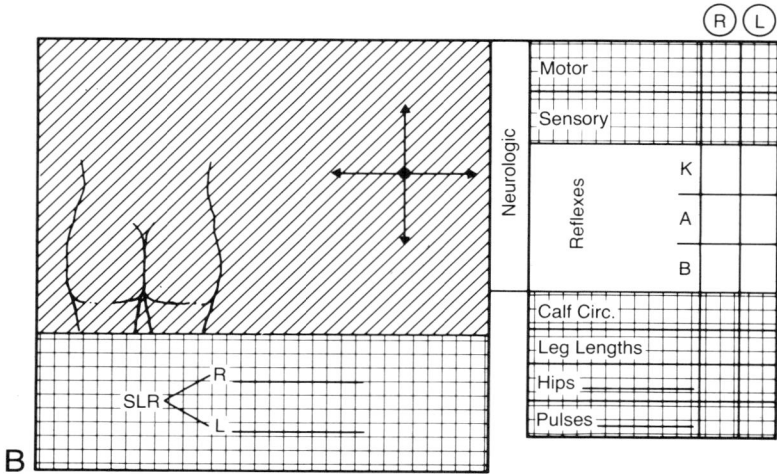

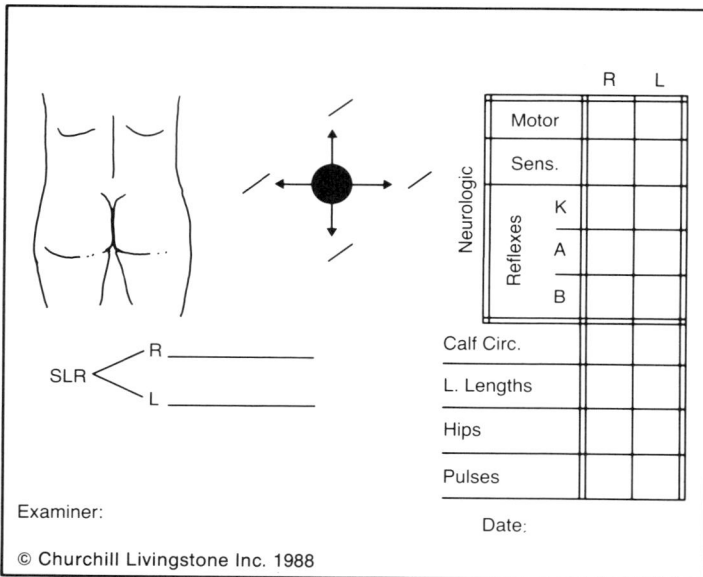

Fig. 7-4. (*Continued*). **(B)** Schematic plan for examination of the low back. ▨ = Portion of examination done with patient standing. ▦ = Portion of examination done with patient lying on examination table. ☐ = Portion of examination done with patient sitting on side of examination table with legs dangling over side. **(C)** A rubber stamp may be created for tabulation of the results of examination of the low back. The various components of the examination are described in the text. The author and publisher hereby grant permission for this illustration to be copied as a rubber stamp to be used in the clinician's office. Serial examinations on different visits are easy to compare if the stamp is used each time.

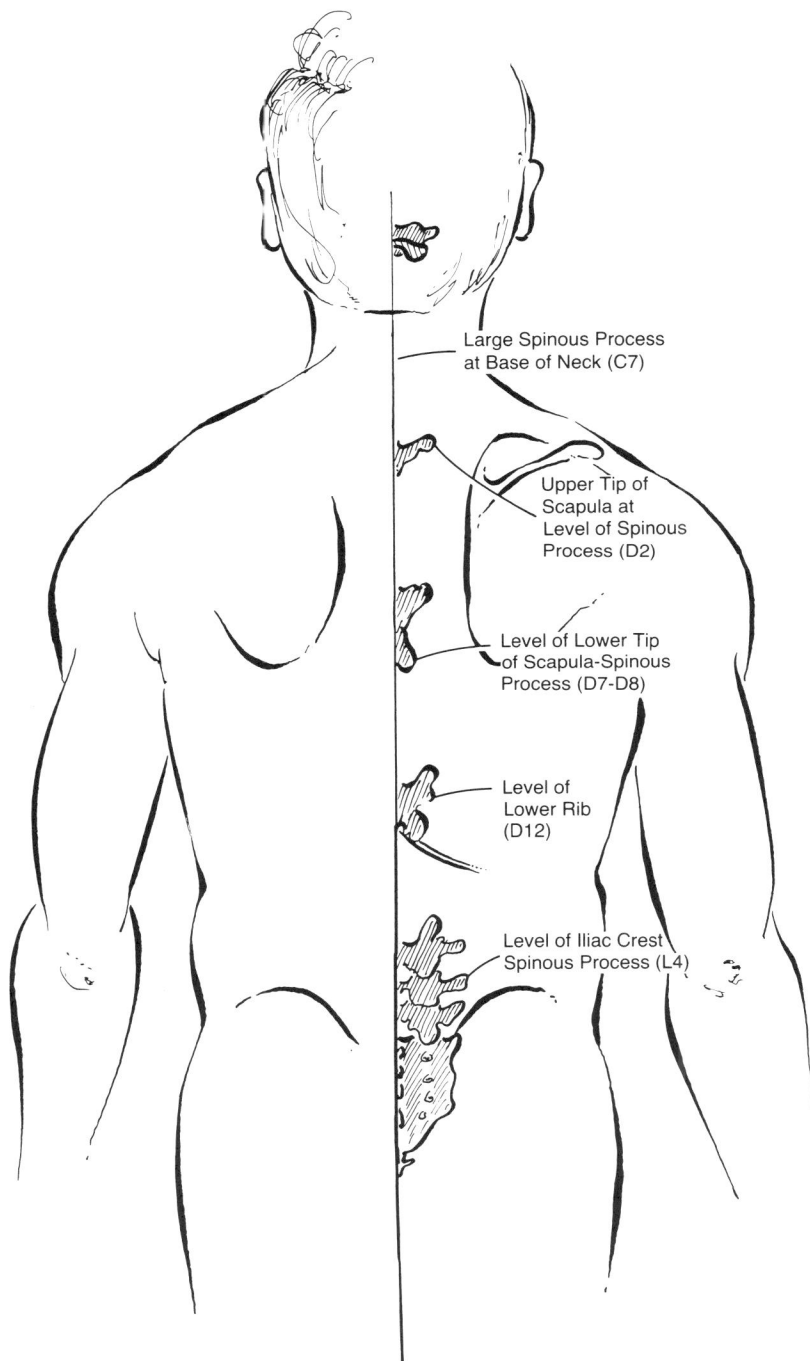

Large Spinous Process at Base of Neck (C7)

Upper Tip of Scapula at Level of Spinous Process (D2)

Level of Lower Tip of Scapula-Spinous Process (D7-D8)

Level of Lower Rib (D12)

Level of Iliac Crest Spinous Process (L4)

Fig. 7-5. Topographical views, as indicated by various other anatomical features. C1 and C2 are very difficult to palpate and lie just under the margin of the occiput. The prominent spinous process at the base of the neck is C7. The level of the lower tip of the scapula is usually at D8. The lower rib cesignates the spinous process of D12. The spinous process occurring at the level of the iliac crest is usually at about L4. The lumbosacral level can be determined by palpating up the body of the sacrum to its upper margin where it articulates with L5.

2. Fixed deformities should be noted; whether or not the patient has scoliosis or whether or not there is any chest deformity, either congenital or acquired. All of these make some difference in the mechanical situation that may lead to low back pain.

3. Increased lumbar lordosis may or may not be congenital, but is without question one of the leading factors predisposing to low back pain. It results in abnormal stress on the lumbosacral articulation particularly. It also allows for a diminution in the size of the neural foramen, which leads to compression of the nerve root going through it with less impingement by a protruded disc.

4. Increased rounded back is important because it usually is associated with an increased lumbar lordosis. This should be noted on the diagram of the low back.

5. Gait: Note whether the patient has a limp, whether he has any difficulty walking, and whether this appears to be related to loss of muscular strength, pain, or some fixed deformity.

6. List: Note whether the patient's pelvis is completely straight or is tilted to one side or the other, such as with inequality of leg length. A list may also be caused by a muscle spasm and this should be noted. In most instances the presence of a list can be noted on the diagram of the low back by making a line in the central portion of the spine that deviates to either side, with an arrowhead on top, to indicate the direction and relative amount of list.

7. The appearance of a rash is important. This is particularly important for recognizing early shingles or it may indicate other types of skin rash related to systemic disease that might cause low back pain.

Palpation

Palpation of the low back at the examination is extremely important. The standing portion of the examination should be done with the patient standing erect in front of the examiner who should sit on a low stool so that his eye level is about the midlumbar area. He is thus much more likely to note abnormalities in this area. Palpation is then quite easy and should be done with one hand on the back and the other hand flattened across the abdomen so that the patient's back can be palpated without shoving him forward, particularly when pressure is applied. Several things should be noted.

Muscle Spasm.   It is sometimes difficult to tell whether the spasm is involuntary, in which instance it is considered an objective finding, or whether it is voluntary and merely related to the patient's tendency to stand with a list. This may be done as a way of relieving pain but more often it is done to impress the examiner, particularly when the patient otherwise has minimal findings.

Muscle spasm may be easily identified, however, by palpating the area on the concave side of the list, if present, or the area where the muscle spasm is suspected and gently tilting the patient backward and hyperextending his spine. In doing this the mechanical advantage of the musculature is diminished and it is very difficult for the patient to maintain voluntary contracture of the muscles. On the other hand, if involuntary muscle spasm is present it will remain and can be palpated even with the patient pulled over passively into a considerable amount of hyperextension of the low back.

Tenderness.   Tenderness over specific areas is important. While the entire low back may be somewhat tender, tenderness elicited by pressing over a small specified area with the examiner's thumb is most important. Again, one hand (usually the right) should be placed in front of the patient's abdomen so that the patient will not move forward as his back is palpated. In this instance, pressure should be applied first over the lumbosacral facet area on either side and then over the sciatic notch area on either side and over the trochanter on either side.

Other areas of tenderness may likewise be noted but these three areas should be specifically identified on the diagram. Even if there is no tenderness in this location the notation "NO" should be recorded, so that the examiner can remember that this particular area was tested for tenderness. Tenderness is graded from 0 to +4. If 0 is no pain and +4 the maximum amount of pain the patient can have with pressure over a single area, the level (1, 2, 3, or 4) will indicate the relative amount of pain, in the examiner's judgment. Small circles can be drawn on the diagram over the facet on either side and the amount of tenderness evaluated here. Over either sciatic notch and finally over the trochanteric bursal area, markings can be made as shown in Figure 7-4A.

Muscle Defects or Masses.   Muscle defects or masses present in the low back area should be noted, particularly if there is a soft tissue mass palpated on either side of the spine. In the low back area these should be noted and an attempt should be made to determine whether they represent a true mass or merely a muscle enlarged with muscle spasm.

Motion

Motion in the lumbar spine should be tested again with the patient standing and his back to the seated examiner. In this position it will be possible to determine the exact amount of motion present and to place a hand on his shoulder to help him in the particular area of motion desired, particularly with hyperextension and lateral flexion to either side. He should be tested in flexion, extension, lateral bending to either side, and rotation. The extension, lateral bending, and rotation all are relatively easy to identify but flexion deserves an additional explanation.

It is possible to flex, with the low back completely straight, by flexing completely through the hip joint areas if the hamstring muscles are not tight. One should observe, therefore, whether a rounded curve is present in the lumbar spine area as the patient bends over as if to touch his toes. He should bend over as far as he can in this direction; note whether the lumbar spine has a gentle curve or remains straight during the flexion. Also note whether the patient's hamstring muscles seem unusually tight. In these instances the small circle with arrows pointing upward, downward, and to either side should be utilized to express the amount of motion and pain experienced on that motion in each direction. As mentioned previously the pain is graded from 0 to 4 and motion is graded in the low back from 0 (normal motion) to −4 (no motion at all). All the gradations between this are as estimated in the judgement of the examiner. No pain present is scored 0; the maximum amount of pain that can be experienced by bending a certain direction is indicated as +4, and the gradations of pain between these two should again be judged by the examiner.

I usually make these notations at the end of the arrows pointing from the circle indicating motion. The arrow pointing up indicates flexion, the one pointing back indicates hyperextension and, of course, lateral flexion to either side. Rotation, if normal, is not usually recorded. If it is diminished, it can be shown as a small, curved rotatory arrow pointing posteriorly (down on the page) on the side where it needs to be represented. At the top of the flexion arrow, for instance, a small slanted line should be made and on top of this line should be noted the amount of pain from 0 to +4. On the bottom part of the slanted line (like a fraction line) the amount of motion should be noted. A moderate amount of pain and moderate limitation of motion would be shown on the forward flexion arrow as +2 and −2. These figures are shown on Figure 7-4A.

Dorsiflexor and Calf Musculature Test

The patient is asked to stand on the tips of his toes and then to stand on his heels and pull the toes up. In a very short period of time this demonstrates whether the dorsiflexors of the toes and feet are active on both sides and whether the calf musculature is strong enough to lift the patient up on the toes on either side. This will be noted in the neurologic examination but is done more efficiently with the patient standing.

Supine

This portion of the examination is done with the patient lying on the examining table on his back, covered by the examination sheet, with the legs exposed.

Measurement

Leg lengths should be measured from the anterior iliac spine to the medial malleolus on either side and recorded in the appropriate place on the examination form.

Circumference of the thigh and calf are both very important since these will indicate muscle atrophy, swelling if it is unilateral, or other abnormalities of size. Usually a transverse line is made across the midportion of the patella. From this line, a second line is made on either thigh approximately 6 inches superior to it. The exact distance above the patella is not important, as long as both legs are marked in the identical position so that this level can be measured on both sides for comparison. Similarly, a mark should be made 6 or 8 inches below the patella on either side, at exactly the same level, to correspond roughly with the maximum circumference of the calf on this side. These circumferences should be recorded on the examination form.

Hip Joint Motion

Hip joint motions should be then tested by lifting the leg up with the knee flexed and checking to see whether normal motion is present.

Motion should be tested in flexion and extension, in external and internal rotation, and in abduction as well as adduction. If normal, these motions should merely be recorded as normal. Any abnormal findings should be shown on the examination form. The presence or absence of pain on hip joint motion should be recorded.

Flexion Contracture

Flexion contracture of either hip is important since this will often increase the lumbar lordosis with the patient standing erect. The hip's flexion contracture is measured by taking the lower extremity on one side and acutely flexing the thigh upon the abdomen, with the knee acutely flexed. This levels the pelvis against the examination table. If a flexion contracture exists in the opposite hip it will be drawn up into a flexed position by the pelvis as it rotates. Likewise, if there is no flexion contracture down the opposite hip it will continue to lie flat on the table even though the pelvis has been rotated somewhat by flattening the lumbar spine against the examining table. This should be done on both sides.

Straight Leg Raising

Straight leg raising tests are important to determine nerve root irritations, but often they will determine only hamstring tightness.

The straight leg raising should be marked on the diagram in the specified locations for either side. The usual technique is to catch the leg under the heel and slowly lift up to the maximum point that the patient will allow. If he does not have much hamstring tightness it may be possible to bring the leg up to right angles with the pelvis. If the hamstrings are tight it may be possible to only bring it up to 45 degrees. In any event, determine whether radicular pain is produced by this maneuver; if it is produced, the area of radiation should be identified by asking the patient to what area the pain is radiating. The test used for meningeal irritation is the so-called "Koernig" test in which the hip is flexed to 90 degrees with the leg flexed and then the leg is straightened while the hip is maintained in the flexed position. Actually, this test is about as good as the true straight leg raising test for determining nerve root irritation, but if the straight leg raising test is done routinely one is always certain of the mechanism being used.

Sensation

Sensation is tested with a pin. This is done over each foot; careful to cover both the L4 and S1 dermatomes on the foot. If an area of diminished sensation is indicated by the patient take care that this has constant borders by repeated testing over the same area in order to be certain that it is an area of diminished sensation and not merely a subjective judgment.

It is then convenient to do a Babinski test on either side by stroking the sole of the foot in the classic manner.

Toe Extensors

This is a good time also to test the strength of the extensors of the great toe on either side.

Toe Position Test

One of the tests used by many veteran examiners to determine whether the patient is attempting to falsify responses is the so-called toe position test. The regular toe position test, of course, is an important neurologic test in the diagnosis of spinal tract disease. In this instance the great toe is grasped on either side so that there is no possibility that the patient can tell whether the toe is being pushed up or down by the examiner.

In this type of true toe position test care is taken to move the toe up or down and the patient is instructed to relate to the examiner what position the toe is held in, when held strictly by the sides. With the type of testing used here, however, it is important for the patient to know exactly where you are pushing so that there will be no question that he should be able to tell the position of the toe. The examiner very elaborately catches the great toe on the nail and the pulp of the toe, between the thumb and forefinger and, while talking to the patient, moves it backward and forward rather briskly before holding it either up or down for the patient to tell him in what position it is held. It is usually customary to do the uninvolved or asymptomatic, side first so that the patient will have little trouble in identifying the position of the toe. Following this, with very elaborate precaution to point out to the patient that "we are now going to do the toe on the involved side," the same test is used.

There are virtually no circumstances in which the patient should not be able to tell whether the great toe is held up or down when the pressure is applied to the undersurface of the toe or to the top portion of the toe when holding it in that position if he has any sensation at all. It will be found, however, that in people attempting to falsify the responses (such as the patient with secondary gain motives, or the so-called malingerer), the position related by the patient will almost invariably be reversed. For some reason people who are attempting to impress the examiner cannot resist the temptation to falsify the toe position test. It is surprising how many times this will happen with the patient who is falsifying information. I believe that it demonstrates unequivocally that the patient is falsifying his response; this can even be so reported in any type of legal report.

Sitting

After completion of the examination done while his is lying down, the patient is asked to sit on the side of the examining table and the knee jerk and ankle jerk are both tested. Finally, the extensor function in the foot and the extensor hallucis longus can be tested, thereby completing the examination.

LABORATORY AND RADIOGRAPHIC EXAMINATION

After the patient has had a careful physical examination, adequate laboratory studies should be ordered.

Plain Film X-Ray

Plain films of the low back should be taken, as previously described. This should include a large antero posterior (AP) and lateral scout film of the low back, extending on up into the thoracic area, taken on a 14 × 17 film.

Next a spot AP and lateral view should be done at the lumbosacral joint, including, of course, the L3 and L4 vertebrae and the sacrum. The lateral film should be taken as a true lateral and the AP should be taken with the tube tilted slightly cephlad to account for the normal lordosis in the lumbar area. The amount of tilt of the tube should be adjusted to give a true AP view of the lumbosacral articulation. Finally, oblique films on both the right and left side should be done. This should constitute the minimal x-ray examination.

Myelography

Myelographic examination is done usually only when surgical intervention is anticipated. There is not much reason to do a myelogram as long as the patient is responding to conservative management. However, when he fails to respond and when there is evidence to indicate a protruded disc with nerve root compression, myelographic examination by the instillation of a radiopaque dye into the spinal sac will often give valuable information about nerve root compression. The dye acts much as a carpenter's spirit level, being heavier than spinal fluid with the patient lying supine on the x-ray table. The table is then rocked with the head down and then head up so that movement of the column of dye can be followed by an image intensifier and appropriate spot films made.

Computed Tomography

Computed tomography (CT) has become the primary tool for diagnosis of lesions in the lumbar spine causing nerve root compression and, for the most part, has supplanted the use of routine myelogram in many institutions. Much can be determined by the CT scan and the cuts can be made at such small levels that the entire level of the neural foramen can be very adequately visualized along with the associated structures at that level.

Laboratory Studies

Patients with low back pain of any intensity or duration should have routine laboratory studies including a complete blood count, urinalysis, and automated tests. The sedimentation rate is a good index of the amount of inflammatory disease present and is valuable in establishing a diagnosis. Likewise, the rheumatoid fixation test and other specialized laboratory examinations may be indicated.

Radioactive Bone Scan

Radioactive bone scan with technetium 99 isotope is valuable in determining the presence or absence of inflammatory bone lesions. These studies are more valuable in determining the presence or absence of inflammatory changes within associated joints or the intervertebral disc spaces and will also show bone lesions such as metastatic disease of the vertebral body or its processes.

Electromyography

Electromyography has long been used to aid in the diagnosis of low back pain. Its use is relatively limited, however, and the interpretation depends upon a very experienced electromyographer to have any real value. For the most part, this particular examination is reserved for instances in which a very difficult differential diagnosis is present.

Thermography

Thermography has become a new tool for use in determining nerve root irritation. Few institutions have the equipment necessary for reliable thermography and the information obtained in other instances is often subject to many artifactual variations. A completely temperature-stable environment is mandatory if one is to place any significance upon the changes in skin temperature. However, when such information is available it may be a valuable adjunct in the diagnosis of nerve root compression syndrome.

CAUSES

Trauma

Low back pain due to traumatic lesions of bone should be relatively easy to identify. When examining the low back, it is important to secure a complete set of films of the lumbar and lumbosacral spine to evaluate the circumstances effectively. These should include a large AP and lateral film on 14 × 17 film. This gives a good scout film and shows, to a certain extent, the general alignment of the lumbar spine. There should be then a smaller oblique film from both the right and left sides taken over the region from approximately L1 or L2 down to the sacrum but centered over the L4 level.

Oblique films, for instance, are mandatory when making a diagnosis of spondylolisthesis or fractures of the pedicles or posterior elements of the vertebra. Finally, a spot AP and lateral radiograph of the lumbosacral articulation should be done and should include L3, L4, L5, and the sacrum. The lateral view should be taken centered over this level while the AP should be the so-called "Hibbs view," taken with the x-ray tube tilted slightly cephlad to allow for the normal lumbar lordosis. Most fractures discovered in the lumbar area should be evaluated and treatment recommended by an orthopedic surgeon.

Infection

Infectious lesions of the spine usually are extremely difficult to diagnose since the majority are not due to common organisms such as staphylococci or streptococci but are related to brucellosis, tuberculosis, and rather rare types of infection. The occasional abscess occurring in the spine, if due to pus-forming organisms, exhibit relatively acute symptoms and the suspicion of some catastrophic condition should be fairly obvious. The majority of the infectious lesions of the spine are seen on x-ray studies and, of course, the accompanying laboratory studies should help in making this diagnosis. These patients, obviously, should be referred to the orthopedic surgeon for diagnosis, the obtaining of material for culture, and appropriate treatment.

Neoplasms

Neoplastic diseases of bone occurring in the spine are relatively rare. The hemangioma has a characteristic x-ray appearance in the vertebral body and most of the time can be diagnosed from the radiograph alone. These lesions ordinarily do not need treatment; as a matter of fact surgical intervention in these very vascular lesions can be disasterous. Other benign lesions that may occur in the spine are osteoid osteoma and aneurysmal bone cyst. All of these are diagnosed from the x-ray appearance and should be referred to the orthopedic surgeon for evaluation and treatment.

Malignant tumors of bone in the spine are somewhat more common because of the great tendency of malignancies in the various parenchymatous organs of the body to spread to the spine. Among those most commonly seen in the spine are metastases from the prostate, breast, kidney, lung, and thyroid, though any of the malignant tumors of the gastrointestional tract may metastasize to the spine. Metastases from the prostate, of course, are usually osteoblastic in appearance and are related to increased serum alkaline and acid phosphatase levels. Other metastatic lesions in the spine are usually osteolytic in appearance and often result in the collapse of the vertebral bodies from destruction of the vertebral body itself.

Most of the lesions have striking x-ray appearance and can be verified with a marked increase in serum alkaline phosphatase level though the acid phosphatase level will, of course, be normal. These patients should probably be sent for a work-up by the oncologist and appropriate treatment recommended by him. The only primary malignant tumor of the spine is the multiple myeloma that quite often involves the vertebral body with an osteolytic lesion and vertebral body collapse. Diagnosis, of course, is related to the finding of cells in the examination of the blood and Bence-Jones protein in the urine. Again, these patients should be seen by the oncologist for appropriate therapy.

Demineralization

Metabolic causes of low back pain are usually related to demineralization of the spine and secondary changes due to vertebral collapse. The most common metabolic cause for low back pain is senile osteoporosis related to the changes of advancing age and hormone deprivation. Other causes such as hyperparathyroidism and calcium metabolism errors, such as seen in osteomalacia, will require a full medical work-up for a diagnosis. Whatever the cause, the collapse may occur gradually and be only mildly symptomatic. These patients, however, will often have interludes of acute pain in the back related to acute collapse. In those instances they should be supported with rigid immobilization afforded by a Taylor or Jewett brace. Patients with excruciating back pain from vertebral body collapse should always, however, be braced with some sort of an appliance that will afford good stability to the spine because only in this way can the acute pain be relieved. Appropriate treatment for the osteoporosis or other metabolic problems does not fall within the scope of this chapter and can be found in publications related to these conditions.

Degeneration

Probably the greatest cause of low back pain in patients past age 50 is *degenerative* joint disease or degenerative disc disease. The most obvious finding is narrowing of the disc space with formation of marginal osteophytes along the vertebral margins. There is a gradual diminution of space width, related to the loss of fluid content in the disc and the gradual collapse of the disc with the development of these changes. The loss of stature of the disc and the narrowing of the disc space results in mechanical derangement of the balance between the two articulations posteriorly and the vertebral bodies anteriorly and in continued strain of the facet joint due to this abnormal position. Patients with degenerative disc disease will ordinarily have chronic low back pain with recurring episodes of acute pain. These patients may even develop radicular symptoms into the lower extremities caused by narrowing of the neural foramen and nerve root compression, usually by posterior osteophytes present in the canal. Most patients with chronic low back pain related to degenerative disc disease fare quite well on a flexion exercise program. These exercises should be demonstrated to the patient for use two to three times daily at home. Descriptions of these flexion exercises can be found in many publications, or designed by a physical therapy department. In the acute stages, support with a canvas corset and more intensive physical therapy by the therapist either on an inpatient or outpatient basis may be necessary to control the symptoms.

Spondylitis

The presence of degenerative joint disease is considered in the last section; however, the arthritic changes that occur in the spine are often those of rheumatoid spondylitis, as discussed in the preceding chapter. The findings are relatively characteristic in the later stages of the disease but, as mentioned previously, they are often very obscure and a diagnosis is hard to make early. Probably one of the earliest physical findings is the loss of chest expansion and diffuse tenderness over the entire spinal area along with limited motion. One of the earliest roentgenographic findings is obliteration of the sacroiliac joint on either side followed, of course, by the typical findings of the "bamboo spine" with ossification of the anterior ligament and complete ankylosis of the spine.

Spondylolysis and Spondylolisthesis

Spondylolisthesis results in a loss of mechanical stability to the low back, generally at the lumbosacral level but occasionally at the L4-L5 level. There is disagreement among various investigators over whether the defect in the pars interarticularis is a congenital abnormality or is in fact related to trauma. Convincing evidence has been accumulated to substantiate both views. It has been my feeling, however, that this represents a congenital abnormality with a defect of fusion across the pars interarticularis and resulting loss of stability afforded by the mechanical placement of the facet joints on either side, which allows the vertebral body above the defect to migrate forward with respect to the vertebral body below. The classic finding on oblique radiographs is the "scotty dog" figure. The superior articular process of the vertebra is the ear of the dog while the pedicle represents the eye. The transverse process represents the muzzle and the pars interarticularis the neck. The spinous process and laminae represent the body and the inferior articular process represents the foreleg, while the opposite inferior articular process represents the hind leg. In most instances only the head, neck, and anterior leg can be seen on the radiograph and the patient with the spondylolysis will show a "collar" across the neck. When the spondylolysis turns into a true spondylolisthesis there will be an actual separation or "decapitation" of the dog. These various findings are shown in Figure 7-6.

Spondylolysis or spondylolisthesis may cause a variation of symptoms from virtually none to incapacitating pain. However, in the patient who complains of low back pain and whose radiographs indicate a defect in the pars interarticularis, one must conclude that that pain is organic and related to this defect as shown. The symptoms are ordinarily of a mechanical nature with pain being made worse by activity, standing, and hyperextension of the back. Improvement is afforded by rest, support with a canvas corset, and attitudes that reduce the amount of lumbar lordosis. Occasionally there may be entrapment of the nerve root with radicular pain down into the leg. This is particularly caused when the fibrous tissue bridges across the pars interarticularis defect and results in a nodule formation protruding into the neural foramen with compression of the nerve. Most of the cases of spondylolysis and many of the cases of spondylolisthesis may be treated conservatively with the flexion exercise program described previously, support with a canvas corset, and other symptomatic measures. However, if the pain becomes severe and is incapacitating or if recurring incapacitating episodes occur, particularly when nerve root irritation becomes a problem, the patient should be referred to the orthopedic surgeon for evaluation and treatment.

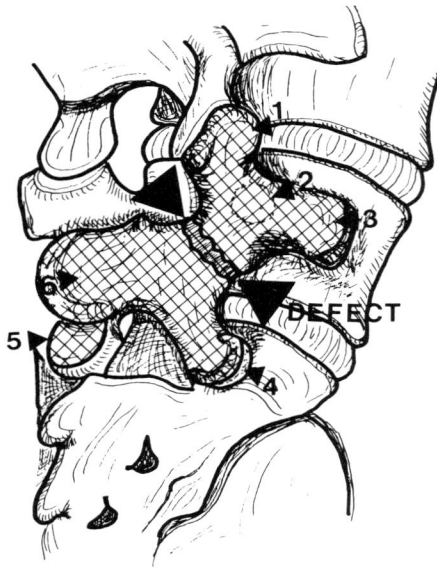

Fig. 7-6. Diagrammatic explanation of structures seen on right oblique examination of the lumbosacral spine in spondylolysis. Note that the hatched figure appears to outline a "scotty dog." (1) The ear is represented by the superior articular facet. (2) The pedicle can be seen in an end-on view as a circular structure and represents the eye of the dog. (3) The transverse process represents the muzzle. (4) The inferior articular facet represents the foreleg. (5) The inferior articular facet on the opposite side represents the hind leg. (6) The body is represented by the lamina and spinous process, seen in the oblique view. The defect is seen as being a collar around the neck of the dog.

Spinal Stenosis

Spinal stenosis designates the encroachment that occurs from marginal osteophyte formation around the facet margins into the neural foramen with a decrease in the size of the foramen and the crowding of the nerve passing through the bony canal. These patients ordinarily have radicular pain into the lower extremity with some back pain related to degenerative changes in the facet joints. For the most part, these symptoms are progressive and do not respond to conservative management. These patients should be referred to an orthopedic surgeon for evaluation and treatment.

Soft Tissue Lesions

Myofascial sprains or strains probably represent the most common causes of low back pain. They result from excess stretching of the supporting ligamentous structures or musculature, with resulting pain. In the case of ligamentous strains an inflammatory reaction occurs around the joint, much as in the sprain of any other joint of the body. This excites the protective muscle spasm response that actually is the cause of the majority of the pain. These patients usually have essentially negative x-ray findings. They have a history of injury by fall or by lifting and their condition responds to conservative management. They should be treated with flexion exercises, by bed rest during the acute state, followed by support with a canvas corset and use of heat, muscle-relaxing medications, and other general supportive measures. The average sprain of the back should clear up in a maximum of 6 weeks if properly treated. However, those that go untreated or are improperly treated may develop into a more chronic type of low back pain. If the patient fails to respond to these conservative measures in a relatively short time, he should be referred to the orthopedic surgeon for evaluation and treatment.

Disc Degeneration

Disc degeneration has been discussed in the previous section related to degenerative changes in the spine and is related to wearing of the disc itself and loss of fluid of content from the disc with gradual narrowing. These findings are quite readily seen on radiographs in the form of narrowing of the disc space with marginal osteophyte formation. This represents the more common type of back disease seen in the aging and the individual who has done heavy work over his lifetime. The pain is usually chronic but is characterized by frequent exacerbations with acute episodes sometimes present. It is treated for the most part by the general conservative measures described previously. In most instances the patient can be maintained in a relatively comfortable condition by the continuation of flexion exercise program, twice daily, over a long period of time. Occasionally leg pain will be a feature, particularly when the neural foramen is decreased in size by the osteophyte formation and marginal lipping along the vertebral body. These patients, of course, should be referred to the orthopedic surgeons as should others who do not respond to properly administered conservative management.

Disc Herniation

If one considers that the intervertebral disc acts much as a hydraulic "shock absorber," one is more likely to understand the pathomechanics of acute disc herniation. The disc is formed of a very hard casing known as the annulus fibrosis. This constitutes the majority of the bulk of the intervertebral disc. Contained within this annulus fibrosis is a small core of gelatinous or mucoid material that acts to create the hydraulic effect of the disc itself. During normal circumstances the nucleus is well-contained within the casing of the fibrous annulus and the action of the hydraulic shock absorber is maintained. That the disc will often undergo the degeneration and dissication with time and use has been described previously. However, in acute disc herniation the annulus actually develops a weak spot in its structure, usually in the posterior lateral quadrant. The material contained within the nucleus then begins to herniate through this weakened area and will often create a small nodule on the margin of the disc as shown in Figure 7-7. This is known as the protruded disc. When the disc is in this condition bedrest, traction, flexion exercises, and support will, many times, allow the material to be sucked back into the normal container in the central portion of the disc. If the patient remains on the flexion exercise program and guards the back during heavy activity, this restored condition of nucleus may remain intact for years. However, with repeated episodes of herniation the small nodule on the surface of the disc posterolaterally becomes larger. When it does this it extends into the neural foramen and entraps the nerve root at that level as it passes through the fibroosseous canal of the neural foramen. If the protrusion

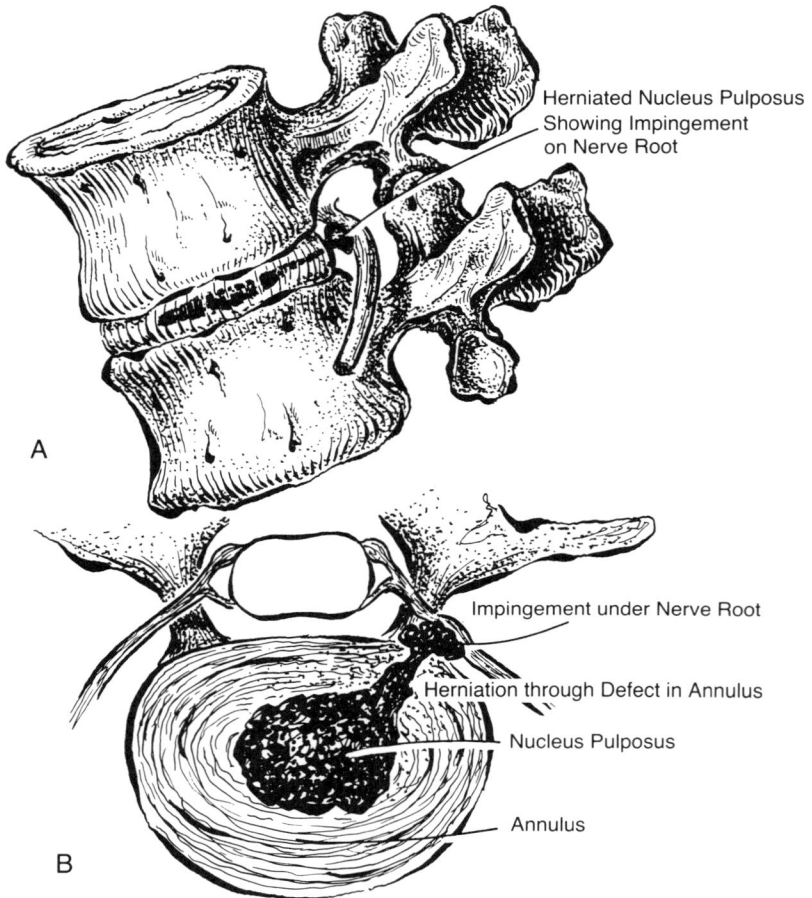

Fig. 7-7. (A) Lateral and **(B)** superior views of typical lumbar vertebrae show the relationships of the vertebral bodies and the interposing intervertebral disc. **(A)** The dorsal elements are seen in the lateral view to extend posteriorly and create the superior and inferior facet surfaces on either side. They complete the tripod type of articulation with the vertebral body lying in front and the two facet joints lying posteriorly. **(B)** The superior view of the typical lumbar disc shows the annulus fibrosis and the nucleus pulposus extruding through a defect in the annulus to impinge on the nerve root as it passes through the neural foramen.

becomes severe enough, the knot on the disc (which simulates the knot often seen on an automobile tire) will sometimes "blow out." When this occurs the material in the disc space actually "spurts" out of the opening into the neural canal. This is known as the so-called extruded disc; once material has been squirted out of the ruptured nodule on the posterolateral aspect of the disc the possibility of sucking this back into the disc by any type of treatment is virtually nil. These patients require surgery.

A further step is the so-called sequestrated disc in which the material has actually come loose in the canal. This may result in a changing clinical picture, occasionally with the patient with acute rupture since the material will move about in the canal and cause various signs and symptoms from compression of various portions of the nerve root.

Patients with suspected disc disease should be treated by the family practitioner for only a limited period of time. If they fail to respond, or if they respond but recurrences of acute syndrome occur often then they should be referred to the orthopedic surgeon for evaluation and treatment.

8

THE SHOULDER

ANATOMY

The shoulder girdle is the point of attachment of the upper extremity to the axial skeleton and is made up by the articulation between the clavicle, the scapula, and the humerus. (Fig. 8-1). The clavicle attaches to the axial skeleton by its articulation at the sternoclavicular joint but is, in fact, more or less floating since it has a considerable amount of motion at the sternoclavicular articulation. The other attachment to the axial skeleton or body is of the scapula to the chest wall. This does not form a true bony articulation: the flat blade of the scapula is attached to the thorax by heavy, strong, musculature. This musculature will hold the scapula to the chest wall and allow a certain amount of rotation in the coronal plane. It also has a small amount of forward motion by the mechanism of winging of the scapula when it is released by relaxation of its supporting musculature, allowing it to move a short distance from the chest wall.

The point of attachment between the clavicle anteriorly and the scapula posteriorly forms the supporting mechanism of the shoulder girdle in the form of the acromioclavicular joint. This joint has a relatively small surface area and virtually no motion at all. The stability of this articulation is related in part to its strong capsule, which surrounds the joining of the acromion process and the clavicle. For the most part, the real stability of the acromioclavicular joint resides in the coracoclavicular ligament. This is a broad, thick, stout ligament that attaches between the coracoid process of the scapula and the undersurface of the

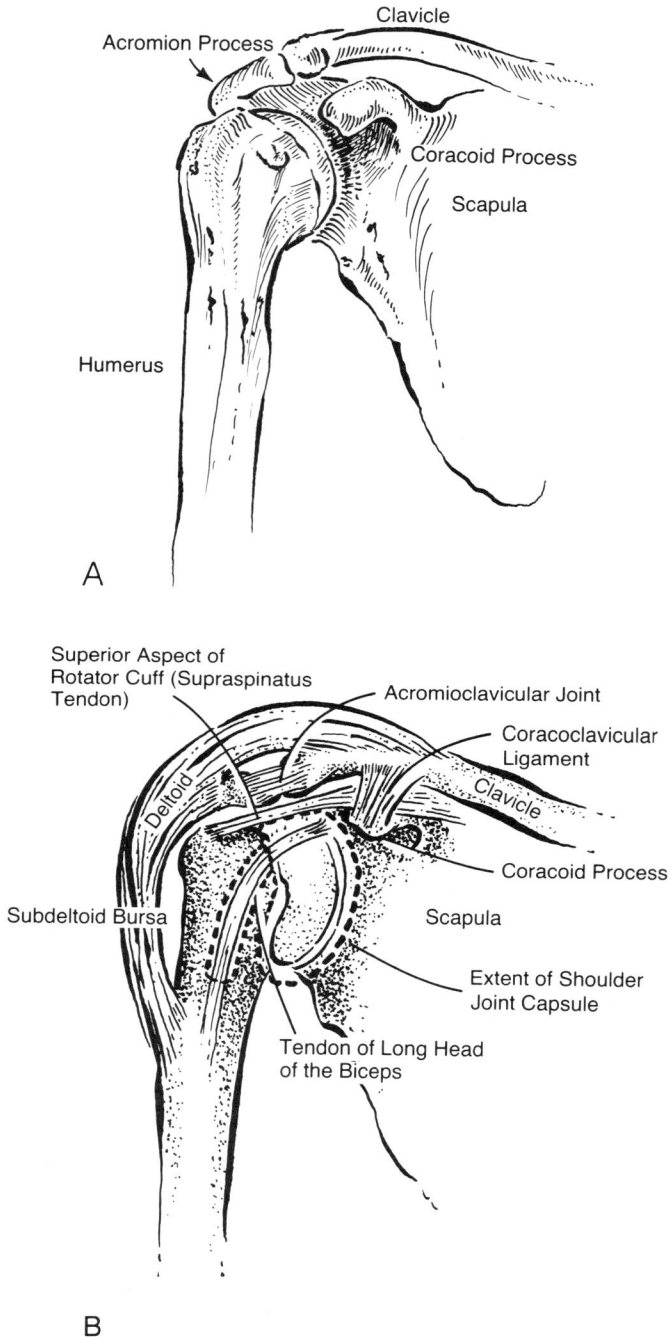

Fig. 8-1. An anterior view of the shoulder shows the attachments of the capsule to the glenoid and to the anatomical neck of the humerus, with extension down the bicipital groove. The close relationship of the superior aspect of the rotator cuff (supraspinatus portion) to the overlying acromion is shown, demonstrating the close space and the likelihood of impingement of the tuberosity on the acromion pinching the rotator cuff when the arm is abducted. **(A)** Without soft tissues; **(B)** Soft tissues added.

clavicle. This arrangement allows for considerable stability of the claviculoscapular articulation, particularly since the coracoclavicular ligament acts mainly to hold the clavicle down and prevent its riding superiorly out of the acromioclavicular mechanism. In fact, as will be discussed later, only by rupture of the coracoclavicular ligament with loss of its tethering effect on the clavicle can a true acromioclavicular separation occur. This demonstrates its importance in maintaining the stability of the shoulder girdle.

The upper extremity attaches to the claviculoscapular mechanism by means of the glenohumeral joint which is, in large part, protected by the superiorly lying acromioclavicular articulation. The glenohumeral joint is relatively instable since it represents the articulation between the rounded medial head of the humerus and the very shallow dish created by the glenoid fossa. Since this articulation must, in the upright position, support the weight of the upper extremity it is surrounded by the very strong fibrous tissue elements and musculature. Along with this rather poor mechanical arrangement the shoulder has a very wide range of motion, which lends further to its instability. Again, this stability is dependent upon the strong fibrous tissue and muscular elements around the shoulder joint. These elements, however, must all act in concert as the shoulder joint moves through its full range of motion in projecting the upper extremity into the various positions necessary for normal function.

Supporting the shoulder joint directly is the very strong capsule, which is redundant in all areas so that it does not restrict glenohumeral motion by tethering it at the extremes of its various positions. This capsule attaches around the articular margins of the glenoid fossa. At the point of attachment to the bone is a very heavy fibrocartilaginous structure called the glenoid labrium, which acts to deepen the glenoid "saucer" and gives the shoulder somewhat more stability from various shearing forces. Damage to this glenoid labrium anteriorly will be discussed in the section on dislocations that allow migration of the humeral head outside of the glenoid fossa anteriorly.

Overlying this capsule, and actually becoming an intimate part of it anteriorly, superiorly, and posteriorly, is a structure known as the rotator cuff. This mechanism forms a heavy, thick, fibrous "hood" that represents the continuation of the fibrous tissue insertion from various muscles that lie attached to the scapula. Anteriorly, the subscapularis provides a powerful internal rotator to the glenohumeral joint and also is important in most types of surgical repair following recurring dislocation of the shoulder. Superiorly, the cuff is made up of the supraspinatus tendon, which is one of the most important portions of the rotator cuff from the standpoint of maintenance of stability. The superior portion of the rotator cuff acts as a stabilizer when the arm is brought out into abduction at right angles from the body in the coronal plane. By contracting, it draws the humeral head into the glenoid fossa and thereby forms the fulcrum necessary to maintain the pivotal action of the glenohumeral joint in this motion.

It will be shown later, in the discussion of tears of the rotator cuff, that loss of continuity of the superior portion of the cuff results in inability to abduct the arm from the side. However, once the arm has been abducted passively and the fulcrum established at the glenohumeral joint with the arm at 90 degrees, the surrounding musculature often will hold the arm in this position even though it cannot initiate the movement in abduction.

The structures forming the posterior part of the rotator cuff are much less important functionally than the superior and anterior components. These are the fibrous insertions of the infraspinatus, and teres major and minor muscles and provide external rotation of the humerus in the glenoid fossa.

In addition to the bony and fibrous tissue elements described above, the musculature around the shoulder girdle gives motor power to the other movements through the shoulder joint. The lateral muscle of greatest importance is the deltoid, which attaches to the acromioclavicular portion of the shoulder girdle and then extends down as a large triangular muscle to attach into a tubercle along the lateral aspect of the shaft of the humerus.

This muscle is the very strong abductor of the shoulder but, as mentioned previously, it can function smoothly only with normal function of the superior aspect of the rotator cuff. The posterior extrensic musculature is again rather inconsequential from a functional standpoint and includes the triceps musculature which has, for the most part, function on the elbow and does not constitute a primary motor of the shoulder joint itself. Anteriorly, however, the large biceps muscle does play an important role in shoulder joint function more than in shoulder joint symptoms.

The biceps arises from a short head originating along with the pectoralis minor and the coracobrachialis muscles from the coracoid process from the scapula. This head seldom gives any great problems clinically. The long head of the biceps attaches to the superior rim of the glenoid fossa and from there courses downward intraarticularly to pass through a groove in the humerus known as the bicipital groove. This tendon then passes down to communicate with the belly of the biceps muscle at about the same level of entrance of the short head of the biceps.

The basic importance of the long head of the biceps in shoulder joint symptoms is the frequent occurrence of bicipital tendinitis. Because this long tendon passes through a bony groove, a mechanical situation occurs that lends itself to wear and tear changes on the tendon. Even though both the tendon and the groove at this level are covered with a synovial membrane a great amount of wear in the tendon still occurs and changes that develop over the years may cause considerable symptoms of pain in the anterior aspect of the shoulder. Furthermore, in some instances these attritional changes become great enough to destroy the internal integrity of the tendon, resulting in rupture. These clinical features will be described in more detail later.

X-RAY EXAMINATION

X-ray examination of the shoulder should be undertaken in the two traditional planes except that the anatomy of the shoulder joint makes it impossible to take a true lateral without taking it in the "axillary" view. This is usually easiest done by having the patient lie on the x-ray table and placing the x-ray tubes so that the major beam goes from caudad to cephalad through the shoulder joint with the elbow outstretched. The x-ray plate lies superiorly above the acromioclavicular joint. Only in this view can the true status of the glenohumeral joint be ascertained. Often a complete dislocation of the glenohumeral joint not immediately apparent on the anteroposterior (AP) film will be dramatically seen on the axillary view. The AP view itself is usually taken with the shoulder both in internal and external rotation, which helps to visualize the various anatomical parts of the humerus more efficiently.

Films to determine whether a separation of the acromioclavicular joint exists require a special technique. In acromioclavicular separations the clavicle does not actually ride up out of the acromioclavicular joint but maintains its normal level and the weight of the shoulder girdle pulls it down relative to its lateral end. This can be accentuated by having the patient stand erect and then applying traction to the extremity: have the patient hold a weight or pull straight down on the upper extremity with the elbow straight. It is usually better to x-ray both clavicles simultaneously and compare the width of the acromioclavicular joint on the two. The key to separation of the acromioclavicular joint, as discussed previously, is the tear of the coracoclavicular ligament. It would follow that an increased distance between the coracoid process and the underside of the clavicle would be seen with complete tear of this ligament. Often it is confusing to look at an AP view of the acromioclavicular joint taken with the patient in considerable pain since it may not be completely true and therefore difficult to interpret. One can never mistake, however, an increase in the distance between the coracoid process and the undersurface of the clavicle, particularly when compared with the same measurement on the opposite side (Fig. 8-2).

ACROMIOCLAVICULAR SEPARATION

As indicated, separation of the acromioclavicular joint results from loss of integrity of the coracoclavicular ligament and the capsular attachment of the joint itself. The mechanism of injury is usually a fall on the "point" of the shoulder; a sudden downward force on the shoulder girdle per se results in a great stress on the acromioclavicular articulation. In the very young individual, and occasionally in many other individuals, ligamentous structure will be so strong that the joint will hold and a fracture of the clavicle will result. More often, however, the ligamentous structures supporting the lateral clavical will not be able to withstand the force and will rupture, resulting in displacement of the acromioclavicular joint. It is, of course, possible to have complete tears of the supporting ligamentous structures and still have essentially normal x-ray findings, if the weight of the shoulder girdle is supported slightly and the joint not disrupted. Similarly, it is possible to have varying degrees of ligamentous damage that are less than complete rupture, so varying degrees of subluxation of the clavicle out of the acromial bed will occur. The prime factor in determining the appropriate treatment of injuries to this joint is whether or not there is significant loss of stability of the joint.

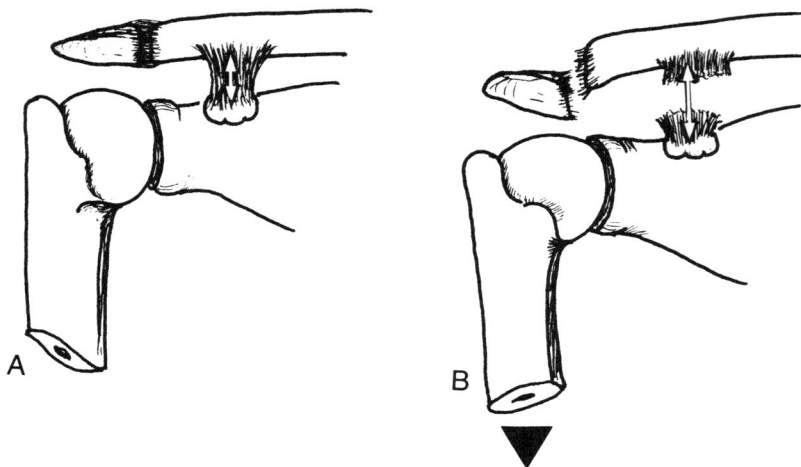

Fig. 8-2. The effects of traction in acromioclavicular separation. **(A)** The normal supporting mechanism of the shoulder particularly with respect to the coracoclavicular ligament, with the capsule of the acromioclavicular joint shown intact. **(B)** The effect of traction, wherein the shoulder girdle is placed under stress that separates it from the clavicle. The acromion, being part of the scapula, rides downward with the humerus; the loss of the supporting mechanism of the coracoclavicular ligament does not pull the clavicle down with the scapula and it is allowed to ride up as shown. Measurement of the distance between the undersurface of the clavicle and the upper surface of the coracoid process is the key to diagnosis. In a true acromioclavicular joint separation the distance will be considerably lengthened compared with the normal opposite side.

In instances of complete separation (a complete rupture of the coracoclavicular ligament and the capsular attachments of the acromioclavicular joint) the course of treatment is clear. The author is not aware of any type of halter, brace, or sling contraption that will hold this joint in the reduced position adequately enough to secure healing. For this reason, some sort of internal fixation must be provided for healing to occur.

If the primary care physician can determine that a complete tear of the ligamentous supports to the joint has occurred, the patient should be referred to an orthopedic surgeon for treatment. Some orthopedists will depend upon closed pinning with percutaneous pins under image intensifier control to provide stability during healing. This will not result in a complete restoration of stability but does restore enough stability to be functionally sound. Often the joint will continue to show symptoms related to a torn meniscus within the joint that has not been removed. Many orthopedic surgeons consider that a complete tear of the acromioclavicular joint requires an open operation, at which time the meniscus can be removed, the joint anatomically reduced and stabilized with fixation pins (which are removed later), and a very stout superior capsulorrhaphy of the joint done with flaps of tissue acquired locally. In some instances, attempts to restore the coracoclavicular ligament mechanism with a Dacron prosthesis, or the like, may be attempted. At any rate, the results following surgery are usually excellent and while some prominence over the joint is likely to be permanent there generally is not much pain in these joints after healing has occurred, and shoulder function is essentially normal.

If one can ascertain from the stress films that less than complete loss of stability has occurred, then whether internal fixation is required or not is a matter of judgment. Certainly acute injuries to the acromioclavicular joint without any demonstrable increase in the distance between the coracoid and the clavicle, as described above, will not require internal fixation. Simple treatment with a sling until the symptoms subside should be enough.

These injuries are often extremely painful for the first few days and an injection of a small amount of steroids into the joint will often do much to relieve the pain. These cases, of course, can be treated quite satisfactorily by the attending physician as can those degrees of ligamentous stretch or partial tear that still have good stability of the joint. Where there is considerable hypermobility of the joint even without a complete subluxation, one might feel safer in requesting an orthopedic consultation since a decision should be made as to whether the amount of instability present is acceptable for a permanent result. If considerable instability exists following partial tear of the supporting structures of this joint, hypermobility will occur resulting in degenerative changes over time. For this reason, if there is much question about the adequacy of the stability the responsibility of the decision probably should be taken by the orthopedic surgeon.

BURSITIS

Patients with a chronically painful shoulder or periodic exacerbations of severe pain in the shoulder have been in the past said to have "bursitis." This term has become well-entrenched in the terminology of shoulder pain. However, most shoulder pain is not caused by bursitis per se, except when the bursa becomes secondarily inflamed as a result of its close proximity to the tendinous structure of the superior aspect of the rotator cuff. As can be seen on Figure 8-1B, the so-called subdeltoid or subacromial bursa actually lies in the interspace between the deltoacromial attachment and the underlying superior aspect of the rotator cuff–humeral tuberosity area. Older surgeons incriminated the bursa as the cause of pain because it did appear to be inflamed when operative procedures were done in the area.

The inflammatory reaction occurs, of course, because the floor of the bursa constitutes the covering of the tendinous structures of the rotator cuff and the bursa becomes inflamed at the time of inflammatory reactions in the rotator cuff. Patients will often understand the term bursitis as an adequate diagnosis for their shoulder pain. It is fine to use this term as a diagnosis, provided that it is accompanied by the explanation that the tendon itself is the mechanical site of injury and that the bursitis is secondary to a more serious condition.

CONDITIONS INVOLVING THE ROTATOR CUFF

As indicated in the section on anatomy, the rotator cuff constitutes an integral part of the "finely adjusted" motions of the shoulder. The superior portion of the cuff in particular is necessary if one is to have normal glenohumeral abduction. Unfortunately, however, the superior aspect of the rotator cuff lies in a hazardous position from the standpoint of injury: during the function of the shoulder it lies in a relatively small gap between the humerus and the undersurface of the acromion process (Fig. 8-3). For this reason, as the shoulder is abducted repeatedly over the years this tendon is repeatedly pinched between the acromion and the humerus, resulting in attritional changes in the tendon substance. These changes will often give rise to a dull aching type of pain in the shoulder and these long-standing symptoms are often punctuated by acute exacerbations of pain following overuse or mild injury. Whether these episodes of injury or overuse result in disruption of some of the fibers or whether a swelling in the tendon itself results, patients usually have acute episodes of pain that are quite disabling and bring them to the doctor's office for treatment.

Examination will usually reveal a full range of motion passively, but the patient experiences considerable pain on active abduction of the arm.

Injections of local anesthetics and steroids can be made periodically, but repeated injections into the tendon will invariably lead to mechanical disruption of the tendon fibers and often act as a prelude to rupture. Occasional injections (one every 6 to 12 months) can usually be accomplished without any real difficulty if done carefully. Once the local anesthetic has dissipated, patients frequently will have an exacerbation of the pain and should be warned of this in advance. For the acute pain the night following an injection usually a pain

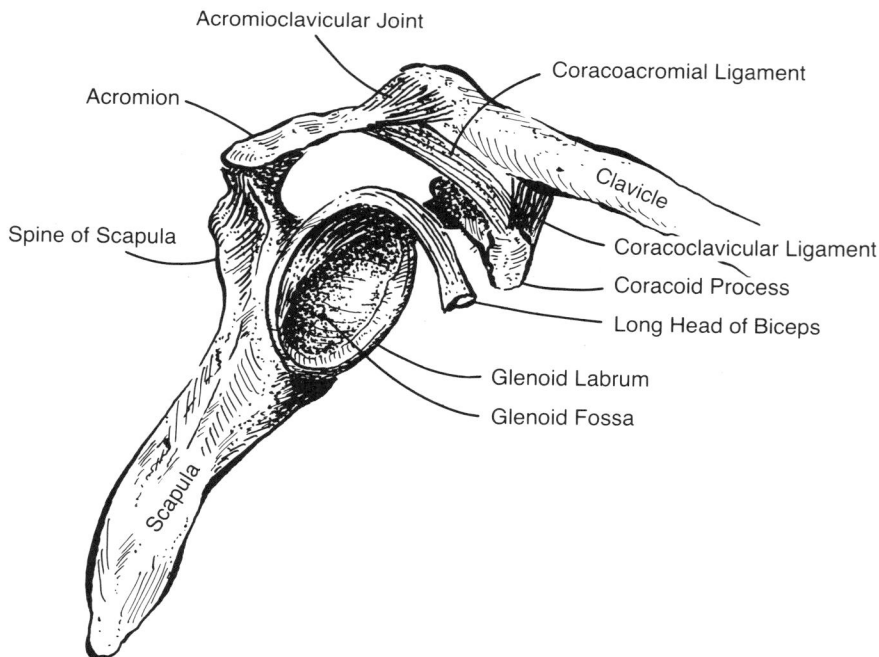

Fig. 8-3. View of the shoulder from the lateral side, demonstrating the glenoid fossa along with the labrum around the rim of the glenoid that deepens it. The superior relationship of the glenohumeral joint to the acromioclavicular joint and to the coracoacromial ligament is demonstrated. The origin of the long head of the biceps and its course through the superior part of the shoulder joint are seen.

medication such as codeine will be required and applications of heat to the shoulder are quite effective.

If the patient's pain persists or is not controlled by the injections, an orthopedic surgeon should be consulted and surgical excision of a part of the acromion to relieve the mechanical pinching on the tendon be considered. If they are responsive to the treatment described, these patients can be treated for long periods of time by the attending physician. Adjunct therapy should, of course, include the applications of moist heat, the use of nonsteroidal anti-inflammatory agents orally, and instructions for range-of-motion exercises for the shoulder to prevent loss of motion.

Tendinitis

Of particular interest is calcific tendinitis of the rotator cuff, in which amorphous calcium is laid down in the area of attritional changes and lies within the tendon itself. This is usually visible on radiographs and has no other implication except that it localizes the area of attritional changes and gives a somewhat different clinical picture.

These patients usually have the periodic aching-type pain in the shoulder characteristic of regular tendinitis. However, the episodes of acute calcific tendinits are unique in their severity and their need for appropriate treatment. These episodes are probably occasioned by the influx of fluid into the otherwise dessicated calcium deposits, causing a relatively sudden increase in the intrensic pressure in the tendon and acute, almost intolerable, pain.

During the acute episodes, a large-bore needle can be used to aspirate some of the liquid amorphous calcium under anesthesia. If the pain persists, however, and continues to be quite severe or if episodes of acute calcific tendinitis recur regularly, surgical evacuation of the calcium by the orthopedic surgeon will be indicated. While the usual calcium seen in this tendon during quiescent stages is quite gritty and dry, the accumulation of calcium during these acute episodes is liquid and has the consistency of toothpaste.

Chronic tendinitis of the rotator cuff that is unresponsive to injection therapy as described previously, or in which recurring episodes are close enough together that repeated injections are not thought to be advisable, will often respond to "orthovoltage" x-ray therapy. Patients may be referred to the radiologist for this type of therapy. The dosage is, of course, determined by the treating radiologist but usually is very low: in the neighborhood of 200 rads, two or three times weekly for a total of four or five doses. The entire dosage is very low: 800 to 1,000 rads. The anti-inflammatory effects of x-ray are well known; before steroid therapy was available this type of x-ray therapy was commonly used and was often quite effective.

Acute Rupture

Chronic tendinitis of the rotator cuff with continued progression of the attritional changes caused by pinching between the humerus and the acromion will often set the stage for an acute rupture of this tendon. The rupture may occur as a sudden episode following a fall on the outstretched arm, resulting in sudden forced adduction of the arm, or following overuse during which the fibers pull apart somewhat more gradually. Whatever the cause, rupture of the rotator cuff requires expert surgical treatment. If their condition is suspected, the patient should be referred to the orthopedic surgeon as soon as possible for treatment. The primary sign of a rupture will be the inability to abduct the arm actively from the body out to 90 degrees. However, as mentioned earlier, the arm can often be held in this position if placed there passively first. Passive motion in the shoulder is ordinarily normal in cases of complete rupture of the rotator cuff.

A diagnosis of complete rupture can be established using an arthrogram, which will demonstrate the leaking of contrast material out of the shoulder joint through the torn tendon. Even partial rupture, which will be seen in cases of long-standing tendinitis without complete rupture, will also show an extravasation of contrast media out of the joint. The radiologist can usually ascertain the degree of tear by the extent and rapidity of this extravasation.

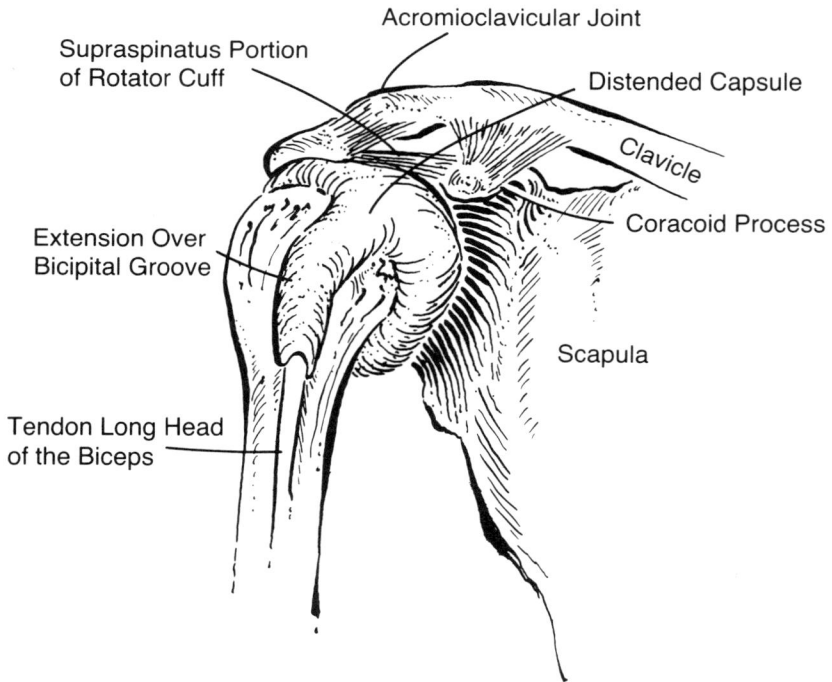

Fig. 8-4. The confines of the shoulder joint are demonstrated as if the joint has been distended with solution. The capsular attachments extend around the glenoid medially and pass deep to the rotator cuff, or supraspinatus tendon, superiorly to attach to the anatomical neck of the humerus. The extension for the tendon sheath of the long head of the biceps is seen.

STIFF PAINFUL SHOULDER

The shoulder beset with long-standing tendinitis or other causes of pain may be stiff and painful. This has been called in the past by various names including adhesive capsulitis, periarthritis, and other similar descriptive terms.

For some reason the shoulder joint is particularly prone to changes in the very lax capsule that limit motion. These may be swelling, formation of adhesions in the many folds of the capsule, or actual shortening of the capsule that prevents its extension in achieving a full range of motion. These changes are related entirely to disuse and therefore may be avoided by active and passive use of the shoulder. This is true even during acute episodes of disease in the shoulder. The patient often cannot torture himself enough to do these exercises without professional help and, therefore, should usually be referred to a physical therapist for aid in regaining motion.

If the shoulder has already become quite immobile when first seen, the patient should be referred relatively early to the orthopedic surgeon. Even though such a patient would probably respond to vigorous physical therapy over a long period of time, many orthopedic surgeons prefer to manipulate the shoulder under general anesthesia in an effort to shorten the time and allow the patient to regain motion earlier. If one is reasonably certain of the underlying diagnosis, the stiff painful shoulder can be quite adequately treated by the attending physician using physical therapy and adjunctive therapy including medication for relief of pain, nonsteroidal anti-inflammatory medication, heat, and the like. If, however, there is any question that the severity of the underlying condition might result in loss of motion, the patient should be referred at an earlier date so that a complete diagnosis may be established.

BICIPITAL TENDINITIS

Bicipital tendinitis is the underlying cause of pain in the shoulder far more often than is realized by many physicians. While many are familiar with the rotator cuff problems discussed previously, often a patient has been seen by several physicians before someone applies pressure over the bicipital groove anteriorly on the upper humerus to cause the exquisite pain characteristic of this condition (Fig. 8-4). As indicated in the section on anatomy, the long head of the biceps tendon, by its anatomical relationship to the upper humerus, is very prone to degenerative changes through wear and tear. This tendon is seldom damaged, while passing through the shoulder joint from its origin at the upper margin of the glenoid fossa. However, once it starts in the fibroosseous canal it has a crowded course and is the site of great mechanical stress as it is brought back and forth through the bicipital groove of the humerus during normal motion of the shoulder and elbow. The friction from rubbing back and forth in the canal, along with the somewhat crowded condition in the canal, results in the relatively early development of attritional changes and resulting low-grade chronic tenosynovitis.

No examination of the shoulder should be complete without palpation of the bicipital groove of the upper humerus. This can be done by having the patient place his entire upper extremity in mild external rotation, which brings the bicipital groove directly forward. In the thinner individual the groove can be palpated quite readily but in one with greater soft tissue covering it is sometimes difficult to feel the anatomical outline of the groove and one must rely exclusively on location. The groove lies at the margin of the articular surface of the humerus anteriorly and medially with the arm in the normal position. In external rotation it is thrown directly anteriorly so that it can be subjected to pressure from the examiner's thumb quite readily. There are no other diagnostic features and treatment consists, as in tendinitis of the rotator cuff, of injections of hydrocortisone. There is, however, somewhat less danger in injecting the bicipital groove with steroids than there is in injecting into the rotator cuff tendon.

In the case of the biceps the greatest inflammatory reaction lies in the tendon sheath surrounding the biceps tendon, so the injection should be made into the sheath rather than penetrating the tendon itself. Usually the symptoms can be relieved by this type of injection. As is true with other similar conditions, repeated injections are not indicated and certainly not at short intervals. The patient who continues to have symptoms despite treatment or who develops episodes at relatively short intervals should be referred to the orthopedic surgeon for possible surgical tenodesis of the tendon in the bicipital groove. This type of surgical procedure results merely in a development of an osseous attachment of the tendon in the bicipital groove that prevents the rubbing of the tendon back and forth in the groove and usually results in a complete and permanent relief of symptoms. An alternative to the injections, as described above, may be low-voltage x-ray therapy.

ARTHRITIS

Arthritic involvement of the shoulder joint is not seen as often as in many of the other joints of the body. Arthritis occurring on a degenerative basis is usually related to changes following trauma. Degenerative arthritis is much less likely to occur on an idiopathic basis without trauma since the shoulder is not a weight-bearing joint. It is a very poorly constrained joint, in which major effort involving the upper extremity results in traction between the two joint surfaces rather than impingement, as in weight-bearing joints. For this reason, this joint seldom wears out unless its surfaces have been made incongruous by previous fractures.

Rheumatoid disease, on the other hand, more often involves the shoulder joint in the course of the development of polyarthritis. Most all people with significant rheumatoid disease at one time or another have had acute synovitis of the shoulder joint. When this occurs over a long period of time, or when these exacerbations with acute synovial reaction occur at frequent intervals, the usual destruction of joint cartilage characteristic of rheumatoid disease occurs. The pain from the rheumatoid joint denuded of articular cartilage can be quite severe, even from the slightest motion. Coughing, sneezing, and even deep breathing that results in a movement of the thorax may cause consequent movement in this painful joint.

In the early stages of either degenerative or rheumatoid involvement of the shoulder joint symptomatic treatment is usually all that is necessary. An occasional injection of steroids directly into the joint may be permitted but this should not be done at frequent intervals over a long period of time. Systemic medication, the use of heat, and of course measures to maintain complete passive motion are the cornerstones of conservative management.

Surgical treatment of the arthritic shoulder is usually unrewarding. State-of-the-art total joint replacement has not resulted in the perfection of a decent total shoulder joint replacement; most not only yield imperfect results clinically but also are fraught with multiple complications and their use is usually ill advised. If the patient's condition has progressed to the point where it is thought that something *must* be done, a hemiarthroplasty with replacement of the humeral joint surface appears to be the procedure of choice. This can be accomplished with any of the prosthetic designs in use today in which the articular surface of the humerus is replaced with a prosthesis extending as a medullary component down the canal of the humerus. It is usually fixed into place with methyl methacrylate cement. A common prosthesis now in use is the Neer prosthesis and it appears to be about as good as any prosthesis introduced thus far. The patient should be warned preoperatively that the prosthesis is being inserted as a salvage measure to relieve pain. However, these patients do not usually develop very good active or passive motion postoperatively and except for the relief of pain, in which the prosthesis is thought to be of paramount value, the insertion of any type of prosthesis is not recommended.

DISLOCATION

Dislocation of the shoulder joint may occur either anteriorly or posteriorly. Less than 1 percent of all dislocations of the glenohumeral joint occur posteriorly, however, so almost all of the dislocations usually seen by the primary care physician will be anterior.

Posterior

Posterior dislocations usually occur in patients who are prone to posterior subluxation of the shoulder and have had this condition more or less since birth. The condition is usually bilateral and these patients are generally thought of as being nervous and emotionally instable. Repeated subluxation of the shoulder joint slipping in and out across the posterior margin of the glenoid becomes, for many of these people a "habit spasm" or "tic." Their anxiety may be manifested by sitting in such a position so that the shoulder can be slipped "in and out of place" repeatedly during these periods. True irreducible dislocation seldom occurs though occasionally in some individuals the humeral head will be caught outside the posterior rim of the glenoid and they will not be able to reduce the shoulder spontaneously. Regular, repeated subluxation of the joint requires no treatment other than that for the patient's anxiety. Reassurance is usually all that is necessary, along with an admonition to try to refrain from doing this voluntarily. However, if laxity of the posterior structures of the shoulder joint becomes great enough that frequent complete dislocations requiring reduction occur, surgical procedures to strengthen the posterior supporting structures (i.e., capsule and rotator cuff structures) may occasionally be indicated. In these instances a thorough evaluation and final decision must be made by the orthopedic surgeon.

Anterior

Since 99 percent of the dislocations of the shoulder are seen as a result of trauma and occur anteriorly, this is the type of dislocation the practitioner can expect to see ordinarily. The arm must be brought into a position of external rotation and abduction for the shoulder to dislocate anteriorly. Anterior dislocation of the shoulder *will not occur with the arm held in internal rotation and adduction.* As the humerus is brought into full external rotation, in most of the people who develop recurring dislocations of the shoulder a flattened surface on the posterior aspect of the humeral head allows the head to slip by the anterior glenoid rim much more easily. This finding is not pathognomonic nor is it absolutely necessary for a patient to develop dislocation. It is, however, frequently seen. The original dislocation usually occurs with a significant amount of trauma. The arm is suddenly brought into abduction with the shoulder in external rotation and the dislocation occurs suddenly, usually with the tearing loose of the attachment of the glenoid labrum to the bone anteriorly. This so-called "Bankhart lesion" is thought to be characteristic of the anteriorly dislocated shoulder but since it occurs in soft tissue elements entirely and does not appear on the radiograph, it is usually seen only at the operating table. As soon as the shoulder dislocates, the surrounding protecting musculature goes into acute spasm so that the humeral head is held outside the glenoid and may occur in a variety of locations on the AP film. The designations subcoracoid or subglenoid indicate the location of the humeral head when the radiograph is taken but these terms have no clinical significance and do not in any way affect the possibility for reduction or the eventual outcome of the dislocated shoulder.

When seen immediately following the injury the patient will be found to have severe pain in his shoulder area, but the most uniquely identifiable physical sign is that he cannot bring his arm down to the thoracic wall. The humerus is held at about 20 or 30 degrees of abduction. The patient who is seen after an injury with severe pain in his shoulder and can bring the arm down to and parallel with the thoracic wall almost never has a dislocated shoulder. This one physical finding can be used many times to make an early clinical diagnosis by physical examination only. Impingement of the humeral head on the axillary vessels and cords of the brachial plexus may occur but this is seldom a problem.

Reduction

Reduction of the acute anterior dislocation of the shoulder requires two basic elements: relief of muscle spasm and longitudinal traction in the long axis of the arm. Manipulation of the joint as described by Kocher is ordinarily not necessary and may actually harm the shoulder or axillary contents. The patient should be placed on his back on the emergency room table and intravenous medication should be administered for sedation and muscle relaxation. Longitudinal traction is then placed, at first gently and then gradually increasing, in the long axis of the arm. Since the arm is usually held about 30 degrees away from the side of the chest the pull is made in this direction. If the pull is made steadily and with increasing force over a period of time usually the patient experiences no great amount of pain and once muscle relaxation has been obtained the shoulder will be felt to reduce suddenly.

If the patient is extremely muscular, additional force and traction may be obtained by bending his elbow to a right angle and passing a sheet or some similar material around the flexed forearm and around the waist of the person attempting the reduction. If the arm has been kept at right angle flexion at the elbow, the forearm acts as a lever and a very strong pull can be made using the additional weight of the physician's body. If the patient is not, for the most part, relieved of his pain, he cannot relax and muscle relaxation cannot be obtained. The chances of being able to reduce the dislocated shoulder in the emergency room are good only if relief of pain and good muscle relaxation can be obtained.

If the reduction cannot be obtained with reasonable ease and without a great amount of trauma the patient should be taken to the operating room for a general anesthetic, since this will relieve the pain and produce relaxation of the protecting musculature. The minute that the patient has been anesthetized and satisfactory muscle relaxation obtained with appropriate medication the reduction can usually be accomplished without much difficulty, using the same method of traction and gentle rotation of the head from side to side as the traction is applied. To facilitate reduction, particularly in the muscular individual, the "Hippocratic method" is usually quite simple and quite effective and serves only to increase the amount of actual traction at the glenohumeral joint. This consists of placing the unclad foot of the operator in the padded axilla of the patient and then pulling, using the pressure of the foot as countertraction at the shoulder and the breadth of the foot as a small lever to ease the shoulder into reduction. Again, if the patient is well anesthetized and complete muscle relaxation has been obtained, the actual mechanism of reduction should not be difficult.

Postoperative Care

Postoperatively the patient should be immobilized in a position of adduction and internal rotation of the shoulder for at least 3 weeks. This is best done by placing the arm in a sling with the elbow at right angles and then wrapping a very loose circular bandage around to hold the arm in the adducted, internally rotated position. A 6 inch elastic bandage will suffice for this quite nicely, except that there is a universal tendency to wrap this too tightly causing increased pain. Actually it is not necessary to have this tight at all but it should give some support to the shoulder and hold the arm in position.

Even after a careful reduction and adequate immobilization of an anterior dislocation of the shoulder, the chances are still significant that the patient will develop a recurring dislocation of the shoulder and he should be made aware of this.

A good rule of thumb uses the age of the patient to determine the probability of recurring dislocation. If the patient is younger than 20 years at the time of the original dislocation, the chances of his developing recurring dislocations are extremely high: probably over 90 percent. Some observers have never seen an individual younger than 18 at the time of his original dislocation who did not develop recurring dislocations. In patients between 20 and 40, the chances are probably in the neighborhood of 50 percent and usually this depends upon the adequacy of the postoperative immobilization while healing occurs. The patient who has his original dislocation when he is past 40 years of age has very little chance of developing recurring dislocation and those past 55 have virtually no chance of developing recurring dislocations of the glenohumeral joint.

When recurring dislocations do occur, they will usually require the same technique to obtain reduction. In some instances the patient will have had so many dislocations in the past that he has developed enough looseness of the supporting structures and enough wisdom about the necessity of complete muscle relaxation that he can facilitate reduction or perhaps even accomplish it without additional help. Those who do have recurring dislocations and have had over three or four documented instances of dislocations requiring reduction should consider a surgical procedure to repair the anterior aspect of the shoulder. Many different techniques are described to accomplish this and each orthopedic surgeon has a technique that he considers to give the most reliable result in his own hands. All of these require a general anesthetic, a hospital stay of 3 or 4 days, and immobilization in the internally rotated position for approximately 6 weeks.

FRACTURE

Except for the clavicle, fractures in the region of the shoulder do not occur often and usually only with rather severe trauma. Older individuals with considerable demineralization of the bone do experience communited fractures of the humerus due to falls on the outstretched arm.

Clavicle

Fractures of the clavicle are extremely common and usually heal satisfactorily without difficulty. There are seldom any indications for open reduction of the fractured clavicle unless the fracture is displaced enough to put pressure on the underlying subclavian vessels or branches of the brachial plexus. When pressure on these structures can be demonstrated, open reduction with decompression of the structures and internal fixation of the fractures are indicated. Other than in these rare instances, the clavicle should be treated by a closed means. If a considerable displacement is demonstrated that is not thought to be compatible with good healing, the patient may be hospitalized and placed flat on his back for a period of time with a sandbag on the point of the shoulder, to achieve a satisfactory position.

Immobilization is generally accomplished with some variation of the figure eight dressing. Many commercial types are available, all with various attributes and all variously recommended by the inventor and the manufacturer. A easy and inexpensive method uses about 3 yards of 3 inch stockinette in a true figure eight configuration. Into the inside of one end of the stockinette can be placed two small sponge rubber pads approximately 3 by 8 inches made from 3/4 inch plastic foam placed at positions so that these fall anterior to the shoulder on either side. The one nearest the end is placed 12 to 14 inches from the end and the other at a distance so that it will fall in front of the opposite shoulder as the figure eight is applied. The figure eight is best applied with the patient standing erect with his hands on his hips.

The stockinette should be rolled up first with the pads in the end to be applied first. As the figure eight is applied, the pad should be kept anterior to the shoulder and *not* within the axilla. The less padding possible in the axilla the better since most of the discomfort from this type of immobilization is due to compression of the axillary vessels and nerves by material contained within the axilla. This dressing is left intact for the first week. Patients are often hospitalized, particularly adults, for the first 24 hours so that adequate sedation can be given since these tend to be extremely painful injuries.

The patient may be allowed to be ambulatory as soon as he desires. He is instructed that if swelling occurs within the arm, he should lie down flat on the back and bring the arms out to the side, thereby relieving the pressure in the axilla. Numerous safety pins are used, particularly in the back, to keep the various layers of the dressing in position. The patient is brought back into the office in 1 week for rewrapping of the immobilization and perhaps change of the stockinette since it will likely have been soiled with perspiration.

It should be pointed out that anatomical reduction of the clavicle is practically never achieved by closed means, but healing of the clavicle almost invariably occurs. Unless there is a considerable amount of shortening (which draws the scapular attachment closer to the midline anteriorly) most of the positions, even with overriding, are acceptable. When overriding occurs with a sharp palpable edge directly underneath the skin, the patient is usually advised that this will smooth off with time. If it continues to be a problem after healing has occurred the procedure to smooth it off surgically through a tiny incision under a local anesthesia is minimal once solid union of the fracture has occurred. Most of the time, however, this sharp prominence will smooth off to the extent that it causes no real difficulty. Immobilization in the figure eight is continued for about 6 weeks. For the last 2 or 3 weeks the bulk of the support can be diminished, and during the last week or so it may even be possible to allow the patient to rewrap the support at home. Healing should be adequate in 6 weeks to allow most activities, however, severe stress on the bone should not be allowed for at least 3 months.

Acromion

Fractures of the acromion are seldom seen and when they do occur are the result of direct trauma, usually in the form of a severe blow directly over the acromion process itself. Fractures of the neck of the acromion process occur but they are seldom displaced. They ordinarily heal with time and simple immobilization of the shoulder in a sling or a sling-and-swathe–type dressing. Fractures of the tip of the acromion usually are stellate. They are seldom displaced and usually heal promptly since this is completely cancellous bone. Damage to the articular surface may occur and be a problem after healing is complete, but there is usually nothing that can be done to prevent this in the early stages and the patient is merely advised of the possibility.

Scapula

Fractures of the scapula are usually the result of violent direct trauma, usually in an automobile accident or the like. Since the scapula is composed of cancellous bone and does not have any great deforming forces acting upon it, fractures will usually not be grossly displaced. Treatment can consist of immobilization with a sling-and-swathe dressing. Healing is usually prompt since the bone is cancellous and active motion of the shoulder can ordinarily be started within the first 2 weeks. If there is significant damage to the glenoid joint surface or displacement of fractures through the neck of the scapula, the patient should be referred promptly to an orthopedic surgeon.

Humerus

Fractures of the upper humerus occur for the most part in older individuals with a considerable amount of bone demineralization. These are usually badly communited fractures but have little displacement, little loss of alignment, and usually do not have any extension into the joint surface. These fractures are ordinarily well impacted so that treatment may consist of simple immobilization with a sling and swathe.

Early motion may be begun in the form of circumduction exercises or other gentle passive exercises, with the patient bent forward from the waist and the arm suspended. If there is a significant displacement, treatment with a hanging cast will usually suffice. Unless one is well experienced in the application of hanging casts and in the margins of acceptance in these fractures, such patients should be referred to an orthopedic surgeon for treatment. Avulsion of the humeral tuberosity may occur when the demineralization of the bone makes it less sturdy than the attached rotator cuff. When this occurs, the large plug of bone is avulsed at the attachment of the rotator cuff to the tuberosity. If this is greatly displaced it will probably require closed reduction by pressure to get it near to its normal location. However, if very little displacement occurred, this can be very satisfactorily treated with a sling-and-swathe immobilization with early passive motion. Active abduction against gravity or against resistance is prohibited for at least 6 weeks. If there is any question about the adequacy of the reduction, the patient should be referred to an orthopedic surgeon. Occasionally these fractures will be quite markedly displaced and so unstable that internal fixation will be required, but this decision should be made by the orthopedic surgeon.

9

THE ELBOW

ANATOMY AND MOTION

The elbow joint should really be considered as comprised of three major joint surfaces. (Fig. 9-1). The most obvious is the joint between the medial distal portion of the humerus, called the trochlea, and the olecranon fossa of the ulna. The normal hinge motion of the elbow joint occurs in this joint and it is usually pictured when one speaks of "elbow joint." The other two joints occur in relationship to the head of the radius. The first of these occurs between the dish shape at the proximal end of the radius and the capitellum. This joint also is related partially to the hinge function of the elbow joint, but the rotatory motion of the radius that occurs in pronation and supination allows for articulation of this dish-shaped surface against the articular surface of the capitellum. Finally, the small joint between the rounded proximal end of the radius and the small joint occurring on the side of the ulna is concerned entirely with pronation and supination.

Flexion and extension motion is primarily a function of the joint between the trochlea and the olecranon. The saddle-shaped impression in the proximal ulna fits quite closely around the trochlear surface. It ends anteriorly in the coronoid process to which attaches the brachialis muscle and ends dorsally in the tip of the olecranon process that, in full extension, passes into a deep fossa in the dorsal surface of the distal humerus known as the olecranon fossa.

Early loss of extension, in degenerative disease for instance, is often related to the filling of this olecranon fossa with either osteophytes or synovial material which impinges when the elbow is placed in full extension, causing the lack of this extension. By the same token, the extremes of acute flexion are often blocked when osteophytes occur along the coronoid process or along the margin of the humeral articular surface anteriorly; blockage occurs as the coronoid

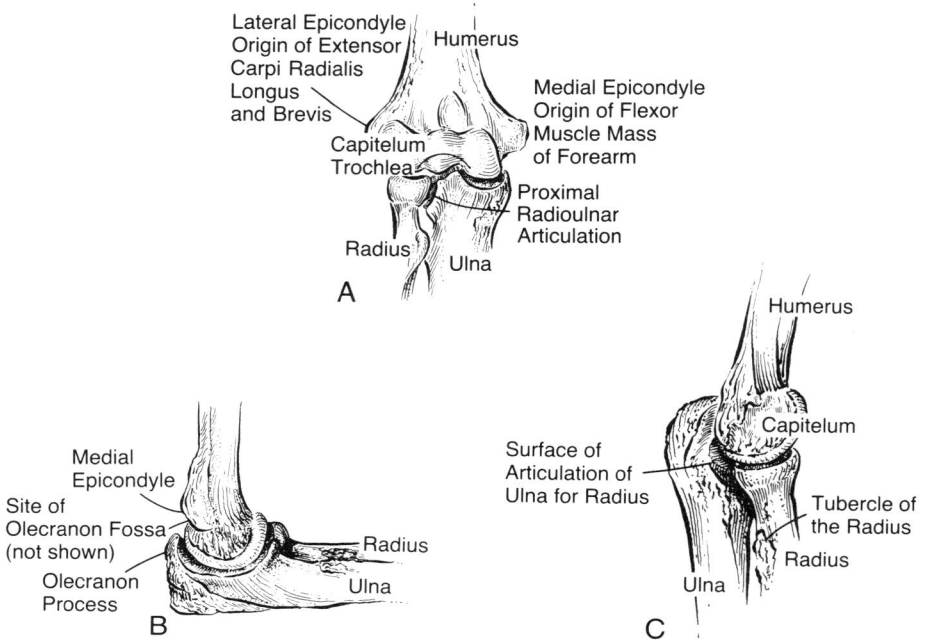

Lateral Epicondyle
Origin of Extensor
Carpi Radialis
Longus
and Brevis

Humerus

Capitelum
Trochlea

Medial Epicondyle
Origin of Flexor
Muscle Mass
of Forearm

Proximal
Radioulnar
Articulation

Radius

Ulna

A

Medial
Epicondyle

Site of
Olecranon Fossa
(not shown)

Olecranon
Process

B

Radius

Ulna

Humerus

Capitelum

Surface of
Articulation of
Ulna for Radius

Tubercle of
the Radius

Radius

Ulna

C

Fig. 9-1. (A) Anterior view: the hinge portion of the joint is made almost entirely of the ulna. Note the articulation between the radial head and the capitellum superiorly and the radial head and the ulna medially, the configuration of the capiellum and the trochlear portions of the articular surface, the lateral and medial epicondyle, and the point of attachment of the radial wrist extensors in the lateral epicondyle (site of inflammatory reaction in "tennis elbow"). (B) Lateral view of the elbow joint. Note the extension of the olecranon process posteriorly, the presence of the bicipital tubercle on the radius, and the medial epicondyle. (C) Oblique view of the radial side of the elbow joint. Note the relationship between the radial head, the capitellum of the humerus, and the articulation with the ulna; and the location of the tubercle on the radius for attachment of the biceps insertion.

process impinges on the lower humerus in deep flexion. Participation of the proximal radius in this hinge function causes considerable difficulties when there is incongruity related to a faulty position or deformity of the radial head.

In fractures or in degenerative disease resulting in abnormal position of the radial head, an incongruity occurs between the finely machined mechanism of the elbow joint that often blocks motion. Normally the saddle-shaped articular surface of the olecranon and the upper surface of the humerus are in exactly the same plane, so that as the elbow is flexed and extended these two surfaces pass in concert with one another to articulate with the two sides of the distal articular surface of the humerus. If the radial head has become mishaped, one can easily see how this mechanism is destroyed and blocking will occur. By the same token, if the proximal end of the radius has been misdirected by a fracture through the neck or upper portion of the radius, blockage likewise occurs. Finally, when fractures occur through the distal articular surface so that the trochlea and capitellum are separated, the more mobile of these two may rotate to such an extent that once again the surfaces are incongruous because of the loss of position of one of the two articular surfaces of the distal humerus. In these instances once again flexion and extension are compromised, usually flexion.

The other motions that occur with participation of the elbow joint are pronation and supination. In normal motion the axis of rotation of the distal radius around the ulna changes so that with the elbow flexed to 90 degrees the wrist may be brought from a position of complete pronation with the palm of the hand facing downward to a position of complete supination with the palm pointing straight upward. This change in relative position of the long axis of the radius and ulna must take into account the articulation between these two bones at the proximal radial and ulnar joints at the elbow and the distal radioulnar joint at the wrist. The proximal radioulnar joint places the circumferential surface of the radial head to rotate in the dishlike depression opposite it on the ulna. Deformity of the radial head causes loss of the finely machined fit between the radial head and the ulnar depression and results in blockage of pronation and supination. The same, of course, is true in incongruities occurring distally at the articulation between the radius and the ulna at the wrist. One will often also see loss of congruity of the proximal or distal radioulnar joint when fracture of the midshaft of one or the other of these bones has resulted in angulation with loss of the normal parallel relationship between the axis of these two bones.

Ligamentous support of the elbow is very strong. The elbow joint, of course, is closed by a housing formed from very dense capsular material completely surrounding the joint. The proximal radioulnar joint is further stabilized with an annular ligament that attaches anteriorly and posteriorly to the margins of the dish-shaped joint surface of the upper ulna and passes around the radial head, holding it securely in articulation with the ulna and allowing the 360 degree rotatory motion necessary in full pronation and supination. Lateral stability of the elbow joint on both sides is provided by very strong collateral ligaments attached from the epicondyles of the distal humerus to the appropriate structures below.

Flexion of the elbow joint is provided by the brachialis muscle, which attaches to the coronoid process and serves as the prime mover in flexion. The biceps brachialis tendon inserts into the tuberosity of the radius so that it acts not only as a powerful elbow flexor but also as a powerful supinator of the forearm. The brachioradialis muscle is not nearly as powerful but does provide some of the flexor power of the elbow, particularly when the biceps or the brachialis is not functioning.

Almost all of the extension of the elbow is provided by the very strong triceps musculature posteriorly. Supination of the forearm is provided as mentioned by the biceps brachii and, to a somewhat lesser extent, by the supinator muscle in the upper forearm. Pronation is provided by two smaller muscles in the forearm; the pronator radii teres in the midforearm area and the pronator quadratus distally.

The ulnar nerve lies in close relationship to the elbow joint medially, passing from its intermuscular position in the distal arm through a small ulnar groove just medial and posterior to the elbow joint and intimately attached to it internally. The implications of this anatomical relation are obvious and will be discussed in some detail later. The radial nerve passes from its intermuscular position laterally across the lateral aspect of the elbow area just above the flare of the distal humerus, to lie in a far lateral and anterior location shortly before it courses into its normal residence in the extensor area of the forearm. Division into its two branches—one motor and one sensory—occurs relatively high in the forearm area. The other major neurovascular structures occur anteriorly and are relatively closely related to the elbow joint when the latter is in complete extension. The flexor musculature acting on the wrist and hand lies on the volar aspect of the forearm and originates from various areas extending from the medial epicondyle down. The extensor musculature lies on the dorsal or posterior surface of the forearm and originates from various locations extending from the lateral epicondyle.

X-RAY EXAMINATION

X-ray examination of the elbow is usually done in only two planes; anteroposterior (AP) and lateral. The oblique projection has very little value in estimating the anatomy of the elbow joint area and, in fact, may often prove to be only confusing.

The AP view should be taken with the elbow in complete extension. If there is flexion contracture with lack of complete extension, two views should be taken: one with the distal humerus directly parallel to the x-ray plate and one with the proximal ulna and radius directly parallel to the plate. An AP view of the elbow in the flexed position has little value. The lateral radiograph should be taken generally with the elbow in some flexion, though for complete evaluation of the joint in certain abnormal states the two lateral films should be taken: one with the elbow in maximum possible extension and the other in maximum possible flexion.

If you are concerned about the function or integrity of the proximal radioulnar joint, particularly with respect to deformities of the radial head, several AP views should be made of the proximal ulna and radius with the forearm in varying degrees of supination and pronation. Likewise, if you are not able to ascertain the condition of the proximal relationship between the two bones, cine studies are often invaluable in determining whether blockage occurs and whether the joint is congruous.

FRACTURES

Massive composite fractures such as those occurring in the so-called "sideswipe" injury must receive expert care and patients should be transferred with all due haste to a center providing specialized orthopedic care. If vascular insufficiency exists due to mangling injury at the elbow, the position in which the best radial pulse is obtained should be elected as the position for immobilization for transfer to the trauma center.

Supracondylar fractures in children pose a special threat from the standpoint of vascularity. As is well known by most practitioners, the vascular problems that can occur from ill-treated supracondylar fractures often will result in the vascular insufficiency syndrome with ischemic changes in the forearm and hand known as Volkmann's contracture.

This fracture is so often related to vascular compromise in the arm because of the relationship between the brachial artery and the fibro-osseous structures around the elbow. Passage of the brachial artery underneath the lacertus fibrosis results in a tethering of the artery at this location distal to the elbow joint. Any deformity of the bone resulting in the projection of a fracture surface toward the anterior aspect of the elbow will often result in impingement of the bone against the artery in this position. Likewise, the great tendency of these fractures to swell voluminously in a relatively short time also results in the tamponade effect. This is particularly true with the artery trapped in the relatively small confines of this fibro-osseous canal through which it passes.

The best treatment of the usual supracondylar fracture in children with vascular insufficiency is early reduction. If this cannot be accomplished by the experienced family practitioner, these patients should be referred immediately to the care of one experienced in this type of injury. If, on the other hand, the fracture can be reduced readily by closed means, the impact on the artery will usually be relieved and circulation restored relatively soon. If the orthopedic surgeon finds that the radial pulse does not return soon after closed reduction of this fracture open reduction must often be done to release the artery from the confines of its small canal.

If the services of an experienced orthopedic surgeon are not immediately available, the usual vascular compromise can be relieved by setting up a traction mechanism, preferably using a small Kirschner wire passed transversely through the olecranon process. With the patient lying flat on his back and the elbow at right angles with the hand extending toward the ceiling, longitudinal traction is placed through this traction pin placed through the olecranon process. Reduction or near reduction of the fracture and release of the deforming features that have resulted in the vascular compromise often occur. If the vascularity can be restored by this mechanism the patient can be left in this traction apparatus until transfer can be accomplished. If reduction is achieved by this mechanism the addition of general anesthetic may allow for complete reduction of the fracture and maintenance of the reduction by continued traction. In these instances the elbow should be left extended past 90 degrees so that the vessels have adequate room for circulation. Also in cases where closed reduction is unstable and swelling is great enough that the elbow cannot be put up at a flexion position greater than 90 degrees, the patient can be left in traction until the swelling subsides enough that the elbow can be flexed to a stable position for the fracture. In other instances the fracture can be stabilized by percutaneously inserted Kirschner wires extending from either epicondyle up across the fracture into the distal humerus to gain enough stability that the arm can be put up in less than 90 degrees of flexion to preserve adequate circulation.

Distal Humerus

Supracondylar fractures in adults are not as likely as in children. When they do occur, however, they are relatively instable and often require internal fixation by either percutaneously passed Kirschner wires or other means of metallic stabilization. If the amount of displacement is not great, immobilization in a posterior shell with the elbow in somewhat less than 90 degrees of extension will allow for healing. Fractures that occur through one condyle or the other require near anatomical restoration for the reasons noted previously. If there is rotation of a smaller fragment of even a minimal amount, the mechanism between the distal humerus and the surfaces of the olecranon and upper radial distally will result in loss of motion. For this reason, most fractures extending into the joint through either of the two condyles should require open reduction with anatomical restoration of position and internal fixation to restore motion early postoperatively. The so-called "T" fracture, in which a supracondylar fracture extends distally through the two condyles into the joint, likewise usually requires anatomical reduction and internal fixation.

Epicondyles

Fractures of the epicondyles require special attention. If the epiphysis has not closed (on the medial epicondyle particularly) it is often avulsed along with the flexor origin. Anatomical restoration of the epicondyle with fixation by transfixing Kirschner wires usually results in a complete restoration of function. If displacement is significant or if the practitioner cannot ascertain from the radiograph whether the fragment has become significantly rotated, the patient should be referred to the orthopedic surgeon for specialized care.

Olecranon

Fractures of the olecranon occurring through the very tip do not result in instability of the joint surface but often do result in the loss of the insertion of the extensor musculature. If this occurs, internal fixation is mandatory. Fractures occurring through the saddlelike articular surface of the olecranon will often be nondisplaced because of the cancellous nature of the bone in this area. If the joint surface is not distorted these fractures can be usually treated by simple immobilization, in about 45 or 50 degrees of extension. Radiographs should be taken often during the first week or so to be certain that separation of these fragments has not occurred. When separation does occur, anatomical reduction and internal fixation by means of some type of olecranon screw should be used. Most of the screws devised for this type of stabilization have a "lag bolt" feature that allows snug reapproximation of the olecranon onto the major ulnar fragment. Relatively early gentle motion can be then started. Fractures of the tip of the coronoid process per se may distract somewhat because of the attachment of the brachialis tendon to it but ordinarily do not compromise the stability of the elbow joint. If the amount of separation is not great these fractures can usually be treated in flexion by immobilization alone and satisfactory functional results will be obtained. If enough of the coronoid process is broken off that instability exists, internal fixation is ordinarily preferable to restore the stability.

Radial Head

Fractures of the radial head are quite common, occurring from falls on the outstretched arm. A fracture of the radial head should always be suspected if the patient has had this type of injury and reports to the emergency room complaining of pain over the lateral aspect of the elbow. The basic problem in radial head fractures stems from the deformity that follows any displacement of the fragments. It has already been pointed out that fractures through the joint surface articulating with the capitellum result in a roughening of the joint surface. If the amount of deformity is great there may be even blocking of motion, particularly in flexion. As a general rule fractures that comprise as much as one-third of the proximal joint surface of the radial head with significant placement should be treated surgically. If it is a single fracture occurring through the joint with displacement, internal fixation may suffice. Many surgeons, however, prefer total excision of the radial head. Fractures that occur around the peripheral margin of the radial head in the area that articulates with the articular facet of the ulna are somewhat more subtle and are often more difficult to see. By the same token, any loss of the complete roundness of the radial head will result in incongruity of the articulation between the radius and the ulna and pain, particularly in the extremes of supination and pronation. A significant displacement of the fractures that distort the roundness of the head will result in blockage of complete supination and pronation of the forearm.

Excision of the radial head is, as mentioned, the procedure of choice for most fractures in this area, particularly those with any degree of comminution. However, fractures that have virtually no displacement may be satisfactorily treated by immobilization of the elbow at 90 degrees of flexion and with near complete supination. Confirming radiographs should be taken with the joint immobilized to be certain that the position of the fragments is still anatomical. Immobilization should be maintained without motion for 3 to 4 weeks. Twice daily gentle active motion in the elbow is then begun with both flexion and extension as well supination and pronation. This is, most of the time, augmented by hot soaks; the motion should be done gently without forcing. The immobilization should be restored each time after the exercise period and total immobilization should be continued for approximately 6 weeks before unrestricted motion is allowed. When excision of the radial head is recommended by the orthopedic surgeon, he will likewise make the decision whether to replace the radial head with a silicone rubber prosthesis. The experience of the author has been quite good with restoration or maintenance of length of the radius by insertion of a silicone prosthesis following radial head removal. The major advantage of this procedure is that it prevents a proximal migration of the entire radius into the defect left following removal of the radial head.

ARTHRITIS

Degenerative joint disease of the elbow is quite common and may occur as a result of years of use, but is more frequently related to trauma. As indicated previously, the finely adjusted mechanism of the articulations between the radius, ulna, and humerus make it very common for degenerative changes to occur in these joints with even minor damage. The first feature of degenerative disease of the elbow is likely to be a loss of complete extension and, later on, loss of complete flexion. Pain may sometimes be a feature of degenerative arthritis of the joint, but the usual complaint is restriction of motion so that function has been diminished. A particularly vexing problem is the loss of flexion that occurs in most elbows with significant disease and precludes the bringing of the hand into relationship with the head and face. Even functions such as eating, shaving, face washing, and hair combing are impossible.

Nonoperative treatment of degenerative disease consists primarily of systemic medication and general supportive measures such as heat. Restricting activities is generally not important, though activities that require a sudden snapping of the joint in extension (such as throwing objects) are to be avoided. Likewise, carrying heavy weights will aggravate the symptoms. On the other hand, judicious exercise to retain motion is permissible and even indicated. It has been learned that exercise against mild resistance is preferable to active exercise alone. This may be done with the help of another person or the opposite extremity using elastic straps and other springlike apparatuses that allow the elbow to be flexed or extended against mild resistance.

Fortunately, most severe "functional" loss due to degenerative disease can be markedly improved by surgical debridement of the joint. Surgical excision of the radial head, debridement of the osteophytes that block the extension, and limited synovectomy will usually result in considerable improvement in function as well as relief of pain. The patient should be cautioned, however, that the convalescence following surgery of this type is prolonged and the necessity for postoperative exercise programs is vital in obtaining a good functional result.

Rheumatoid disease quite often involves the elbow joint and there is likely to be considerable synovial reaction present here, with pain on motion and even at rest when the joint becomes distended with synovial fluid. As in all instances of rheumatoid disease, an occasional injection of hydrocortisone into the joint is permissible provided this does not constitute the only treatment and is not continued at short intervals over a long period of time. Early synovectomy will sometimes delay the course or progress of the disease in the elbow joint and may be considered if the acute synovial reaction persists despite systemic treatment and the occasional injection of a local steroid.

Otherwise, the general supportive measures of heat, gentle exercise, and the like are about all that can be offered. If the joint becomes badly deformed or distorted so that continual pain even at rest becomes a major factor, consideration may be given to total joint replacement. The average total joint replacement using methyl methacrylate cement is not generally successful from a functional standpoint, since in the very active individual who uses the elbow excessively the torsional forces acting on the humeral stem will usually result in loosening of the stem from the humerus. However, in individuals with rheumatoid disease with markedly weakened musculature and whose life is sedentary and does not require excessive strain on the elbow, a total joint replacement will often completely relieve the pain while maintaining a degree of function with reasonably good flexion and extension as well as supination and pronation. A total joint replacement of the elbow should be reserved only for this type of individual and should be used very judiciously in the treatment of other conditions of the elbow joint.

EPICONDYLITIS

Lateral epicondylitis, or the so-called tennis elbow, is caused by the abnormal pull on the insertions of the radial wrist extensors to the lateral epicondyle. These muscles extend above the elbow for their origin and distal to the wrist for their insertions so that their function is related to both joints. Abnormal stress occurs on the origin of the extensor carpi radialis longus when the wrist is suddenly flexed with the elbow in extension. This particular movement occurs quite often during a forehand volley; thus lateral epicondylitis is relatively common in tennis players and hence the name. While many patients develop lateral epicondylitis without any known cause, people in certain occupations, such as carpenters, and other individuals who use the wrist and elbow in stereotyped repetitive motion are much more inclined to have lateral epicondylitis.

The diagnosis is usually made based on the history of the patient's symptoms coupled with the finding of acute tenderness directly over the lateral epicondyle of the humerus. Even though the pain may appear to occur up in the arm per se and extend down into the forearm, the area of acute tenderness is still pinpointed over the lateral epicondyle.

These patients can be very successfully treated with methylprednisolone injections of 40 to 80 mg diluted with some lidocaine for better dispersion. The injection can be done quite easily in the office under lidocaine anesthesia but the area should be thoroughly infiltrated with lidocaine prior to the injection of the steroid so that "needling" of the area may be done without causing pain. The entire injection should be done with a very minimal amount of discomfort to the patient. During the 12 to 24 hours following the injection, however, the patient may experience very severe pain and should be warned of this and given an appropriate medication to take. The application of moist heat seems to have a surprising effect in relieving the postinjection pain and the patient should be instructed in its use. The patient generally should receive oral nonsteroidal anti-inflammatory medication to augment the effects of the local steroids. When repeated episodes of epicondylitis occur at intervals so short as to preclude repeated steroid injections into the area, consideration should be given to surgical release of the muscle attachment to the lateral epicondyle. The patient should then be referred to the orthopedic surgeon, since this procedure usually can be counted on to give a very high chance of complete and permanent relief of symptoms.

Similar symptoms occasionally occur over the medial epicondyle at the point of origin of the flexor mass on the volar aspect of the forearm. These cases are not nearly as common and most of the time respond readily to the single injection and/or systemic nonsteroidal anti-inflammatory medication.

TARDY ULNAR PALSY

The close anatomical proximity of the ulnar nerve to the posterior medial aspect of the elbow joint makes it very liable to damage from conditions involving the elbow joint. The motor and sensory loss of the ulnar nerve related to these conditions around the elbow joint is known as "tardy ulnar palsy." The fibroosseous canal occupied by the ulnar nerve is quite small and does not allow a great amount of room for the passage of the nerve. Conditions resulting in marginal lipping, synovial thickening, or capsular thickening of the elbow are likely to compromise the space enough to cause symptoms distal to this area. Likewise, old injuries or degenerative disease that results in a significant cubitus valgus or increased carrying angle of the elbow will often additionally stretch the ulnar nerve at this point and cause symptoms of functional loss into the hand.

Patients are usually not aware that the symptoms originate from the elbow region and present with symptoms mainly of numbness and tingling in the little finger and adjacent ulnar side of the ring finger. First there is generally loss of sensory acuity in this area that will progress to total anesthesia if pressure on the nerve is continued over a long period of time. Motor loss is not as common but will definitely follow the sensory loss and sometimes may become profound, with intrinsic atrophy and even early clawing of the hand when pressure on the nerve has been maintained. For the most part, however, the sensory symptoms seldom are neglected by the patient enough to allow significant motor paralysis before treatment is sought. Treatment consists of surgical release of the fibroosseous canal ordinarily with a transfer of the ulnar nerve to the anterior aspect of the elbow. In this location it can be buried in the flexor muscle mass and usually the symptoms will subside promptly. Other surgeons prefer excision of the medial epicondyle, which allows the nerve to migrate anteriorly out of this canal. These decisions, of course, are left to the discretion of the consulting surgeon.

OSTEOCHONDRITIS DISSECANS OF THE CAPITELLUM

The articular surface of the capitellum or the lateral humeral articular surface at the elbow is often the site of avascular necrosis of the articular cartilage, known as osteochrondritis dissecans. The origin of this condition is obscure but it is certainly related to the occlusion of subchondral vessels, which result in loss of nutrition to the articular cartilage and subsequent death and dehiscence into the joint. This is very similar to the condition seen in the knee joint except that in the elbow joint the mechanism is not aggravated by weight-bearing and is usually slower to progress. The eventual picture seen in the elbow is multiple loose body formation from the dehisced avascular cartilage into the joint. The patient will often present with locking of the elbow. Unfortunately this is associated with considerable destruction of the articular surface on the lateral aspect of the elbow joint and degenerative changes almost invariably are quick to follow.

In early cases, where only a low-grade synovitis is present without actual extrusion of cartilaginous pieces into the joint, the elbow should be treated by rest, a single hydrocortisone injection if acute, and general supportive measures. This, of course, should improve the current symptoms but will usually not effect any permanent change in the disease process. When loose bodies have formed in the joint, surgical removal is mandatory. It is usually possible to smooth off the articular surface of the capitellum and perhaps drill multiple small holes through the subchondral bone in hopes that additional blood supply may be created and a fibrocartilaginous surface restored. If, however, the changes have become great over a period of time and marked incongruity of the joint occurs, ultimate excision of the radial head will be required to relieve symptoms. These cases should, for the most part, be referred to the orthopedic surgeon if seen past the early stage of synovitis before detachment of loose ossicles in the joint occurs.

10

THE WRIST

The wrist is one of the most frequent areas of injury since it comes under the greatest stress when an individual falls on the outstretched hand. The force delivered onto the wrist, which in most instances is acutely extended, causes longitudinal loading on both the carpus and the distal radius. Extreme force is applied to the radiocarpal joint ligament and varying amounts of force to the carpus itself and the ligaments supporting the intercarpal articulations. Fractures of the radius with or without concomitant fracture of the ulna, fractures of the scaphoid, and various ligamentous disruptions in the radiocarpal and intercarpal systems may occur. While many of the intercarpal mechanisms are relatively complicated and poorly understood even by many orthopedists, fractures of the radius, ulna, and, occasionally, the scaphoid bone constitute a relatively high percentage of the injuries to the upper extremities seen by the primary care physician.

ANATOMY

The two bones of the forearm unite at the distal radioulnar joint and create here an unusual articulation between the head of the ulna and a dished-out articular surface on the ulnar side of the radius. The radius articulates with the carpus, particularly with the scaphoid and lunate bones. The ulna articulates with the proximal carpal row only through the triangular fibrocartilaginous complex that extends from the radial margin over the ulnar styloid (Fig. 10-1).

129

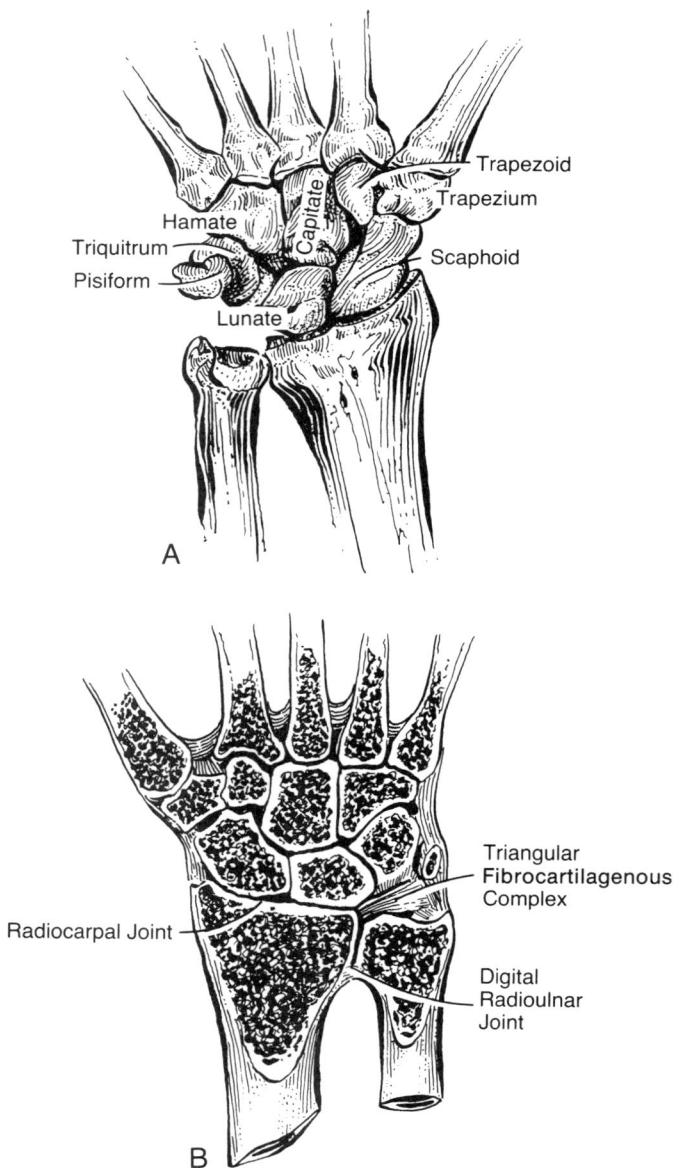

Fig. 10-1. (A) External volar view of the carpus with the various carpal bones labeled. Note multiple overlaps, which should be remembered when interpreting x-ray films. **(B)** Coronal view showing the carpal bones and their articulations between one another, between the radius proximally and the carpal bones distally. The distal radioulnar joint is also shown along with the triangular fibrocartilaginous complex that separates this small joint from the remainder of the carpus.

The major motion of the wrist joint is flexion and extension at the radiocarpal joint and this motion is what most people think about when speaking of "wrist motion." The radiocarpal joint also has the ability to deviate either to the radial or ulnar side for a few degrees in either direction but complete extension and complete flexion of the wrist joint occurring through the radiocarpal articulation are normally about 90 degrees in either direction.

Distal radioulnar articulation is seen only in supination and pronation, at which time the rounded head of the ulna acts as a pivot and the radius articulates in an arch of 180 degrees extending from one side in complete supination to the opposite side in complete pronation.

Theoretically, the ulna stays in a single position and only the radius rotates backward and forward during pronation and supination. The stability of the distal radioulnar joint is maintained by a series of ligamentous structures that constitute a ring around the ulna to allow this wide excursion of the radius. The radioulnar articulation is a very finely adjusted mechanism. Disturbances by injuries to either or both bones result in pain and sometimes the development of degenerative disease.

A frequently occurring example of this is the shortening of the radius that occurs following a fracture of the distal end of the radius. This causes a relative lengthening of the intact ulna, which results in a subluxation of the distal radioulnar joint and is a frequent cause of pain. This relative ulnar lengthening (termed an "ulnar plus variant") also results in abnormal impingement of the ulna on the triangular fibrocartilaginous complex and thus upon the ulnar side of the carpus. If this disassociation is severe, surgical treatment is often indicated and the patient should be referred for orthopedic consultation.

The distal joint surface of the radius faces distally and slightly ulnarly. The ulnar facing is related to the extension of the radius on the radial side to form the styloid process. The proximal carpal row then articulates proximally but also on the radial side with the styloid. This mechanism gives some stability to the radiocarpal joint but, by the same token, it also restricts motion, particularly in radial deviation. The distal joint surface also has a volar facing of about 10 degrees when measured in the sagittal plane with relationship to the long axis of the radial shaft. This degree of volar inclination allows for normal wrist function; however, variations up to 0 degrees or even as much as 10 degrees dorsally may be compatible with normal function. Therefore, after fractures of the distal radius, anything within this 20 degree range (from 10 degrees volar to 10 degrees dorsally) is acceptable. Since the usual distal radial fracture results in a dorsal inclination of the distal fragment, the usual abnormality seen following fractures of the distal radius is an abnormal amount of dorsal facing. This gives rise to the well known "silver fork" deformity characteristic of a Colles fracture, in which the exact position of the distal fragment has not been restored.

The proximal carpal row presents a wide horseshoe-shaped combined surface for articulation with the radius and with the extension ulnarly in the fibrocartilaginous complex. As long as the ligamentous structures are intact, this tends to move as a unit both in flexion and extension as well as in ulnar and radial deviation. It is well known, however, that much interarticular motion occurs during these various wrist motions, particularly with respect to the scaphoid, which undergoes a rotatory movement between its two poles in most all motions of the wrist. This becomes important with ligamentous injury, particularly to the scapholunate ligament since its disruption allows for a rotatory instability of the scaphoid. When this disruption is complete there results a separation between the lunate and scaphoid which can be seen in the anteroposterior (AP) projection. This is the so-called Terry-Thomas sign, which usually is indicative of instability at the scapholunate articulation (see Fig. 10-5A). A small amount of separation may be normal, but if this exceeds 3 or 4 mm the patient should be referred to the orthopedic surgeon for evaluation and appropriate treatment.

FRACTURES
Radius

As mentioned earlier, fractures of the distal radius are among the most common fractures seen and most likely to be encountered by the primary care physician. The so-called Colles fracture resulting from a fall on the outstretched arm that causes a fracture across the distal portion of the radius with a dorsal displacement of the distal fragment is probably the most common fracture seen. It is also probably one of the most often mistreated fractures and certainly even when well treated many times results in considerable loss of function.

Scaphoid

The other fracture of particular importance is the scaphoid. Fractures of the scaphoid are common, particularly in the younger individual and particularly in young male athletes. The fracture usually occurs from a fall on the outstretched arm and probably occurs more in this younger age group because it is the structure of least resistance compared with the ligamentous structures and the distal radius. It becomes involved before ligamentous tears or fractures of the distal radius occur. A few instances of fracture of both the distal radius and the scaphoid have been seen but they are not common since usually if the distal radius fractures, the pressure is relieved on the scaphoid and it does not break.

Fractures of the scaphoid are unusually difficult to treat because of the poor blood supply. This blood supply is provided basically by a single nutrient artery that enters the bone in the midsection across the wrist and then extends to the substance of the bone to either end. Fractures that occur across the wrist area are likely to damage this blood supply irreparably. This is particularly important on the proximal or ulnar fragment, which undergoes complete avascular necrosis much more freely than the distal or radial fragment, which has an additional blood supply from other vessels. Nonunions are also likely because of this faulty blood supply and the difficulty in immobilizing the scaphoid.

Treatment

Though they occur at all age groups fractures of the distal radius are much more common in the older individual who has some demineralization of bone that renders it more susceptible to fracture. The fracture that occurs in the child with the open epiphysis usually occurs at the epiphyseal line and with a small segment of the diastasis broken off dorsally. This is the so-called Salter II type fracture. Because of the inclusion of the diaphysis in the dislocation of the epiphyseal plate, anatomical reduction is mandatory to prevent growth disturbance.

This is not usually difficult to obtain, since the fracture is easily reduced by traction and by forcing the wrist into flexion. However, the fracture will be stable only in fairly marked flexion and must be put up in this position for the relatively short period of time required for the fracture through the dorsal diathasis to heal, thereby locking the epiphyseal plate back into its normal position (Fig. 18-7).

Fractures of the distal radius in the adult may appear in all different forms and degrees of severity. The simple fracture occurs through the distal radius, does not involve the joint surface, and does not have a great amount of comminution. The distal fragment is ordinarily displaced dorsally and is often associated with an avulsion fracture of the ulnar styloid. This fracture is not difficult to reduce nor is reduction difficult to maintain once it has been achieved. (Fig. 10-2). Some of these in which the displacement is not great can be treated by simple infiltration of a fracture hematoma and reduction in the emergency room. For the most part, if there is any degree of displacement the patient should be treated in the operating room with a general anesthetic, an axillary block, or a Bier-type of intravascular block.

In all three of these types of anesthesia, complete muscle relaxation is obtained; this is a factor of major importance in securing an adequate reduction, particularly if displacement is great. Once anesthesia and muscle relaxation have been obtained the fracture can generally be manipulated quite well after longitudinal traction is first applied on the long axis of the forearm with counter traction at the elbow for several minutes. This results in a disimpaction of the fracture and relaxation of the associated musculature. It is then easy for the operating surgeon to force the distal fragment down over the end of the radius and, once it passes over the end of the radius, to bring the entire wrist and distal fragment into the flexed position. The force required for reduction of this fracture may sometimes be relatively great and generally is provided by the thumb of the operator pressing against this distal fragment, which has been slightly increased in this dorsal displacement first and then forced over the end of the distal radius. Once reduction has been obtained it is usually easy to palpate the dorsal radius and to determine whether it has returned to its normal smooth condition. The wrist, however, should be held in flexion while radiographs are taken in the AP and lateral projections.

The use of a portable x-ray machine is mandatory but the technique of taking the film without loss of reduction is unique. The x-ray tube should be turned horizontally so that the beam is horizontal to the floor. The tube should

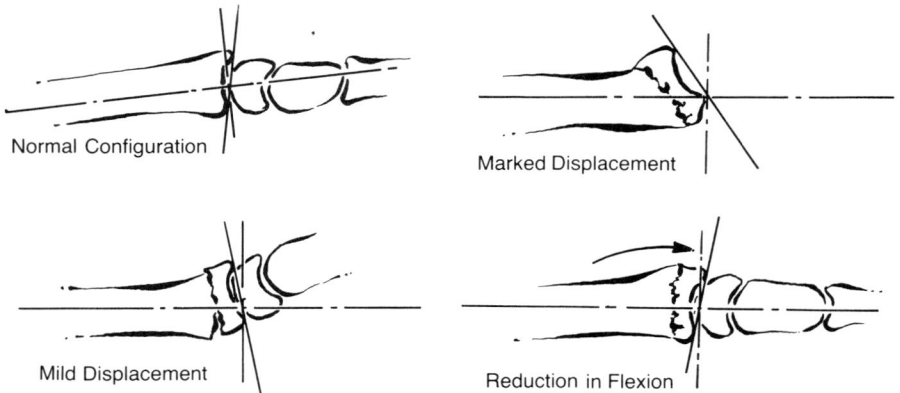

Fig. 10-2. The normal wrist viewed from the side has a 10 degree volar angulation. With a Colles-type fracture of the distal radius there may be varying degrees of dorsal placement of the distal fragment. No matter what the degree, a complete reduction will require that the joint surface be brought back to a 10 degree volar placement.

lie adjacent to the lower part of the body and the beam should be shot toward the head. A lateral view can then be taken quite readily by holding the plate up against the forearm with the elbow flexed at 90 degrees and the flexion of the wrist and the fracture maintained. Then, merely by rotating the shoulder up toward the head the forearm can be brought into a position so that the volar aspect of the wrist is presented to the x-ray tube. The x-ray film can then be placed adjacent to the dorsum of the wrist facing the x-ray tube and the hand extended just slightly so that a perfect AP view can be obtained of the distal radius. By taking the films in this manner the excessive rotation necessary in taking the films from above is prevented and very minimal stress is placed upon the reduced fracture.

In the average case, reduction should be obtained on the first attempt. However, little short of anatomical reduction should be accepted and if this has not been achieved originally then the fracture should be remanipulated until it is. Once reduction has been obtained immobilization with a sugar tong splint is satisfactory.

There is no place for the short arm cast in treatment of wrist fractures. To start with, a circumferential cast is to be avoided because of the possibility of swelling of the wrist that is already being maintained in a flexed position. Secondly, a short arm cast does not control supination and pronation, which are not only prone to be very painful but also are likely to disrupt the stabilization of the reduced fracture. Long arm circumferential casts are satisfactory since they include the elbow but they have the disadvantage again of being circular around an area that is very likely to swell. They have the added disadvantage of holding the elbow completely immobilized for a period of several weeks. With the sugar tong splint, flexion and extension of the elbow to a certain degree are still possible and only the undesired pronation and supination are prevented. The sugar tong splint should be placed with the elbow at 90 degrees of flexion and the wrist in fairly marked flexion. The plaster splint should extend from the metacarpophalangeal joints dorsally around the elbow joint to extend up to the metacarpal phalangeal joints in the palm. This splint can be cut out slightly in the thenar area so that the thumb can have fairly normal motion. It is likewise satisfactory to include a small amount of pronation with the flexion of the wrist since this tends to give additional stability to these fractures that ordinarily occur in supination.

The amount of flexion should not be extreme but should be great enough to hold the distal fragments securely in place (Fig. 10-3). This amount of flexion is ordinarily left in the sugar tong splint for 3 to 4 weeks. At that time, if progress is satisfactory, the splint may be changed and the wrist joint be brought up into a few degrees more of extension. The fracture is then stable enough to allow motion at the joint rather than the fracture. If healing can be seen on the radiograph, a short arm splint may be substituted for the sugar tong. After 4 weeks the motions in supination and pronation are not likely to dislodge the fracture and at that point should not cause a great amount of pain. The fracture should be maintained in this position for a minimum of 6 weeks total time depending upon the x-ray appearance at the end of this time.

Ordinarily, at 6 weeks the patient is allowed to begin removing the splint once or twice daily for short periods of hot soaks and gentle active exercises. Then the splint should be reapplied for an additional 2 weeks before leaving it off entirely. Variations in the time frame will occur, related to the rapidity of healing. Though these times are average they should be directed by the appearance of the progress of healing on serial x-ray films. During the entire healing period the patient should be instructed to wear a sling to prevent edema of the exposed fingers. The patient should also be instructed to put the shoulder through a full range of motion several times daily to prevent stiffness of the shoulder from disuse. Likewise, the patient should be encouraged to exercise all digits many times daily. If much swelling occurs in the fingers, massage two or three times daily from distal to proximal will help milk out some of the edema fluid and allow for a greater amount of motion.

Once motion has been restored in the fingers, edema is not nearly as likely to occur. Many times the disuse symptoms relate to stiffness in the shoulder. Symptoms occurring from a stiff painful shoulder or stiff painful fingers prolong the convalescence over the time necessary for the fracture itself to heal. One should also watch for reflex sympathetic dystrophy. This is quite common following treatment of fractures of this type and usually is manifested by stiff, swollen, and painful fingers that do not limber up with simple measures. At the first sign that reflex dystrophy is occurring the patient should be referred to the orthopedist for vigorous measures to counteract this sometimes catastrophic complication. Similarly, numbness over the finger tips should cause alarm and possible referral for specialized care since this may represent a carpal tunnel syndrome with median nerve compression precipitated by edema in the volar canal as a result of the fracture.

Fractures of the distal radius with a great amount of comminution, and particularly with a great amount of separation of articular fragments, usually

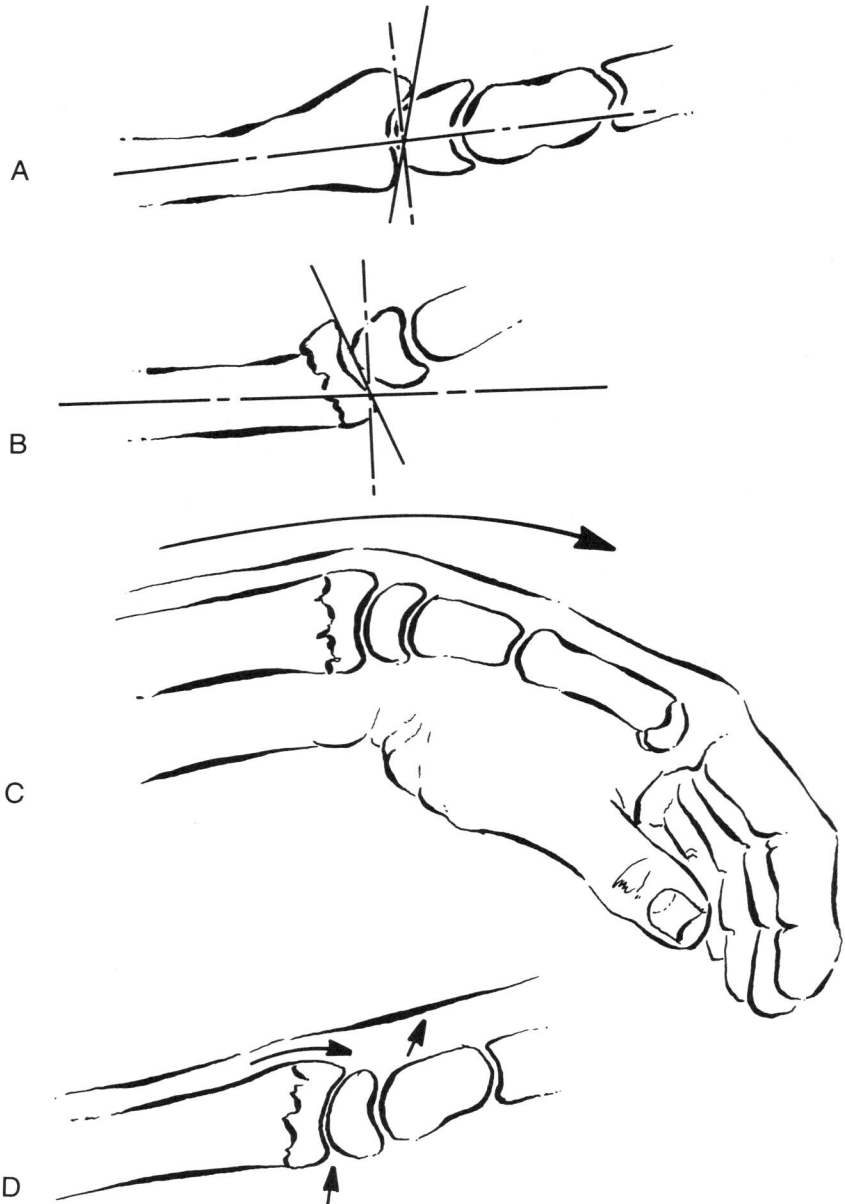

Fig. 10-3. Normal displacement and the method of reduction in a fracture of the distal radius (Colles type fracture). (**A**) Normal alignment in the lateral view showing a 10 degree volar angulation of the distal joint surface in the normal wrist. (**B**) Usual displacement in a Colles fracture with the distal fragment and the carpus displaced dorsally, so that the distal joint surface points dorsally a varying amount depending upon the amount of deformity. (**C**) To hold this fracture in reduction, the wrist must be put up in a fairly marked flexion. (**D**) This position must be maintained for 3 weeks for the fracture to become somewhat healed. Then the wrist joint may be brought back in neutral position to the radiocarpal joint, and the fracture of the radius will stay in a relatively volar-deviated position.

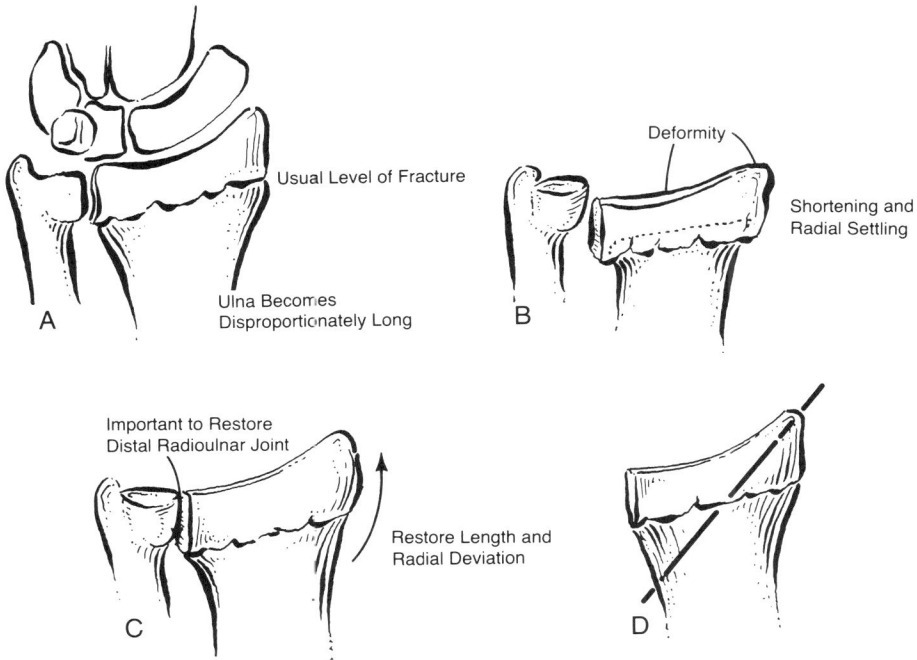

Fig. 10-4. Mechanism of reduction of fractures of the distal radius (Colles type fractures). (**A**) The usual level of the fracture is near the distal radius, often at the lower margin of the sigmoid fossa articulation with the ulnar. (**B**) The type of deformity usually seen is radial shortening along with the dorsal angulation, as shown on the previous figure. Reduction then must not only include a restoration of the normal inclination of the distal articular surface but also must correct the radial shortening. (**C**) These should then be placed in flexion, slight radial deviation, and slight pronation. (**D**) However, it may be necessary to use fixation pins or an external fixator to maintain length.

require expert care and such patients should be referred to the orthopedic surgeon or hand surgeon. Reduction in these cases can often be obtained by the measures described above; a considerable amount of traction with gentle manipulation of the distal fragments and molding of these fragments by the operator results in a near anatomical restoration of these fragments. Occasionally it is not possible to reduce the joint surface anatomically by closed means, but for the most part these comminuted fractures do surprisingly well by closed manipulation. The problem, however, is that they are extremely difficult to maintain. Settling of the fracture is very likely with radial shortening and relative ulnar lengthening as a final result. For this reason, once the fracture has been reduced, some additional fixation is mandatory (Fig. 10-4).

The author's preference is a percutaneous fixation pin inserted under image intensifier control from the radial styloid area and from the dorsum across the comminuted fragments into the stable shaft fragment of the radius. (Fig. 10-4D). External fixation has become popular in the last few years and can often be used to maintain the length of the radius once reduction has been obtained. These measures, however, require a considerable amount of expertise not only to use but also to monitor. These patients with markedly comminuted fractures, particularly with interarticular extensions, should be referred to the orthopedic surgeon for care.

Fractures of the distal ulna are almost invariably associated with fractures of the radius. When the fracture is complete the reduction of the ulna can usually be obtained when the radius is reduced. Stability of the ulnar reduction is ensured if the radial reduction remains constant. Reduction of both bones rather than the radius alone, however, is a procedure of somewhat greater magnitude and may require an orthopedic surgeon, particularly if the reduction is attempted and anatomical reduction of both bones cannot be obtained. Even slight degrees of angulation of the ulnar fragment will result in mechanical deficiencies in the distal radioulnar joint with the resulting problems previously described.

Fractures of the ulnar styloid that occur with the usual distal radial fracture do not need treatment. These will sometimes heal without much deformity but will sometimes heal with a considerable amount of elongation deformity. Occasionally they will not heal and a pseudarthrosis is formed. Most of these abnormalities, however, do not give any symptoms and treatment is ordinarily not necessary. An occasional nonunited fracture will develop enough instability because of the attachment of the ulnar collateral ligament to it and surgical treatment may be necessary. For the most part, however, the ulnar styloid fracture is of no consequence when treating the usual Colles fracture.

Fractures of the scaphoid and the difficulty in their healing have been discussed previously. The most important and fundamental responsibility of the primary care physician is to make the diagnosis, since many scaphoid fractures are not seen on the original films and the diagnosis is not made until considerable time has passed. If a great amount of time has passed before immobilization is started, the chances of nonunion are greatly increased.

The basic method of finding a nondisplaced fracture of the scaphoid is to suspect it. In an individual who has fallen on the outstretched hand and complains of severe pain over the anatomical snuff box (the interval between the abductor to the thumb and the long extensor of the thumb), one should suspect a scaphoid fracture. Scaphoid fractures may not be seen on the usual AP and lateral projections. If, however, there is point tenderness over the anatomical snuff box and pain on motion of the wrist without any other obvious deformity, special projection should be taken so that the scaphoid can be better visualized. Often a fracture not seen on plain films will be identified. If the patient has signs and symptoms that point to a scaphoid fracture and if one can still not be identified on the x-ray film, most orthopedists believe that the patient should be treated by the application of a cast anyway. If his signs and symptoms are suspicious enough, there is very likely a fracture with minimal displacement that may not be identified even on special projections. This fracture, however, will be immediately apparent 3 weeks after the beginning healing stage, which is manifested by demineralization around the fracture line. In 3 weeks the fracture will be very obvious on the x-ray films and if the patient has been already immobilized for these 3 weeks he is already well established in his treatment program and his chances of securing a solid union are greatly enhanced. If, on the other hand, when the patient is seen in the office in 3 weeks, the cast removed, and further x-ray films fail to reveal a fracture, the cast can be removed and he can be started on an active exercise program. One then need not fear missing an occult fracture of the scaphoid. Three weeks of immobilization in a cast is a small price to pay to prevent missing a fracture of the scaphoid. Actually, casting is a good treatment for an acute sprain of the wrist which is what the patient had if there is no fracture.

Once the fracture has been diagnosed, a gauntlet type of cast should be applied from the metacarpophalangeal joints of the fingers up to the proximal forearm with the thumb included out to its tip in a position of some abduction. Some orthopedists apply a long arm cast with the thumb included but it is the author's opinion that the gauntlet cast is adequate as long as the patient refrains from excessive use of the extremity. Cast changes should be done at 1 month to 6 week intervals to ascertain the extent of healing and the maintenance of good position at the fracture.

The patient should be warned in the beginning that a minimum of 12 weeks is required for healing of the scaphoid fracture. Occasionally a delayed union will occur that requires longer immobilization, but if the fracture does not show healing at 12 weeks the patient should be referred to the orthopedic surgeon for follow-up.

INSTABILITY SYNDROMES

In 1972 Linscheid and associates, at the Mayo Clinic, classified and outlined the pathomechanics of traumatic instability of the wrist. Largely due to the insights gained from this study, much research has been conducted during the past 15 years on these instability patterns. The pathomechanics of the wrist joint and the interrelationships of the various carpal bones are extremely complicated and not within the scope of this chapter. It is important, however, for the primary care physician to recognize the possibility of wrist instability patterns, since these indicate disruption of intercarpal ligament stability; early referral and diagnosis is important for institution of appropriate treatment. Failure to diagnose these instability patterns will result in the patient developing a chronically painful wrist and degenerative joint disease.

Though there are a number of variations, three distinct syndromes should be considered by the primary care physician when confronted with a wrist that continues to be symptomatic for some time following an injury; in all three, a diagnosis can be made relatively early, usually with plain radiographs.

Disassociation of the Lunate and Triquetrum

Disassociation of the lunate and triquetrum leads to a volar intercalated segment instability (VISI) pattern. This is a relatively rare condition and is suspected when volar facing of the lunate on the lateral view exists (Fig. 10-5D),

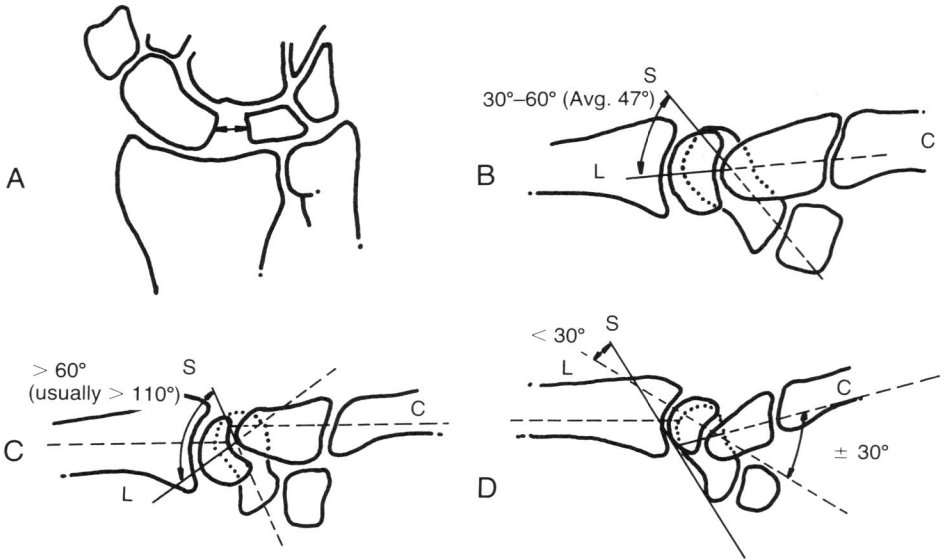

Fig. 10-5. The radiographic findings in instability syndromes. (**A**) The "Terry-Thomas" sign with separation at the scapholunate articulation. To be significant this separation should be greater than 3 mm and comparison with the normal opposite side should be done often. (**B**) The normal attitude of the lunate as compared with the distal radial surface and the remainder of the carpal bones, as seen on lateral x-ray projections. Note that the long axis of the radius and the midaxis of the lunate are the same. (**C**) The dorsal-facing lunate with the obvious changes in the position of the scaphoid and an increase in the angle created by projection of the long axis of each of these two bones indicate the dorsal intercalated wrist instability syndrome (DISI pattern). This ordinarily suggests scapholunate disassociation and often is associated with the findings in Fig. A. (**D**) Note the volar facing of the lunate with respect to the lateral projection of the radius and the obvious collapse of the normal architecture of the carpal bones with a marked decrease in the angle created between the long axis of the lunate and scaphoid.

instead of the straight-forward facing seen in the normal lateral wrist joint projection (Fig. 10-5B). The finding of this abnormality on the radiograph, particularly in association with a click on motion of the wrist in flexion, extension, and ulnar deviation and tenderness over the ulnar aspect of the wrist, should lead one to suspect this diagnosis; and referral to a hand or orthopedic surgeon should be made.

Disassociation of the Scapholunate Articulation

Disassociation of the scapholunate articulation leads to two primary findings.

1. The dorsal intercalated segment instability (DISI) pattern, which is identical to that seen with the VISI wrist except that there is a *dorsal* facing of the distal lunate surface on the plain lateral film (Fig. 10-5C). The DISI pattern almost invariably represents a loss of stability at the scapholunate articulation.

2. A visible separation between the scaphoid and the lunate on the AP projection – the so-called Terry-Thomas sign (Fig. 10-5A). Separation of up to 3 mm may be normal; if a great amount of separation is seen, a plain AP radiograph of the opposite wrist should be taken for comparison.

These findings along with tenderness over the dorsum of the wrist overlying the scapholunate articulation should warrant a referral to a hand or orthopedic surgeon.

Damage to the Triangular Fibrocartilagenous Complex

The triangular fibrocartilagenous complex (TFCC) attaches the distal radius to the ulnar styloid. The TFCC, triangular in shape, has its base across the distal extremity of the sigmoid fossa on the ulnar side of the radius and tapers off so that the apex of the triangle attaches to the ulnar styloid. It is several millimeters in thickness and tends to separate the carpus from the distal radioulnar joint. Continued pain over this area, particularly during supination and pronation, and an audible click felt with movement to the area often indicate TFCC damage. Often the distal ulna will be hypermobile with respect to the radius. These findings should create enough suspicion of an injury to the TFCC that referral to an orthopedic or hand surgeon is indicated.

Use of Radiopaque Dye

The wrist instability patterns are well demonstrated on arthrograms of the wrist with radiopaque dye. The material is injected into the radiocarpal joint, and if all structures are intact the dye will remain only in this proximal joint. If, however, tears in the intercarpal structures occur, the dye can be seen to leak through this interspace into the midcarpal space; and the finding of dye in the midcarpal space is strongly suggestive of intercarpal ligament damage. By the same token, dye is not ordinarily extruded from the proximal "radiocarpal" joint into the distal radioulnar joint unless there is a tear of the TFCC. When such a tear exists the dye extrudes through it into the joint filling it with dye, which is readily visible on the arthrogram.

OTHER CONDITIONS

Synovial Cysts of the Joint Capsule

The so-called ganglion cyst seen on the dorsum of the wrist joint represents a disease of the wrist joint capsule itself in which cystic degeneration occurring in the capsule ruptures through into the joint. Because of this communication with the joint, the cyst begins to distend and create a cystic mass extruding from the dorsal wrist joint capsule. These cysts may be relatively small or may sometimes assume quite large proportions. It is not mandatory that they be removed, however, just because they are present. Indications for removal are pain, limited motion because of the size of the cyst, or the poor cosmetic appearance created by the protrusion of the cystic mass on the dorsum of the wrist.

When excision is done it should be treated as a procedure of some magnitude and performed in the operating room under general or regional anesthesia using strict aseptic conditions. In this manner the dissection can be carried out and an avascular field created by tourniquet control and the entire process removed, including the segment of dorsal wrist joint capsule that constitutes the origin of the cyst and the communication of the cyst with the wrist joint. The defect created in the wrist joint capsule can be closed with small absorbable sutures unless it is extremely large. Procedures done in the physician's office under local anesthesia result in a very high percentage of recurrence and the rate of complications is great.

Cases that are thought to be multilocular or in which a recurrence has followed an initial simple removal should most likely be referred to the hand surgeon or orthopedic surgeon for removal. The recurrence rate is extremely high and the amount of material resected must be great, usually including the entire wrist joint capsule.

The second most common site of synovial cysts around the wrist joint is on the volar radial side of the wrist. These cysts are usually very closely associated with the radial artery and may arise from the capsule of the flexor carpi radialis tendon as well as from the capsule of the radiocarpal joint. These should, again, be removed in the operating room under regional or general anesthesia, under tourniquet control so that the cyst may be dissected out without damage to the adjacent and often adherent radial vessel. Care must be taken to remove all tissue-bearing synovial cells since residual cells in any number will usually form a focus for recurrence.

Dorsal Joint Capsulitis

Inflammatory reaction in the dorsal wrist joint capsule may or may not be a companion condition to that described above with the occurrence of synovial cysts. Often, however, the patient has a continually painful wrist with acute tenderness dorsally over the capsule but no cysts ever occur. Besides the usual program of immobilization with a splint, hot packs applied over the area, and the systemic use of nonsteroidal anti-inflammatory agent, the judicious injection of steroids into the capsule may be used *once*. An injection should be done very carefully and an attempt made to avoid acute distention of the capsular fibers, since this often results in attritional changes and advancement of the disease process. If all other measures fail the patient may be referred to the radiologist for possible "orthovoltage" radiation over the area. Many times the administration of small (200 rads administered four times over 10 to 12 days) doses will result in dramatic improvement of symptoms. There have not been any deleterious effects of this treatment. Finally, if all measures have failed to result in improvement, the patient should be referred to the orthopedic surgeon for some sort of surgical resection of the involved wrist joint capsule with reconstruction, perhaps utilizing the dorsal carpal ligament. The decision, of course, should be left to the consulting orthopedist.

De Quervain's Stenosing Tenosynovitis

The patient with de Quervain's disease usually present complaining of severe pain over the radial styloid area. This area is acutely tender, it may be sometimes slightly swollen, but the characteristic picture is that any movement of the wrist that causes a tension or pulling on the tendons lying over the radial styloid causes an acute exacerbation of pain. These two tendons, of course, are the extensor pollicis brevis and the abductor pollicis longus and pass through a very small fibro-osseous tunnel overlying the radial styloid area. The classic clinical test for de Quervain's disease is the so-called Finkelstein's test (Fig. 10-6). This test is done by having the patient clasp his thumb in his closed fist, thereby, tethering the long abductor and short extensor tendon. With the thumb thus tethered the wrist is moved quickly into ulnar deviation, pulling these two tendons suddenly through the canal. This usually causes exquisite pain and is more or less diagnostic of de Quervain's disease.

Nonoperative treatment of de Quervain's disease includes the applications of moist heat, immobilization in a splint, and the administration of nonsteroidal anti-inflammatory medication. Methylprednisolone should be injected into the canal and will usually result in a dramatic improvement of symptoms. The problem arises from the fact that if the canal is extremely crowded by the inflamed tendons the symptoms will not be completely relieved or they may be relieved for a period of time only to recur after the effects of the steroids have diminished. In these instances repeated injections are not indicated but the patient should be referred for surgical excision of the tight roof of de Quervain's canal.

At surgery, the tendons are often found to be quite swollen, to have a considerable amount of reactive material around them, and to crowd the small canal considerably so that movement of the tendons through it is not possible. It is also often found that there has been a reduplication of the abductor pollicis longus tendon so that the canal has always been a little more crowded than normal but with time, use, and perhaps a superimposed injury the swelling

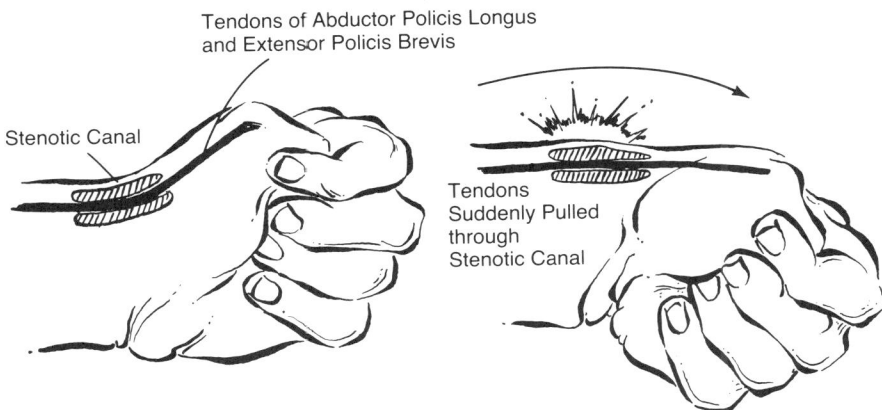

Fig. 10-6. Finkelstein's test. See text for description.

becomes an irreversible process that requires surgical intervention. The surgery should be done by one experienced in surgery in this area since damage to the superficial radial nerve is often seen and on occasion incomplete unroofing of the canal may occur when a small accessory canal is undiscovered and continues to give symptoms postoperatively.

Subluxation of the Distal Ulna

Subluxation of the distal ulna at the distal radioulnar joint is a relatively uncommon condition but is quite distressing when it does occur since it almost defies any type of conservative management. Most of these cases follow trauma and many are related to fractures of the distal radius with some distortion of the distal radioulnar mechanism as was described in the section under fractures of the distal radius. Occasionally a congenital weakness in the restraining structures will result in a gradually increasing amount of symptoms as the restraining ligament gradually stretches out. The subluxation usually occurs only with the wrist in pronation since this is the position of greatest stress to the distal radioulnar joint. With the wrist in complete supination, the distal radioulnar joint is quite stable and does not require any additional ligamentous support.

There is seldom any nonoperative treatment for the congenital variety since some sort of reconstruction must be done surgically to restore stability. However, in the cases of the acute stretch or tear of the ligament a period of immobilization in a sugar tong splint with the wrist in complete supination may allow enough healing of the injured ligaments to restore stability. If, however, the symptoms continue to be a problem even after this type of splinting the patient should be referred to the orthopedic surgeon for treatment.

11

THE HAND

Conditions involving the hand are different from those involving the rest of the musculoskeletal system because the hand is so specialized and has such a specialized anatomical arrangement. It requires, therefore, a careful analysis of the anatomical features before one can expect to examine it adequately or diagnose conditions. Conditions involving the hand usually result in a loss of function so that the objective of treatment is to restore that function. Less often do conditions of the hand present with a primary complaint of pain. The physicians may be extremely objective in the evaluation of the hand and its function. It should be remembered also that the hand represents different things to different individuals, depending upon their life style and their occupation, so that some consideration should be given to these factors. Likewise, there is a difference between the dominant and the nondominant hand from the standpoint of restoration of function and, therefore, the identity of the dominant hand should always be carefully noted.

ANATOMY

Skin

The skin on the dorsum of the hand is quite loose, being separated from the underlying tissues by a loose areolar tissue. For this reason the skin on the dorsum of the hand quite often is the site of considerable swelling since there is no limiting factor and edema fluid can collect in the areolar tissue separating the underlying structures from the skin. That the dorsal veins lie on the dorsum of the hand has considerable importance since the dorsal veins represent the primary mechanism for return of blood from the hand. Disruption of these dorsal veins therefore results in swelling of the entire hand since the venous return is almost entirely dependent upon their patency.

Palmar skin is different, being thick and bearing no hair follicles. The palmar skin is tethered to the underlying tissues at frequent intervals, particularly at the flexion creases. This has considerable clinical importance in that lacerations or puncture wounds that occur in the flexion creases of the finger are likely to extend directly into the flexor tendon sheath since there is no subcutaneous fat in these regions. Between the flexion creases there is a considerable amount of subcutaneous fat separating the skin from the underlying flexor tendon sheath. Injections into the tendon sheath, for instance, should be made through the area that contains fatty tissue since this is much less likely to create a fistula than injections made through the flexor crease. The palmar fascia lies deep to the skin and is often the site of a proliferative response known as Dupuytren's disease. This contracture of the palmar fascia often results in loss of extension of the fingers by the tethering effect of these Dupuytren's bands.

The nails are very specialized structures occurring in the epidermis. They are produced by the cellular matrix lying at their base. As the nail is produced from the matrix it extends out and is attached to a nail bed underneath. The proximal margin of the nail is covered by a skin fold known as the ungual fold. Bacterial infections in this region that give rise to the common perionychia. The nail is attached to the underlying bed completely out to the end of the bed and at this point it usually grows out or extends past the nail bed for a variable length depending upon periodic cutting or wear. On either side the nail extends into a gutter wherein the nail margin lies down in a fold of skin with the margin of skin folding over it. Injuries that result in a detachment of the nail from underlying bed create difficulties since once the nail has become detached it is not likely to reattach. If there is damage to the nail bed the new nail grown from the matrix extends out only to the line of detachment of the old nail and is not attached from this point further distally. Likewise, damage to the nail matrix may result in various deformities of the nail including areas where no nail will grow if damage to the matrix has resulted in death of specialized cells that create the nail.

Any type of injury that results in an avulsion of the nail will require careful repair of lacerations across the nail bed so that the new nail will grow out over the area of injury. Likewise, either the old nail should be used as a splint or a splint should be created from sterile material such as the foil covering of suture packs and inserted underneath the ungual fold so that the fold will not seal over and prevent advancement of the new nail. Subungual hematomas occurring from trauma should, of course, always be drained, preferably with a hole through the nail, either bored with a small #11 Bard-Parker blade or burned through the nail with a hot paper clip. Drainage of these hematomas not only reduces damage to the matrix of the nail bed but also relieves the intense pain that usually follows crushing injuries of the nail.

Bones and Joints

There are a total of 8 carpal bones, 5 metacarpal bones, and 14 phalanges, making a total of 27 bones in the skeleton of the hand (Fig. 11-1).

Carpus

The carpus is comprised of a total of eight bones of various odd shapes that fit together very snugly and are divided into two rows (see Fig. 10-1). The proximal row contains the scaphoid, lunate, and triquetrum and constitutes a curved surface that articulates against the radius in the "radiocarpal joint." The distal row includes the trapezium, trapezoid, capitate, and hamate bones which all are articulated with the proximal ends of the metacarpal bones in various ways.

The first metacarpal–trapezium joint is quite specialized since it constitutes the major articulation for movement of the thumb into its various positions for pinch and grasp. Because of this, injuries to this joint should be carefully treated so that the joint surface is maintained. Likewise, this joint is very early the site of degenerative disease in many individuals since it sustains the most trauma from use. Often with arthritic changes the ligamentous support becomes lax with loss of stability and a gradual subluxation of the first metacarpal bone out of the joint. The remainder of the carpometacarpal joints are all quite stable and a small amount of motion occurs there with strong ligamentous support.

Metacarpals

The five metacarpal bones are somewhat different in their anatomical arrangement and function. The first metacarpal bone, as previously described, articulates with the trapezium to give a very wide range of motion in delivery of the thumb into the opposing position for action against the various fingers. The other four metacarpal bones, however, are relatively stable in their position. The

Index
Middle
Ring
Little
Distal Joints
Middle Joints
Proximal Joints
Thumb
Distal Joint
Proximal Joint
Radiocarpal Joint

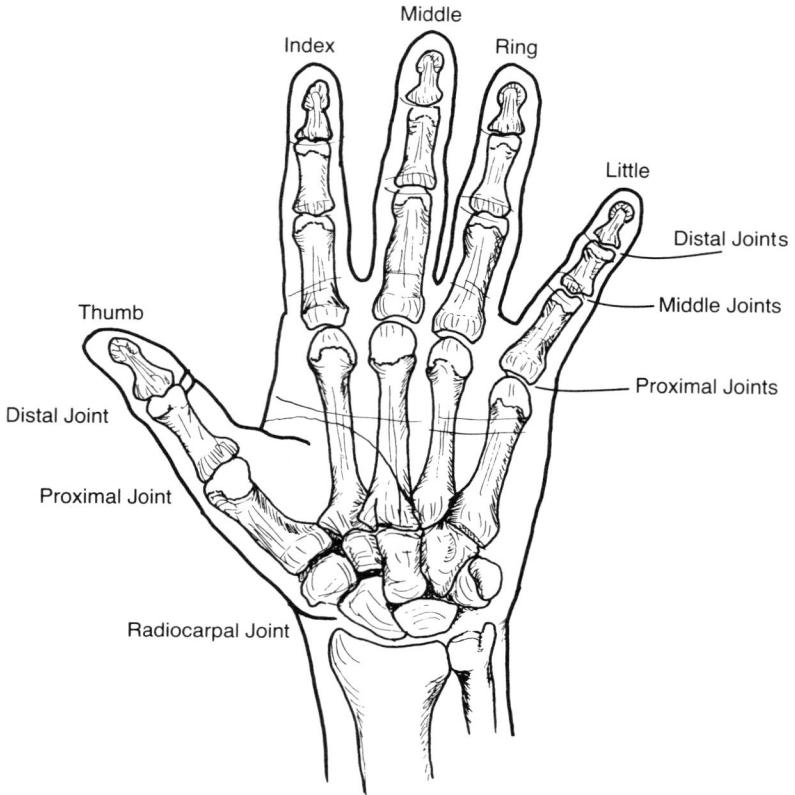

Fig. 11-1. The skeleton of the hand and wrist. There are three joints in each finger but only two in the thumb (proximal and distal). The digits should be named instead of numbered: thumb and index, ring, middle, and little fingers. The joints should be identified as proximal, middle, and distal to avoid confusion with other nomenclature. The proximal joints of the fingers lie well within the palm but can be identified dorsally by the metacarpal heads. The entire carpus acts as a unit and articulates with the radius so that movement in the wrist joint is present for the most part in the radiocarpal joint.

second and third comprise the portion of the hand considered the fixed unit. The mobile two metacarpals are the fourth and fifth and have a considerable increase in motion at the carpometacarpal joints over the second and third. This allows the more mobile ring and little fingers to be brought across into the palm to a greater degree so that articulation with the thumb and the grasp of small objects is made more functional. The proximal joint of the thumb (metacarpophalangeal) is somewhat different from the metacarpophalangeal joints of the four fingers: it has two collateral ligaments that completely restrict lateral motion so that the motion is entirely limited to extension and flexion in the sagittal plane. The other four metacarpophalangeal joints have a much greater degree of lateral motion with the joints in extension since the collateral ligaments in this position are relatively loose and allow for this type of motion. With the metacarpophalangeal joints of the four fingers in flexion, however, there is a considerable amount of lateral stability.

Phalanges

There are three phalanges in each finger—separated by two joints—the middle joint (proximal interphalangeal) and the distal joint (distal interphalangeal). The middle and distal joints of the fingers are similar to the joints of the thumb: they have very little lateral motion and act as true hinge-type joints with flexion and extension occurring in the sagittal plane. All of the joints of the digits, however, have very strong volar plate mechanisms to prevent a great amount of recurvatum. Certain individuals have a normal laxity of the volar plate so that a few degrees of recurvatum are possible. However, all of the digital joints have stability on the volar side, which allows for stability from the standpoint of hyperextension.

Musculature

The musculature that promotes hand function for the most part does not lie in the hand but in the forearm, with tendinous extensions into the hand that create motion into the wrist and digits. The extrinsic muscles in the forearm may be roughly divided as far as function is concerned into the extensor and and flexor surfaces.

Extrinsic Muscles

Extrinsic muscles lie in the forearm and move various portions of the wrist or hand by means of tendinous extensions into the hand.

Extensor Muscles.   The extensor muscles lie on the dorsum of the forearm with extension into the hand by means of tendons that pass through six extensor compartments at the wrist (Fig. 11-2). It should be fairly easy to locate possible extensor tendon injuries by the location of the laceration or the injury itself. All extensor muscles are innervated by the radial nerve.

The *first extensor compartment* contains the adductor pollicis longus, which extends the first metacarpal, and the extensor pollicis brevis, which extends the metacarpophalangeal joint of the thumb. Both of these functions can be fairly easily tested. The long extensor does not pass through the number one, or radialmost compartment, but along through the third compartment.

The *second extensor compartment* contains the two radial wrist extensors that insert into the bases of the second and third metacarpal bones and, therefore, barely extend into the hand itself. They are, however, the most powerful muscles in extending the hand at the radiocarpal joint.

The *third extensor compartment* contains the long thumb extensor, which courses at an angle around Lister's tubercle and extends over the thumb where it results in extension of the distal phalanx only. Lacerations over the dorsum of the hand, even overlying the second metacarpal bone, should be suspected of

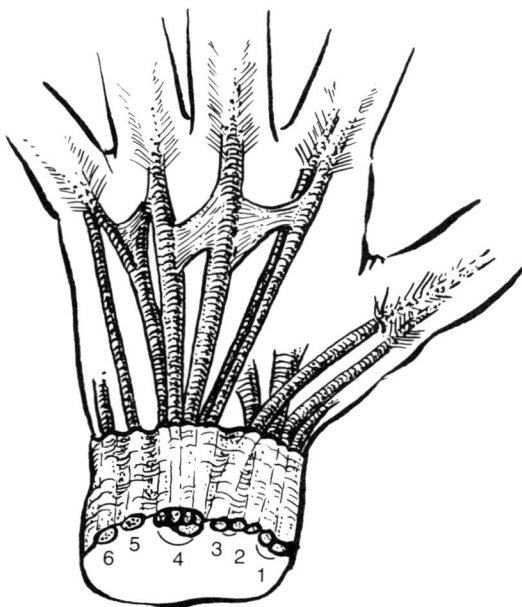

Fig. 11-2. The extensor compartments of the dorsum of the hand and wrist. There are six separate compartments passing underneath the dorsal retinaculum and containing specific tendons. Compartment 1 contains the abductor pollicis longus and extensor pollicis brevis. Compartment 2 contains the extensor carpi radialis longus and brevis. Compartment 3 contains the extensor pollicis longus before it deviates radially to insert into the thumb. Compartment 4 contains all of the common extensors to the fingers as well as the extensor indicis proprius. Compartment 5 contains the extensor digiti minimi and compartment 6 contains the extensor carpi ulnaris.

lacerating the extensor pollicis longus. Any dorsal laceration on the radial side of the wrist or hand should alert the examiner to test for extensor pollicis longus function (Fig. 11-3.)

The *fourth dorsal compartment* contains the major finger extensors, including all common extensors to all four fingers and the extensor indicis proprius. These can be easily tested since they merely extend the joints of the fingers. The only exception is the extensor indicis proprius, which will extend the index finger alone with all of the rest of the fingers flexed into a fist. The extensor digitorum communis extends the proximal joint of all the fingers and the middle and distal joints may be extended by the intrinsics.

The *fifth extensor compartment* contains a single tendon, the extensor digiti minimi, which, like the extensor indicis proprius, will extend the little finger with the remainder of the fingers clinched in a fist.

The *sixth extensor compartment* contains only the extensor carpi ulnaris, which extends the wrist but also deviates it ulnarly in extension. This function is relatively easy to test.

Flexor Muscles.   All of the flexor muscles lie on the volar aspect of the forearm and are innervated either by the median or the ulnar nerve (see section on nerve supply). These functions may be quite easily tested.

Flexor pollicis longus.   This flexes the distal joint of the thumb and may be tested by stabilizing the remainder of the thumb and seeing if individual flexion is present.

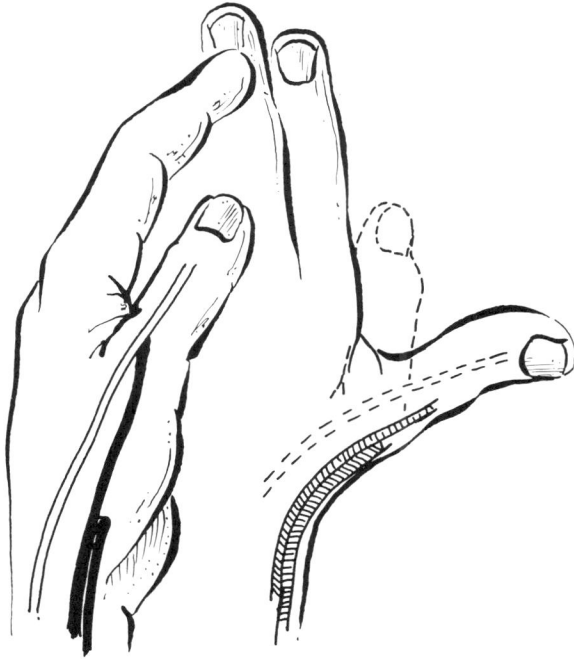

Fig. 11-3. The first extensor compartment contains the long abductor and short extensor of the thumb. The extensor pollicis longus runs through the third compartment, indicating how far to the side the longus runs before entering the extensor hood at about the point of insertion of the extensor pollicis brevis. This tendon courses from its position passing around Lister's tubercle on the dorsum of the wrist, and injuries in this area, even though relatively far removed from the thumb per se, may often include injury to the extensor pollicis longus.

Flexor digitorum profundus. This muscle can be tested for all four fingers by stabilizing the various fingers in extension and asking the patient to flex the distal joint of the finger actively. This should be done holding the wrist in neutral position (Fig. 11-4A).

Flexor digitorum superficialis. These muscles to all four fingers are tested individually by holding the other three fingers in the extended position while asking the patient to flex the middle joint of the finger being tested. Holding the remaining fingers in extension locks profundus action and allows only the superficialis to work on the finger being examined (Fig. 11-4B).

Flexor carpi ulnaris, carpi radialis and palmaris longus. These are all evaluated by asking the patient to flex the wrist actively against resistance. All three of these tendons can be palpated with this maneuver. Approximately 20 percent of patients examined will not have a functioning palmaris longus and, therefore, the absence of this tendon does not constitute a real abnormality.

Intrinsic Muscles

The intrinsic muscles are those that are wholly contained within the hand, having both their origin and insertion in the hand proper. These include the thenar and hypothenar muscle groups, the adductor pollicis, the four lumbricales, and the seven interossei.

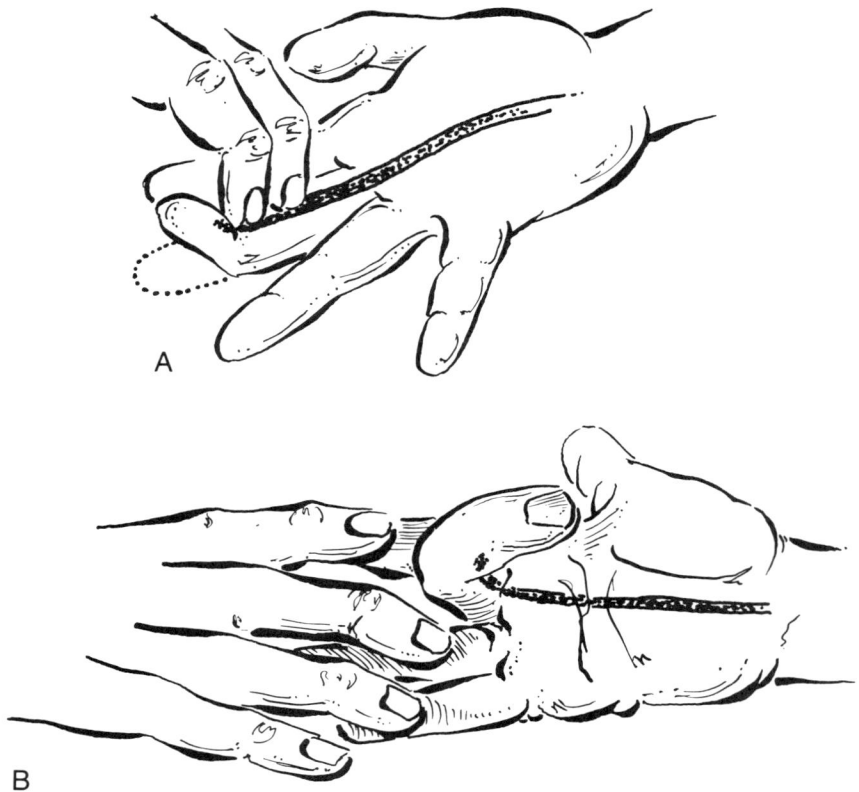

Fig. 11-4. **(A)** When testing the function of the flexor digitorum profundus, the finger should be held in an extended position out to the distal joint. The patient is then asked to flex the distal joint independently and ability to do so indicates the presence of a functional flexor digitorum profundus tendon to this finger. **(B)** Testing for superficialis tendon function is done by holding the other three fingers in complete extension. This locks the profundus tendons in the extended position (since they come from a common muscle belly) and will not allow the profundus to function in the finger being examined. Since the superficialis tendons all act independently, the function of the tendon in this finger can be determined by active flexion at the middle joint. (*Figure continues.*)

Thenar Muscles.   These overlie the palm on the radial side at the base of the thumb and bring the thumb into the opposed position opposite the fingers. They include the abductor pollicis brevis, the opponens pollicis, and the flexor pollicis brevis. All are innervated by the median nerve. Testing is done by asking the patient to oppose the thumb to the little finger with nails parallel and feeling whether these muscles contract. Pulling against the thumb, likewise, will give some idea of the relative strength of these muscles.

Hypothenar Muscles.   These are composed of the adductor digiti quinti, the flexor digiti quinti, and the opponens digiti minimi. All are evaluated as a group by asking the patient to bring the little finger away from the other fingers in

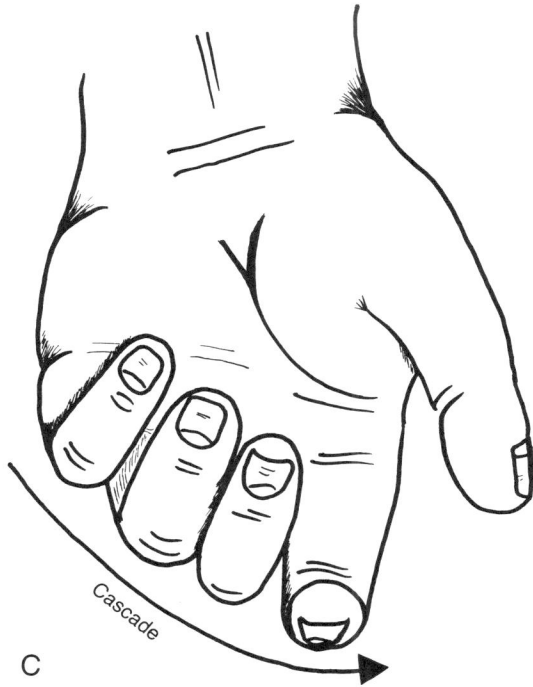

Fig. 11-4. (*Continued*). (**C**) The normal cascade of the fingers in the resting position. This cascade is caused by the tethering of the flexor tendons; injury to the flexor tendon results in a loss of this position so that the finger with the injured tendon lies completely straight as compared with the flexed condition of the other fingers. Disruption of this cascade appearance is extremely important.

C

abduction and palpating the muscle for function and strength. The muscles are ulnar-innervated.

Adductor Pollicis Muscle. This is tested functionally by having the patient hold a card or piece of paper between the thumb and the radial side of the index finger at the level of the proximal phalanx. This muscle is innervated by the ulnar nerve.

Lumbricale and Interossei Muscles. There are four lumbricale muscles each lying on the radial side of the respective finger, taking origin from the flexor pollicis longus tendon and inserting into the side of the extensorhood into the lateral band on the radial side. These muscles are basically responsible for flexion of the proximal joints. Loss of lumbricale function usually renders the patient incapable of strong flexion of the proximal joint even though, if the interossei are intact, he may still be able to flex down reasonably well. In ulnar paralysis, of course, with loss of the interossei and the two ulnar lumbricales the patient assumes a characteristic position in which he can extend the proximal joints of all four fingers but can actively extend the middle joints in only the index and middle fingers. The two lumbricales to the index and middle fingers are from median nerve distribution and retain their function with ulnar palsy. The interossei are entirely ulnar in innervation. The volar interossei bring the fingers all together and the dorsal interossei spread them apart. This is easy to remember by recalling that to cup the hand, such as in receiving something, the hand is turned up and the volar interossei work to pull the fingers together.

Circulation

The hand is served by two arteries that combine to make up two arches with the palm of the hand. The superficial volar arch has major contribution from the ulnar artery with less contribution from the radial. The deep volar arch, which lies underneath the palmar structures, has its major contribution from the radial and a lesser contribution from the ulnar artery. This establishes an excellent collateral circulation for the hand: if either the radial or the ulnar artery is intact both arches have adequate blood supply (Fig. 11-5). By the same token, each of the arteries contributes a segment to form the common digital artery that supplies the inner space between each of the two fingers. Therefore, occlusion or damage to either the superficial or deep volar arches will not result in vascular insufficiency to the fingers as long as the other arch is intact. To carry the idea of a generous collateral circulation somewhat further, each digital artery divides into two branches that serve the adjacent sides of each web space. Each finger, therefore, has blood supply from two separate common digital arteries (Fig. 11-6). It will follow, then, from this brief description that only if both arteries are occluded in the wrist, or if both arches are destroyed in the palm, or if both digital arteries in a single finger are destroyed will the finger have insufficient blood supply for survival. This concept of collateral circulation is extremely important when one is evaluating the circulatory condition of a hand following injury.

Testing Patency

The *Allen-Barker-Hines test* (usually called Allen's test) for patency of the radial and ulnar arteries is important in evaluating an injured hand. If the examiner catches the patient's wrist so that his fingers may press on both the ulnar and radial arteries at the wrist these arteries can be both occluded simultaneously. This results in loss of blood supply to the hand. If the fist is clinched and opened, the blood is squeezed out of the palm. Since no blood returns, the hand remains cadaveric in appearance. If either the radial or the ulnar artery is released while the other is held, the palm will promptly "pink up," indicating that the circulation has been reestablished through patency of that particular artery. The procedure can then be done for the opposite artery and the patency of both arteries can be determined. A similar modification of this test can be done with a single finger to determine whether both digital arteries are patent.

Distal-Based Flap

Of particular importance to the injured hand is the *distal-based flap*. The flap of any great length that has its base towards the distal end of the extremity is suspect from the standpoint of circulation. With a sectioning of vessels forming the proximal blood supply and the deep blood supply to the flap, it must depend

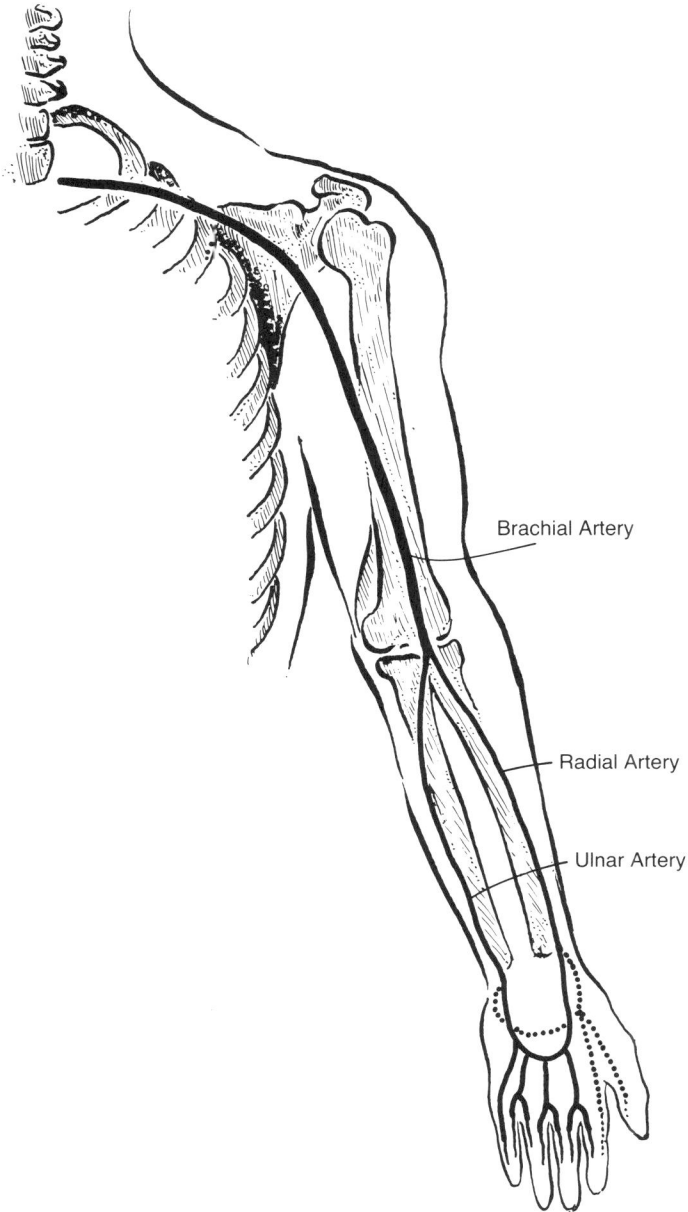

Fig. 11-5. Arterial supply of the upper extremity. The axillary artery becomes the brachial as it passes into the arm and then in the upper forearm divides into the radial and ulnar arteries. These two arteries pass into the hand and form two deep palmar arches that, in turn, form various divisions to serve all of the digits of the hand with arterial supply. See text for full description.

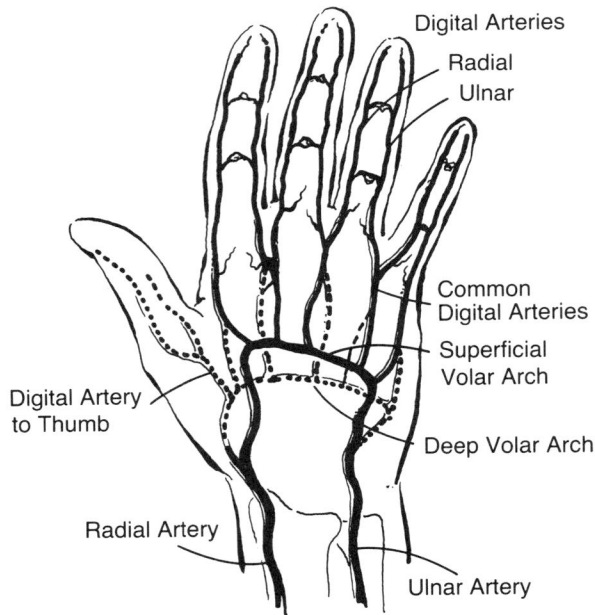

Fig. 11-6. Arterial circulation in the hand. Note that the divisions of the radial and ulnar arteries create two volar arches. A major contribution to the superficial arch is from the ulnar artery, with the deep branch of the ulnar artery entering into the deep volar arch. The major contribution to the deep volar arch is from the radial artery. The single artery to the thumb rises from the deep volar arch and separates to form the radial and ulnar digital arteries to a point that makes the collateral circulation in the thumb much more precarious than to the other digits. The other common digital arteries are formed from contributions from the deep and the superficial volar arteries. The common artery then divides to create two digital arteries that serve the adjacent sides of the web space.

upon circulation going ''around the corners'' to extend in from the distal direction. Since this will not occur to any great extent, distal-based flaps will usually not survive. This, of course, is not invariably the case. Since one cannot always estimate the exact amount of flap that will be lost (some will most certainly survive near the base), it is best usually to repair distal-based flaps. It is important, however, to warn the patient and his family that the circulation is poor to this flap and that it very likely will not survive in its entirety and may require a secondary skin grafting procedure.

Revascularization

Recent advancements in microsurgical anastomosis of small arteries have made it possible to consider *replantation* or revascularization in amputated extremities and digits. While the ultimate decision as to whether a replantation is feasible or should be done remains that of the treating surgeon, the primary care physician should know the protocol for care of the amputated part and the stump so that the patient can be transferred to the replantation center for evaluation and treatment.

Treatment of the stump basically involves control of bleeding. It is preferable to not use hemostats to clamp vessels since this destroys additional vessels and makes the repair more difficult. By the same token, most bleeding can be controlled by pressure. Even if the pressure must be maintained during the trip from the point of injury or the primary treating facility to the replantation center, this is preferable to clamping vessels. Since arteries and nerves run so close together blind clamping of the artery is very dangerous and many times will include the nerve in the clamping instrument.

Since the possibility of replantation is very closely related to the "warm ischemia time," it is extremely important to cool the amputated part early. Replantation is only feasible for about 1 or 2 hours if the amputated digit has not been cooled. Proper cooling of the digit extends this possible time for replantation to 16 or 18 hours.

Another factor of importance is hydrolysis in the amputated part. If the part is immersed in a solution (even saline), considerable shriveling occurs that results in a tissue dehydration, making replantation much less likely to succeed.

Freezing the digit destroys the tissue and makes the replantation doomed to failure. For this reason, the proper method of preparing an amputated digit or part for transportation is to place it in a water-tight container such as a plastic bag that has been sealed, and then to immerse this plastic bag in ice water. The temperature should be from 0 to 4°C; iced water is therefore, the appropriate vehicle. Salt or saline solution should not be added to the ice since this tends to lower the freezing temperature. In the case of amputated fingers or thumbs, an excellent vehicle that is always immediately available in the emergency room is a surgeon's glove. This is sterile and, of course, once the digit is placed in the glove and a knot tied in the wrist the container is waterproof and can be placed in the iced water for transportation.

The surgeon may choose not to replace a single digit that has been amputated, unless it is a thumb, particularly if the site of amputation is proximal to the middle joint. No mistake can be made, however, by properly transporting the patient and the amputated part to the replantation center so that the decision can be made there by the treating surgeon.

Vasospastic Disease

Vasospastic disease is often manifested by circulatory insufficiency in the hand. Pure spasm alone resulting in the so-called Raynaud's phenomenon is common and, carries a relatively poor prognosis. It is imperative that the patient stop smoking, refrain from exposure to cold for long periods of time, and avoid other injuries to the hands. The patient should be referred to an anesthesiologist for stellate ganglion blocks. More recently, an intervascular block similar to the Bier block technique for regional anesthesia has been devised in which guanethedine is used for its beta-blocking effect. Since this technique has some danger, it should be done only by those experienced in its use. The use of guanethedine seems to have rather long standing effects, so that instead of the relatively short effect of the stellate ganglion blocks, the results may last for several weeks. In addition, some anesthesiologists have used 6 percent phenol to try to obtain long-standing effectiveness of a stellate ganglion block. This procedure apparently has some merit. The use of vasodilating drugs and other adjunctive therapy is questionable but usually is tried out of desperation.

Nerves

Three primary nerves serve the musculature and provide sensation to the hand. The radial nerve does not have a motor component in the hand but has only the sensation over the dorsum of the thumb, index, and middle fingers. The ulnar and median nerves both have motor components in the hand as well as sensory components over the touchpads of the fingers.

Radial Nerve

The radial nerve divides relatively high in the forearm into motor and sensory branches (Fig. 11-7). The motor branch serves all of the extensor musculature going to the hand as well as the supinator, anconeus, and the abductor pollicis longus. The sensory branch (superficial radial nerve) arises in the proximal forearm and courses down the entire length of the forearm underneath the brachioradialis muscle. It emerges from the muscle 1.5 or 2 cm proximal to the tip of the radial styloid and soon divides into two major branches. These then divide several times to serve the entire aspect of the dorsum of the hand, as previously described.

An important point concerning the superficial radial nerve is that injury often results in neuroma formation with symptoms that are quite severe and often defy treatment. It is also important to recognize that since the long extensors to the fingers extend primarily to the proximal joints, if these are held passively flexed, the middle and distal joints may be extended quite easily with the intrinsic musculature. This must not be misconstrued to represent some residual radial function.

Median Nerve

The median nerve courses down the volar aspect of the forearm, crossing over in the midportion of the elbow and extending through a rather straight course down into the wrist (Fig. 11-8). It serves most of the flexor muscles in the forearm including the radial wrist flexor, the pronator teres, palmaris longus, all of the flexor digitorum superficialis muscles, and the flexor digitorum profundus muscles to the index and middle fingers. The long thumb flexor is likewise served by the median nerve as is the pronator quadratus. The nerve passes into the hand and at this point gives off a small motor branch that extends into and innervates all of the muscles in the thenar eminence, with the exception of the flexor pollicis brevis, which may have ulnar innervation. The common digital branches extend down to supply sensation to the radial aspect of the hand, including the thumb, index, middle fingers, and the radial half of the ring finger. The two common digital nerves extending into the palm have small motor branches that supply the two radial lumbricales.

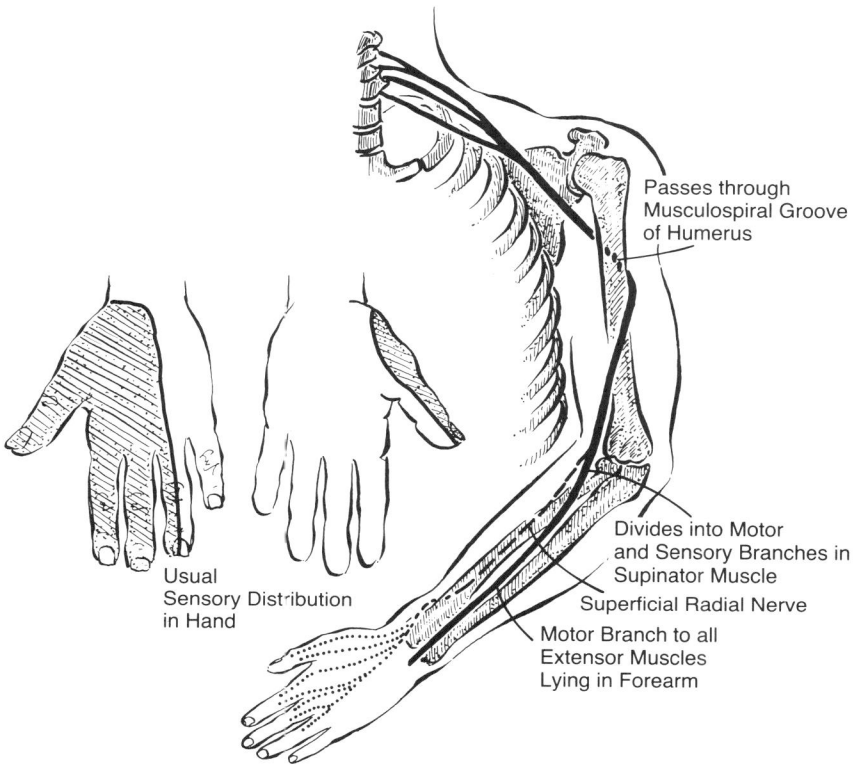

Fig. 11-7. The radial nerve's course from its origin down into the hand. The very close relationship of the humerus as it passes through the musculospiral groove makes it very prone to injury with fractures of the humerus in this area. The division occurs in the upper forearm, where the superficial radial nerve courses down into the hand and the motor branch extends to innervate all of the extensor muscles of the forearm that act to extend the wrist, all fingers, and the thumb. Note the sensory distribution shown in the small diagrams of the hand. The superficial radial nerve courses from its origin within the supinator muscle down underneath the belly of the brachioradialis to emerge just proximal to the radial styloid and pass subcutaneously from there downwards.

In the region of the wrist the median nerve is surprisingly superficial. Most of the time it is less than 1 cm beneath the skin and in the interval between the flexor carpi radialis and the palmaris longus.

The location of the motor branch as it divides from the main nerve trunk is usually indicated by a point touched by the middle finger as it is flexed down into the palm. This is variable, but gives a good indication as to the general level of the origin of the motor branch.

Ulnar Nerve

The ulnar nerve enters the forearm from the cubital canal, which lies posterior to the medial epicondyle where it is quite easily injured (Fig. 11-9). It is often the site of recurring trauma resulting in the classic tardy ulnar palsy. This may be related to scarring, repeated trauma, or encroachment in the canal by

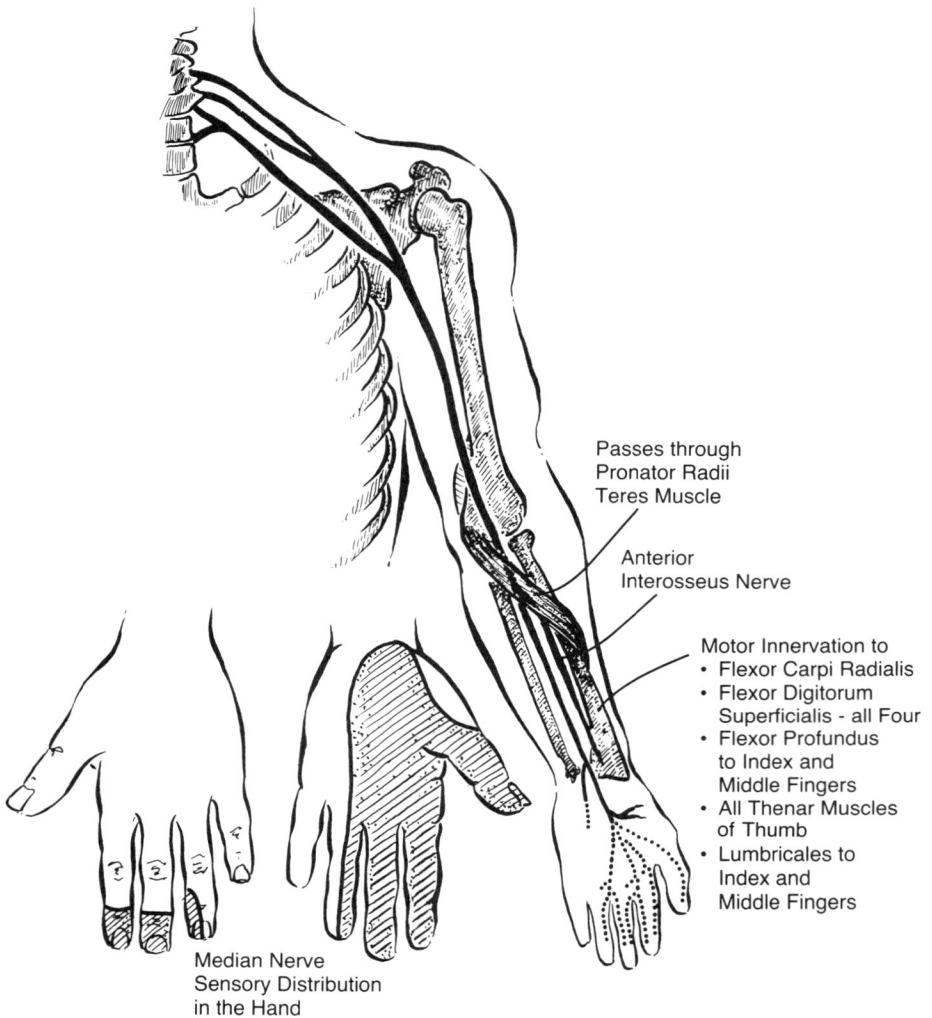

Passes through
Pronator Radii
Teres Muscle

Anterior
Interosseus Nerve

Motor Innervation to
• Flexor Carpi Radialis
• Flexor Digitorum
  Superficialis - all Four
• Flexor Profundus
  to Index and
  Middle Fingers
• All Thenar Muscles
  of Thumb
• Lumbricales to
  Index and
  Middle Fingers

Median Nerve
Sensory Distribution
in the Hand

Fig. 11-8. Median nerve distribution in the upper extremity. The median nerve has most of its innervation in the forearm and hand. It passes beneath or through the pronator teres muscle and divides into the anterior interosseus and the main median nerves. It furnishes motor innervation to the flexor carpi radialis, the flexor digitorum superficialis of all four fingers, the flexor profundus to the index and middle fingers, all thenar muscles of the thumb, and the lumbricale muscles to the index and middle fingers. The sensory distribution is as shown involving the palmar aspect of the thumb, index, and middle fingers, and radial half of the ring fingers and in the dorsal distribution as shown.

osteophytes that occur in degenerative disease of the elbow joint. In the forearm the ulnar nerve has only two motor responsibilities: to the flexor carpi ulnaris and to the ulnar two of the profundi muscles. The remaining portion of the ulnar distribution is to the intrinsic musculature with the exception of the superficial

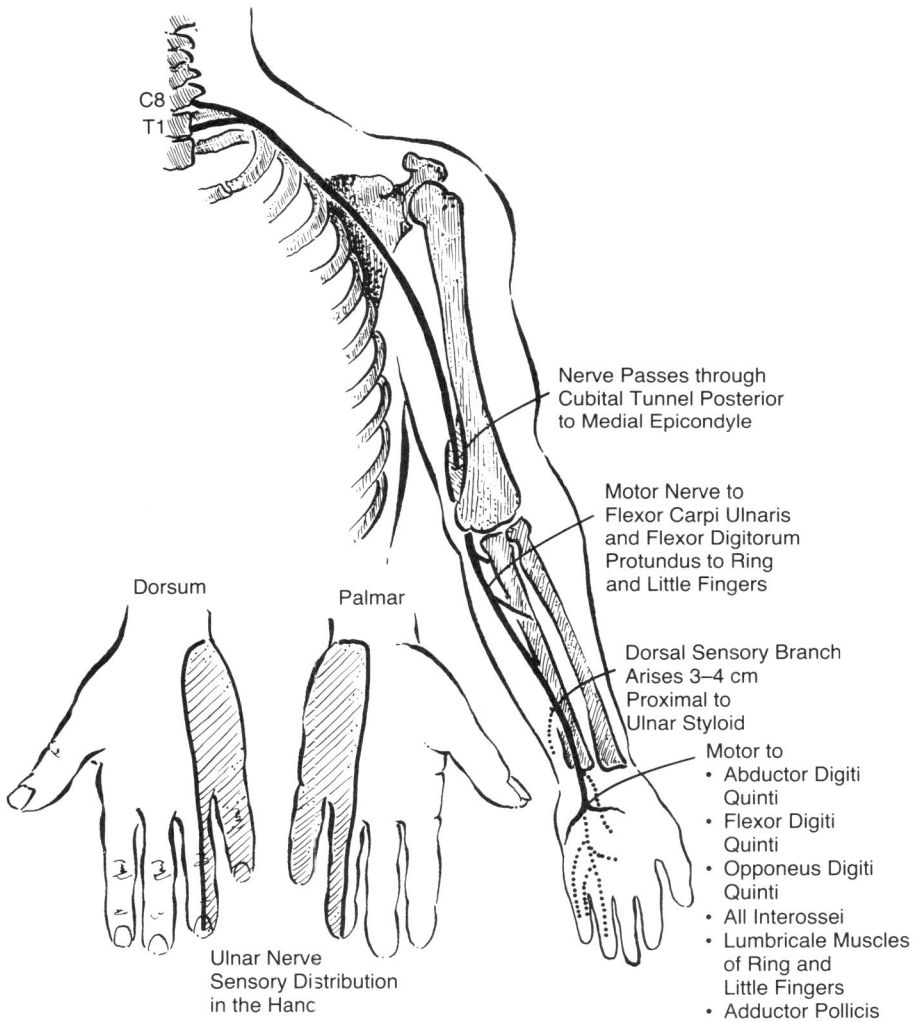

Fig. 11-9. Course and distribution of the ulnar nerve in the upper extremity. The nerve passes through the cubital tunnel posterior to the medial epicondyle and is subject to injury or irritation at this level. In the upper forearm it supplies the flexor carpi ulnaris and the flexor digitorum profundus muscles to the ring and little fingers. In the hand it serves as the motor innervation to the abductor digiti quinti, the flexor digiti quinti, and the opponens digiti quinti—all of the hypothenar muscle group. It then passes into the hand and serves all seven interossei and the two lumbricales on the ulnar side (to the ring and little fingers). It courses over and innervates the adductor pollicis muscle, which is the major muscle for strong pinch. The sensory distribution is as shown. The dorsal branch arises several centimeters above the ulnar styloid so that both the palmar and dorsal surfaces of the hand are furnished with sensation symmetrically.

head of the flexor pollicis brevis, the opponens pollicis, abductor pollicis brevis, and the two radial lumbricales. For this reason injuries to the ulnar nerve can be quite devastating due to the loss of power in pinch and grasp. The sensory innervation, which includes the entire surface of the little finger, has considerable importance from loss of its function and may account for undetected injury to the totally anesthetic digit. The dorsal branch to the ulnar nerve arises relatively high, usually at the junction of the middle and distal thirds of the forearm. Injuries to the nerve distal to this result in anesthesia only of the volar side of the little finger, with sensation being retained over the dorsal aspect.

X-RAY EXAMINATION

X-ray examination of the hand is usually done in three standard projections: anteroposterior, (AP), oblique, and lateral.

Lateral x-ray examination of the hand is difficult because of the multiple overlying structures. It should be done with the fingers flexed at varying degrees so that the individual joints of the individual fingers may be visualized effectively. This results in an overlay of the metacarpal heads. However, the metacarpal heads as well as the metacarpophalangeal joints can be reasonably well marked out, identified, and studied with care. If difficulty is experienced it may be necessary to resort to tomograms to get decent projections of the metacarpophalangeal joints of the fingers. By the same token, lateral views of an individual finger require that this finger be done separately, since it should be placed directly on the film to obtain a nondistorted view.

Dental film are often used to obtain true lateral films of the joints and this may be preferable in some instances. The middle and distal joints can usually be well visualized on the lateral. The primary problem is that one should be careful to be certain that this is a true lateral. The best method to determine this is to see if there is a single condylar shadow or if both condyles can be seen in the lateral. If both condyles can be seen on the lateral, a slightly oblique position has been obtained; the condyles should completely superimpose on one another and only one image be seen. This "double condyle" sign was described several years ago and is more or less indicative of rotation in the joint at the time the radiograph was taken (whether by rotating the entire finger or by a rotatory deformity in the bone).

Additional studies may be necessary, including flexion and extension films of the fingers, to determine whether joint blockage occurs and whether free excursion of the joints is possible. Special views of the first metacarpal–trapezium joint may be necessary to get a true AP and a lateral view of this joint. Both views must be taken by spotting directly over the joint and holding the joint in these desired positions when the film is taken.

Body sectioning films such a tomograms or computed tomograms may be used in difficult instances when better visualization of structures is necessary. Both hands, of course, should be taken for comparison.

Occasionally arthrograms can be of value, particularly in evaluation of the proximal joints of the fingers and thumb. The joint must be anesthetized thoroughly by injecting lidocaine and distending the joint with the local anesthetic first. The injection of dye will point out the integrity of the joint capsule, with extravasation usually present at points of ligamentous damage and capsular tears.

Occasionally, cine studies are necessary and the radiologist can make video tapes of the cine studes for further evaluation. This, however, is usually ordered by the orthopedic surgeon and their interpretation should be reserved for him and for the radiologist.

Stress films may be taken to determine ligamentous integrity, particularly when evaluating the collateral ligaments of the joints of the fingers and thumb. This is particularly necessary in rupture of the ulnar collateral ligament of the proximal joint of the thumb (gamekeeper's thumb). Often it is necessary in evaluating instability after injury to the collateral ligaments in the middle joints of the fingers. Care must be taken that the stress films are done with a slight amount of flexion to remove the stabilizing effect of the volar plate if it is intact. Also be certain that the fulcrum for bending the finger lies just at the joint, so that the true integrity of the collateral ligament on the opposite side may be evaluated.

EVALUATION AND TREATMENT OF LACERATIONS

The primary care physician should establish some sort of routine for examination of the injured hand, particularly where lacerations occur without other obvious injury. It is the usual practice of the inexperienced to focus immediately on the wound. In doing this, many times, important associated injuries are missed. To start with, the laceration should not be injected primarily since this will make it difficult to evaluate sensory loss, discovered later distal to the point of laceration (Fig. 11-10). If a local anesthetic solution has been injected into the laceration it is difficult to tell whether anesthesia over the touchpad of the finger distal to the laceration has resulted from a cut of the digital nerve or from the local anesthetic.

For this reason the wound should never be injected with anesthetic until a thorough examination has been done. By the same token, when excessive bleeding is occurring from the laceration the temptation to use a hemostat to clamp the bleeder within the wound should be resisted. Ordinarily, peripheral nerves run in close approximation to the vessels in the hand and fingers; indiscriminate blind clamping of the vessel may result in damage to the associated structures as well. If the patient can become calm and lie down on the examining table with the injured hand elevated, and pressure is applied to the laceration, bleeding will usually stop in a short time and the examination can be accomplished without further difficulty.

The structures in the hand should be visualized and an estimation made of the structures possibly cut by a laceration in this position. Remember that the location of the structures cut in a laceration depends to a certain extent upon the position of the hand at the time of the injury. Lacerated flexor tendons with the fingers in the flexed position are usually due to a laceration far distal to the point of the obvious skin wound, since the tendon has been pulled down into this

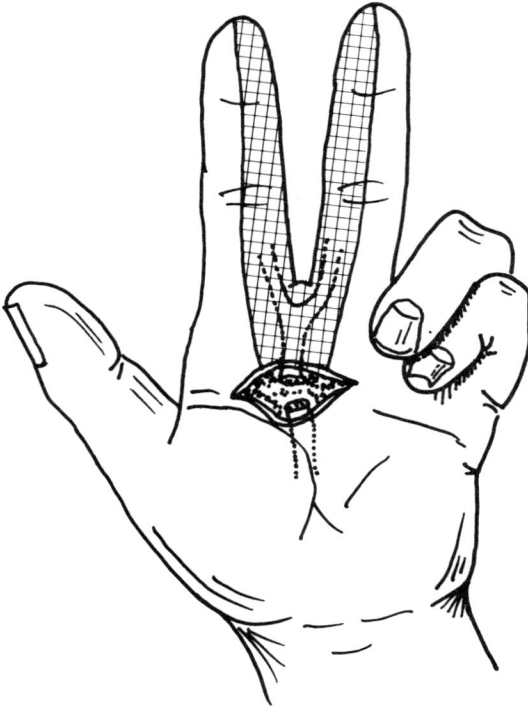

Fig. 11-10. Lacerations in the palm must always be suspect for injuries to the structures that pass through this area into the fingers. Caution should be given concerning the insertion of a local anesthetic agent into a wound without first evaluating the sensory status of the fingers distal to the wound, since it is impossible to tell whether a nerve is injured or not once the local anesthetic agent has been administered.

position in the flexed finger. By the same token, if the finger is cut while in extension the skin laceration will usually overlie the lacerated tendon. Both the profundus and the superficialis must be tested separately for function. Slight resistance should be placed against the finger as flexion occurs since partial lacerations will be apt to cause pain when stressed in this manner; uninjured tendons will not. The hand can be observed from a distance and usually evaluated as to whether both flexor tendons to any single finger are lacerated. With the hand lying at rest on its dorsum, all fingers are slightly flexed and a gradual "cascade" of position will be noted. The little finger will be more flexed than the ring and so forth over to the index finger. If, however, both flexor tendons have been lacerated at any level this particular finger will lie out straight while the rest of the fingers remain slightly flexed in a neutral position. By the same token, lacerations over the dorsum can better be evaluated by supporting the hand and asking the patient to extend all fingers simultaneously. Lacerated tendons, of course, will result in the inability of the patient to extend that particular finger in relationship to the others.

Likewise, it is important to remember that the long extensor to the thumb courses over from the midportion of the wrist around Lister's tubercle (palpable on the dorsum of the distal radius) and obliquely over to the thumb. Lacerations across the dorsum of the hand, even though they lie over far ulnar to the thumb, may result in a laceration of the long thumb extensor. The function of this tendon should always be included in routine examination.

Following observation of the hand and the evaluation of function in the tendons, the sensation distal to the laceration should be evaluated. Simple pinprick is usually a reliable gross test for sensation. To be certain that the patient understands the response expected, the examiner should first demonstrate the normal sensation over an obviously unaffected touchpad and allow him to compare this sensation to that over the area in question.

A special mention should be made of the laceration over the fifth metacarpal head sustained in the "clenched fist" injury (Fig. 11-11) resulting from one individual striking another with his closed fist and the hand becoming lacerated on a tooth. The laceration will be relatively small and the severity or seriousness of the situation may be unrecognized by the inexperienced examiner.

Since the extensor tendon is pulled forward with the fist clinched, a laceration that occurs through the skin, then through the tendon, the joint capsule, and into the joint, may be unrecognized with the finger extended since the

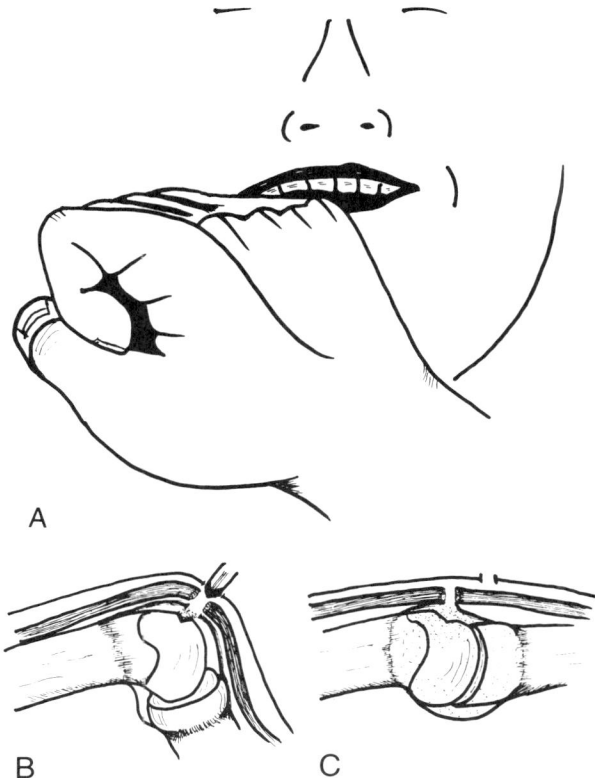

Fig. 11-11. (A) The clenched fist injury commonly results from the striking of one's hand (usually the fifth metacarpal head) against the tooth of another individual. **(B)** The importance of a thorough inspection of the wound. The tooth enters with the fist clenched and extends through the skin, tendon, and capsule and into the joint. **(C)** Once the finger is extended, the skin opening does not overlie the tendon and joint opening and thereby camouflages the entry into the joint with the finger extended. These wounds must be explored.

laceration of the tendon will not be apparent through the small skin opening. For this reason these wounds must be inspected much more carefully. The routine in most hand surgery services is that these injuries should be inspected through a larger incision.

The hand is exanguinated by wrapping it tightly with an elastic bandage and then a pneumatic tourniquet is inflated. A blood pressure cuff may be substituted for this since the procedure will not require any great length of time. The patient can usually tolerate a tourniquet around the extremity for the 30 minutes or so required to explore the wound without undue pain, particularly if he is given an intravenous narcotic injection before the tourniquet is applied. With bleeding controlled by the tourniquet, the wound can be thoroughly scrubbed and be lengthened slightly at each extremity so that the area may be inspected.

A good practice is to extend the wound several millimeters proximally on one end and several millimeters distally on the other end, resulting in a Z-type exposure. One can then be certain of whether the tendon has been violated. If an opening is found through the tendon, the patient should be taken to surgery where, under strict aseptic conditions and a regional anesthetic, the area can be completely exposed and the joint opened, cleaned of all debris, thoroughly lavaged, and a primary closure of the structures done. Only in this way can this joint be salvaged if an inoculation has been made into it with the types of organisms usually encountered in the mouth. If, on the other hand, no violation of the tendon or joint capsule can be demonstrated, the wound can be thoroughly cleansed, the two extensions closed, and the central portion packed open with a small gauze pack that can be removed in 24 hours to allow for complete wound healing. These patients can then be allowed to go home and use oral antibiotics but should be examined carefully at frequent intervals for the next several days to be certain that no evidence of infection is seen.

EVALUATION AND TREATMENT OF FRACTURES
(Fig. 11-12)

While most markedly displaced fractures will create enough deformity that their presence is easily determined by the examiner, many times fractures will have only minimal or no displacement. For this reason radiographs should be taken in most all injuries severe enough that a fracture may have resulted. Open fractures are those in which an open wound in the skin communicates with the fracture itself. These have in the past been called "compound" fractures but "open" is a more significant and realistic term and the one customarily used today. The implications of the open fracture are the same as in other parts of the body: that the fracture has been contaminated and care should be taken to be certain that it is completely clean before the wound is closed. Patients with open wounds are generally taken to the operating room where completely aseptic conditions can be created. The wound can be completely cleansed, debrided, and

Fig. 11-12. Composite description of general methods of treatment.

1. Fractures of the tuft or ungua are usually stellate. It is impossible to reduce them well in most instances, but splinting alone suffices.

2. Fractures in the waist of the distal phalanx can usually be reduced by closed methods. They are stable in extension.

3. Avulsion of the extensor insertion when containing only a small fleck of bone may be reduced by holding it in extension with a "Stack" splint. If the joint surface is disrupted, if the fragment constitutes over one-third of the joint surface, or if the joint is subluxated, open reduction must be done.

4. Fractures in the distal shaft past the level of insertion of the superficialis (5) can be reduced by closed manipulation and are stable in flexion.

6. Fractures proximal to the level of insertion of the superficialis (5) can usually be reduced by closed methods and are stable in extension.

7. Intraarticular fractures of either the base of the middle phalanx or of the condylar portion of the proximal phalanx if articular and displaced must be carefully reduced by open means and with internal fixation.

8. Fractures of the proximal phalanx, if transverse, may be stable and treated by immobilization alone. If not stable, internal fixation should be used so that early motion may be started.

9. Fractures in the midshaft of the proximal phalanx, if of a long spiral type, should be open and internal fixation done to maintain length and start on early motion. Fractures in this area that are badly comminuted should not be opened but should be reduced as well as possible and stabilized with percutaneous pins.

10. Fractures involving the joint surface of either the proximal phalanx or the metacarpal head if displaced with distortion of the surface should be open for anatomical reduction and internal fixation.

11. Fractures of the metacarpal neck if angulated may be difficult to hold, particularly in the fifth metacarpal. Percutaneous pinning is often necessary for stabilization and is usually adequate.

12. Shaft fractures of the metacarpal bones should be treated by open reduction if there is marked shortening, particularly with a long spiral fracture. If they are not displaced they may be treated by splinting alone. Metacarpal shaft fractures that are badly comminuted may need percutaneous pinning to maintain length.

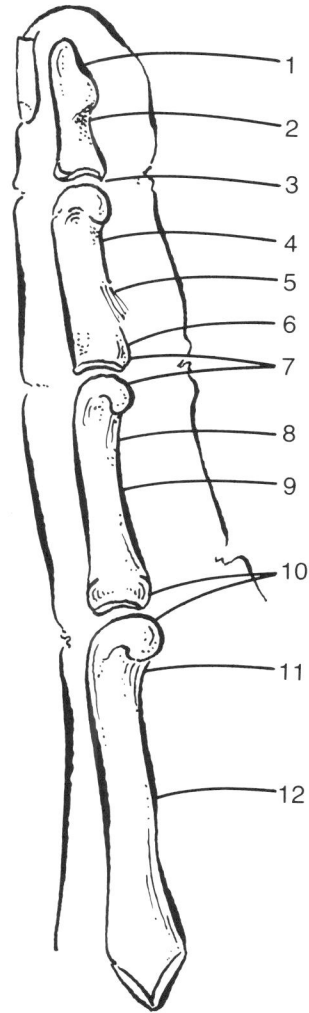

the fracture reduced manually. The use of internal fixation is open to question and probably should be left to the discretion of the orthopedic surgeon to whom the case is referred.

In cases where open fractures are to be treated by the primary care physician, be certain that a stable reduction has been obtained and adequate fixation established. Instability with motion at the fracture site is one of the greatest causes of failure of the fracture to heal and development of infections in the fracture site. Closed fractures may be successfully treated in the emergency setting. Many of these can be done under a regional block type of anesthesia

(Fig. 11-13). Care must be taken when splinting the fractures, after reduction has been obtained, since pressure areas in the finger caused by the fixation device are common. They can be avoided only by careful padding, careful fitting of the splint to the part, and careful attention to position of the part.

Distal Phalanx

Fractures of the distal phalanx are usually seen from crushing injuries and usually are markedly comminuted. Fractures of the distal phalanx almost always involve the nail bed since it normally lies directly on the bone. Nail hematomas, of course, should be evacuated either by using a hot paper clip to burn a hole through the nail at the point of the hematoma or by drilling with the sharp end of a #11 Bard-Parker blade. Drilling has been better in the hands of most surgeons since the size of the hole can be controlled and the opening can be made larger for better evacuation of the contained blood. If the nail has been disrupted it may be left in place. If it is completely loose, removal may be necessary. However, if a nail is removed a small splint should be placed underneath the ungual fold to keep it open so that a new nail may grow through. We find the foil package that contains suture to be ideal for creating a splint to go under the subungual fold. The foil can be folded so that the paint is not exposed and can be cut to slip easily under the subungual fold and maintain its patency. If difficulty is experienced in keeping it in the fold, a small mattress suture may be passed from a point 2mm proximal to the nail margin underneath the ungual fold through the splint and back. This can then be used to guide the splint underneath the fold and tied to hold it securely in place for the 2 or 3 days necessary to establish the patency of the ungual fold. If the nail bed has been split or lacerated it should be repaired with tiny 5-0 polyglycolic acid sutures on a very small cutting needle. To leave the nail bed open invites a deformity in the nail bed with subsequent nail deformity.

Comminuted fractures of the distal phalanx do not need to be reduced. Unless one of the comminuted fragments is extruded from the soft tissue no treatment is indicated other than simple splinting. Nonunion of some of these small fragments is common and has not been seen to be of any great importance in the average case. Occasionally a fracture will occur across the small waist of the distal phalanx that may remain dislocated. In the usual case this will cause considerable deformity and so these separations should be reduced. Once reduced, they are ordinarily quite stable since they are usually transverse.

Middle Phalanx

Fractures in the shaft of the middle phalanx ordinarily are not markedly displaced. There is ordinarily volar buckling at the fracture site caused by the pull of the superficialis insertion if the fracture occurs distal to this tendinous insertion. There is usually a dorsal buckling of the fracture if the fracture occurs proximal to the superficialis insertion, since the central slip mechanism will ordinarily angulate the proximal fragment dorsally. These fractures are usually

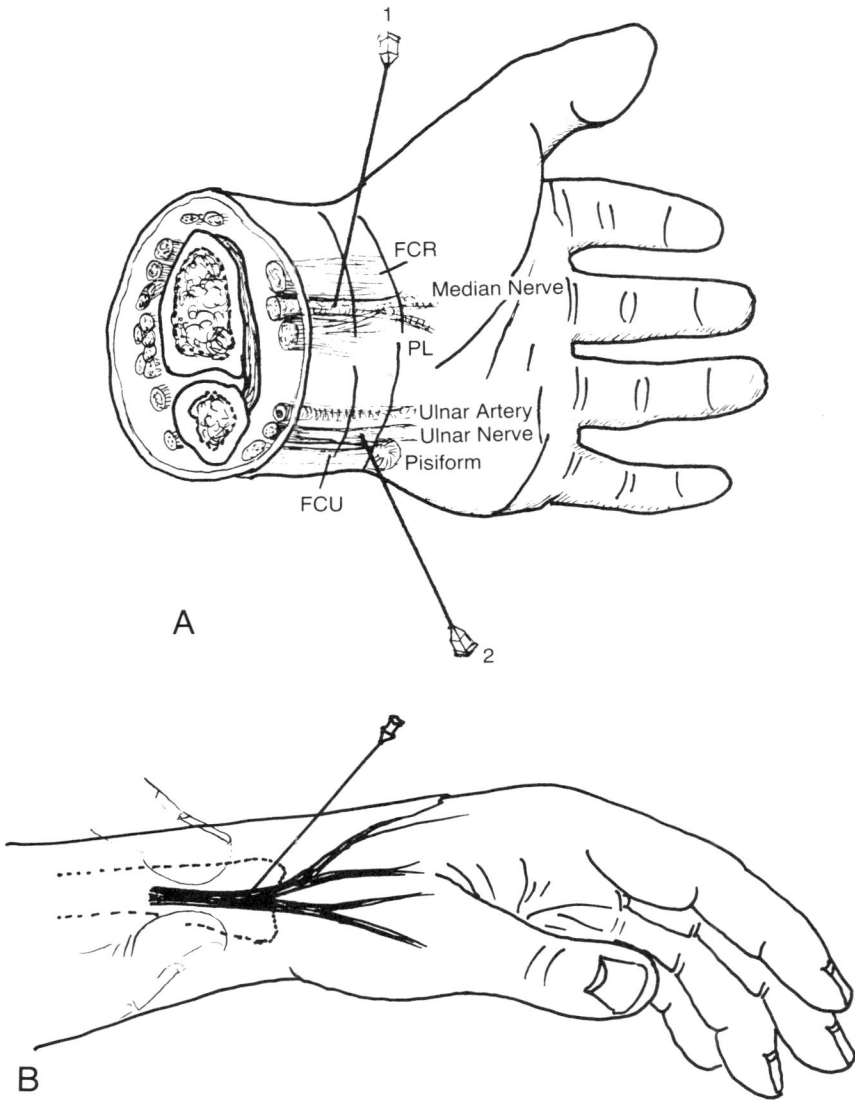

Fig. 11-13. (A) The appropriate side for injection of the median and ulnar nerves. (1) The median nerve lies between the tendons of the flexor carpi radialis and the palmaris longus. It lies only 5 to 8 mm deep to the skin margin, and the injection should be made about 1 cm proximal to the flexion crease of the wrist. The usual mistake is injecting too deeply after going through or around the nerve. (2) Injection of the ulnar nerve is shown at the level of the nerve's entrance into the hand. The nerve runs just underneath the flexor carpi ulnaris tendon alongside the ulnar artery, which can often be palpated. The nerve is relatively mobile as it lies underneath the tendon but becomes much more fixed as it passes underneath the margin of the pisiform bone, and injection in this area can usually be done easily with 2 or 3 ml of 1 percent lidocaine. **(B)** Injection of the superficial radial nerve should be done overlying the radial styloid. Careful palpation by rubbing the examining finger back and forth across the styloid will reveal its presence; the nerve can then be trapped between the thumb and index finger of the opposite hand, and in this position a very sharp short needle can be placed directly in the nerve for anesthetization with 1 or 2 ml of lidocaine. Paresthesia will be felt by the patient as the injection is made.

relatively easy to reduce under a local anesthetic. They are quite easy to maintain either in the slightly flexed position, if volar angulation is present, or in the more extended position, if dorsal angulation is present.

Proximal Phalanx

Fractures of the proximal phalanx constitute one of the really difficult fractures to treat since angulatory deformities are found so often and are usually so subtle that they occasionally go undetected. Fractures of the proximal phalanx often require open reduction.

Specific cases requiring open reduction are:

1. Intraarticular fractures involving one condyle or the other with rotation of the condyle.

2. Fractures at the base of the condyles with marked rotation of the condylar fragment (very common).

3. Long oblique fractures usually require open reduction since rotatory deformity is very difficult to control and shortening is likewise difficult to control in these fractures without internal fixation.

4. Fractures that are markedly comminuted usually will require internal fixation, perhaps with fixation pins.

5. Fractures that are markedly displaced require open reduction and internal fixation.

If there is any doubt about the adequacy of the reduction or the fixation when seen by the primary care physician, these cases should be referred to a hand surgeon or orthopedic surgeon familiar with the management of this type of fracture. In rare cases where reduction can be obtained and stability maintained, splinting should be done with the two adjacent fingers incorporated in the splint. Splinting in the mildly flexed position will usually be necessary to maintain position. There has been some increase in the tendency for hand surgeons to fix these fractures internally in the past several years since internal fixation allows for early motion and prevention of permanent stiffness in the associated joints. For this reason if there is any question in the mind of the examining physician these patients should be referred to the specialist for treatment.

Metacarpal Shaft

Special features of certain metacarpal bones requiring special treatment will be discussed in the next section. Fractures of the metacarpal shaft, however, are often unstable and may require internal fixation. As in the case of the proximal phalanges, there has been some increasing tendency in recent years for hand surgeons to fix metacarpal fractures internally so that early motion can be established and joint function maintained. This is particularly true of long oblique fractures, which almost invariably shorten, and for markedly angulated fractures. Except in the very simplest of these fractures with minimal or no disloca-tion, reduction and internal fixation should be considered. If there is any ques-tion, these patients should be referred to the specialist for this evaluation.

There is seldom any place in the current concept of fracture management in the hand for the use of traction. Traction, particularly in the case of metacarpal fractures, must be applied with the metacarpophalangeal joints in the extended position, which will invariably result in an extension deformity of these joints since the collateral ligaments become contracted in this position. Traction, there-fore, is generally ill-advised in fractures of the metacarpal bones. Instead, some type of internal fixation should be considered if there is difficulty in maintaining the position of these fractures.

Special Features

Some fractures that occur in the hand are unique in their features and require special consideration and special treatment.

Intraarticular Fractures

Intraarticular fractures usually require open reduction so that the joint sur-face can be reestablished and maintained. In the case of marked comminution, this is sometimes impossible. However, in most fractures with marked distortion of the joint surface an attempt should be made to reestablish the joint surface so that degenerative joint disease in a markedly distorted joint surface can be pre-vented. These fractures are complicated and usually require the services of one specialized in their care.

Bennett's Fractures

Bennett's fractures, require special treatment since they represent a special situation. The first metacarpal bone is maintained in its position with respect to the trapezium by means of a constraining ligament attached to its base on the internal side. This ligament, which extends from the adjacent bony structures to the base of the first metacarpal bone, maintains the base of the first metacarpal in its normal position. Bennett's fracture is the name given to a small intraarticular fracture in the base of the first metacarpal bone that occurs in a diagonal manner so that the ligamentous attachment is included with the small fragment. The base of the metacarpal bone is therefore left without its normal constraints. It then has a tendency to dislocate and there usually will be a separation of the fracture with a subluxation of the base and the body of the first metacarpal caused by the pull of the abductor that attaches to its base. These fractures are therefore considered to be extremely unstable and require pin fixation to main-tain position of the metacarpal–trapezium joint. Unless this fracture can be totally reduced easily and pin fixation established by the primary care physician, the patient should be referred to the specialist since this complicated type of fracture requires expert treatment.

Fifth Metacarpal Fracture

The so-called fifth metacarpal Bennett's is a similar fracture occurring at the base of the fifth metacarpal and its relationship to the base of the fourth metacarpal and the hamate bone. Fractures that involve the restraining ligament in the smaller fragment result in an instability of the fifth metacarpal in its joint with the hamate. Subluxation will usually occur, as with a true Bennett's. Patients with these fractures therefore also require adequate anatomical reduction with pin fixation to ensure healing and maintenance of function.

Boxer's Fractures

Boxer's fractures occur at the distal end of the fifth metacarpal bone and usually result from a direct blow of the closed fist against another object.

A mild amount of angulation (up to 25 or 30 degrees) may be tolerable and good function will be seen in the hand even if this amount of angulation is left and the fracture allowed to heal. However, if further angulation exists malunion will occur, with an abnormal deviation of the metacarpal head into the palm and a destruction of the mechanism of the metacarpophalangeal joint of the little finger. The badly angulated distal fragment results in a permanent hyperextension deformity of the joint of the little finger and disrupts the ligamentous support between the fourth and fifth metacarpal heads, as well as disrupting the mechanism of the intrinsic musculature that has action through this joint. There also occurs a painful prominence in the palm of the hand at the point of the fifth metacarpal head. This is particularly troublesome when grasping objects such as a hammer or the steering wheel of an automobile. For this reason, angulation of any great amount should be corrected and fixation established.

It is possible to manipulate these fractures under a local anesthetic, the main difficulty occurs in the stabilization. The old practice of applying some sort of splint that required pressure against the middle joint of the finger with the proximal and middle joints both flexed to 90 degrees, resulted in much damage to the middle joint and often in pressure sores over this area. This type of splint is not generally recommended. Unless the fracture position can be maintained by a splint that immobilizes the joint in flexion, but applies pressure mostly to the volar side of the fifth metacarpal head, consideration should be given to internal fixation by percutaneous pinning. This requires specialized ability and these patients should be referred if there is any question of whether the position can be maintained.

DISLOCATIONS OF THE INTERPHALANGEAL OR METACARPOPHALANGEAL JOINTS

Distal Joint

The distal joint is seldom dislocated. When it is, usually it is the result of violent trauma and is ordinarily associated with an open wound on the volar side of the finger. They are quite easily reduced and usually can be maintained by simple splinting. Of course, the usual precautions related to open wounds should be observed.

Middle Joint

Dislocation of the middle joint is probably the most common type seen in the hand and often results in functional loss even when treated expertly. Those that are improperly treated, however, almost always result in very serious functional loss due to pain and stiffness. Structures of the collateral ligaments and volar plate are such that it is almost impossible to dislocate this joint without tearing at least two or three structures, including the collateral ligament and volar plate mechanisms. Dislocations that occur when the distal joint surface dislocates dorsal to the condyles of the proximal phalanx may occur without disruption of supporting structures. Usually simple reduction, with splinting for 3 or 4 weeks in the flexed position, will suffice. In these instances a splint can be applied that blocks extension past about 30 degrees and the patient can be allowed to use the finger in the remaining degrees of flexion, even during the healing stages. The basic problem with dislocation in the middle joint occurs when the volar plate attachment to the volar lip of the middle phalangeal joint surface is disrupted. This results in a total instability of the joint, so that dorsal dislocation of the middle phalanx on the condyles of the proximal phalanx occurs and stability of the volar supporting structures is lost completely.

If a large amount of bone is avulsed and the joint surface is seriously distorted, these joints must have open reduction and internal fixation of the articular fragment. If the amount of bone avulsed is not great and the finger can be shown to be stable in flexion, it may be treated by immobilization using a splint holding it in at least 30 degrees of flexion and allowing use of the finger in the degrees of flexion past 30 degrees. Dislocations of the middle joint may occur if the condyles of the proximal phalanx rupture through the restraining ligaments and become entrapped between the ligaments and the associated tendinous structures. If reduction cannot be accomplished easily after anesthesia has been obtained by digital block, irreducible dislocation should be suspected and the patient promptly referred for an open reduction.

Proximal Joint

Proximal joint dislocations occur fairly often, particularly at the base of the thumb and the ligamentous structures, which may be torn so that repair will be necessary. This is particularly true if the ulnar collateral ligament has been torn, since this ligament is prone to dislocate into the joint, thereby blocking complete reduction and preventing healing of the ligament without surgical repair. If, after a reduction of the proximal phalanx of the thumb, one finds instability of the collateral ligaments the patient should be referred for evaluation by the specialist. The same is true for volar plate injuries resulting from hyperextension of this joint. These injuries can occasionally be treated by immobilization in flexion but usually require surgical repair of the volar plate to restore stability. Dislocations of the proximal joints of the fingers can be splinted after reduction has been obtained by taping to the adjacent fingers for 3 weeks to allow healing.

If symptoms persist in the finger following this stress, X-ray films should be taken to determine the presence of collateral ligament avulsion. Surgical reattachment probably will be necessary. If radiographs reveal the avulsion of small bony fragments near the proximal joints of the fingers, one can be certain that avulsion of the collateral ligament occurred along with its bony attachment. If separation of these fragments from the major bone is very great, surgical reattachment will be necessary. Irreducible dislocations of the proximal joints of the thumb and index finger are seen occasionally due to herniation of the metacarpal head through the ligamentous structures and tendon attachments. These should be suspected if reduction is not easy once anesthesia has been obtained. These cases should be referred to the specialist for open reduction. Even with open operation, considerable difficulty may be experienced in reducing the so-called complex dislocation seen particularly in these joints.

Tear of the ulnar collateral ligaments in the thumb has been described previously as the "gamekeeper's thumb." It is relatively common and occurs from a sudden strain on the proximal joint with a loss of integrity of the ligament. This is commonly seen in ski pole injuries, in which sudden force results in a disruption of the ulnar collateral ligament of the proximal joint. If a complete separation is suspected, stress films will demonstrate the laxity quite well. Even with an intact ligament it is possible for the base of the proximal phalanx to slide over laterally on the metacarpal head as stress is applied. However, if the ligament has been torn the side of the joint will open up like a book and can be easily identified. Care should be taken in obtaining stress films to flex the joint slightly to overcome the effect of the tight volar plate, if this still is intact.

Repair of these lesions is considered the primary choice. Data suggest that the ligament overlaps to lie within the joint occurs with some frequency. This so-called Stinner's lesion has been described as being a reason to proceed with surgical repair in all of these injuries. If no bony avulsion is seen, some surgeons feel justified in applying a gauntlet cast for immobilization for 6 weeks to determine whether healing might occur. If the laxity is found to persist in spite of this immobilization, surgical reconstruction is indicated. The investigators who believe that early open reduction is necessary usually find the ligament is torn from the bony attachment at the base of the proximal phalanx. Reattachment can be done relatively easily with excellent results. For this reason, most of these injuries should be referred to the specialist for open repair.

JOINT DEFORMITY AFTER INJURY

Several other joint deformities that fit into no real classification are relatively common and should be discussed here.

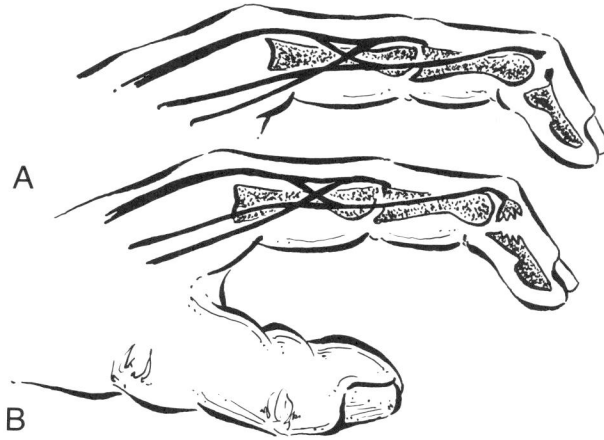

Fig. 11-14. Mallet finger deformities may be of two types. (**A**) Avulsion or laceration to the common extensor insertion, which allows the distal joint to drop forward into acute flexion because the distal phalanx is not stabilized by the effect of the extensor tendon. (**B**) A fracture through the distal phalanx, ordinarily intraarticular and resulting in an avulsion of the portion of bone to which the extensor insertion is made. This results in a flexion deformity of the distal phalanx because, again, the stabilizing effect of the extensor tendon is lost. Cases in which fractures exist often demonstrate subluxation of the remaining portion of the distal phalanx from its articulation with the middle phalanx. With release of the common extensor insertion distally, over-pull of the central slip mechanism at the middle joint will often result in recurvatum of this joint, causing the so-called Swan neck deformity.

Avulsion of the Extensor Insertion

Avulsion of the extensor insertion at the distal joint results in the so-called mallet finger deformity (Fig. 11-14). Acute hyperflexion of the distal joint occurs often with a compensatory recurvatum at the middle joint to give the so-called swan neck deformity. These are quite often associated with an interarticular fracture avulsion of the bony attachment occurring along with the detached tendon. Many times, however, the radiographs will be found to be completely normal. When no x-ray changes are seen and the deformity results from a simple rupture of the extensor tendon the patient can be treated with splinting, with an extremely high percentage chance of reattachment and no need for surgical intervention.

The commonly used splint that seems to be most applicable today is the Stack splint. This small plastic splint gives excellent forceful maintenance of the distal joint in complete extension and will allow for healing in most cases.

The general routine is to apply the splint as soon as possible after the injury and have the patient wear it continuously, without allowing the joint to drop, for 3 weeks. The patient is then examined, the splint gently removed, and the possibility of reattachment assessed. In most instances one can see that the attachment of the tendon is underway and that some stability has been restored.

If so, an additional 3 weeks are allowed for complete healing and then the splint is removed permanently. If, at the 3 week period, no evidence of reattachment has occurred, the patient should be referred for surgical repair. Likewise, if after 6 weeks significant deformity recurs after the splint has been removed, the patient should be referred for surgical repair.

Mallet Finger Deformity

Mallet finger deformity is rather disabling and most people are not happy with leaving it untreated (Fig. 11-14). For this reason every effort should be made to correct the deformity, either by nonoperative or operative means. If a small segment of bone is detached and can be reduced by closed reduction and splinting with a Stack splint established, healing should occur without difficulty. If there is marked displacement of the bony fragment that does not reduce, or if the bony fragment constitutes a considerable portion of the articular surface and is not anatomically reduced, consideration should be given to an open reduction and internal fixation with a Kirschner wire. Stabilization of the distal joint in extension with an intramedullary Kirschner wire usually should be carried out for 6 weeks. If, however, there is any question, these patients should be referred to the hand surgeon or orthopedic surgeon for evaluation and treatment.

Boutonniere Deformity

Boutonniere deformity occurs when there is detachment of the central slip mechanism so that active extension of the middle joint of the finger is not possible. This is seen after lacerations through the area but may often occur from simple rupture due to trauma. This deformity will also frequently be seen as a result of rheumatoid involvement of the joint with disruption of the ligament by invasion with rheumatoid pannus. The term boutonniere (French for "button-hole") signifies the major pathology present. With the disruption of the central slip attachment to the base of the proximal phalanx, an opening in the extensor hood allows for a volar migration of the lateral slips on either side (Fig. 11-15). This results in a "buttonholing" of the joint through this opening in the hood.

When seen early and when there is no evidence of severe rheumatoid destruction these patients can be treated satisfactorily by splinting. The middle joint should be splinted in 0 degrees of extension with motion allowed at the proximal joint and the distal joint left free to allow flexion and extension. If the splint extends out to the distal joint but does not include it, the patient is likely to be able to flex and extend this joint, which has the effect of moving the lateral slips back up into their normal relationship. The splint must be maintained for 6 weeks. If healing does not occur during that time consideration should be given to surgical repair. Likewise, in cases of lacerations across this level with sectioning of the central slip, or in rheumatoid disease with disruption of the slip from

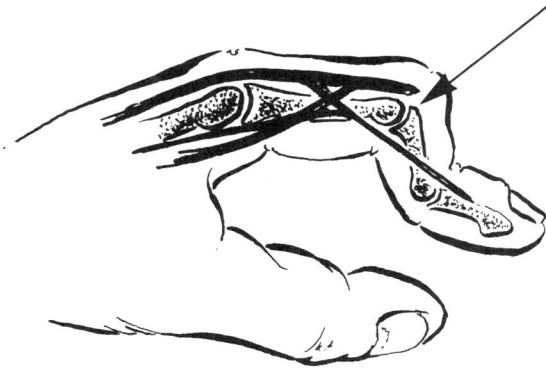

Fig. 11-15. The boutonniere deformity results from a loss of the function of the central slip mechanism in maintaining extension of the middle joint. This joint becomes hyperflexed by an unrestrained action of the flexors so that a hyperflexion deformity of the middle joint occurs. The lateral slips of the extensor hood then are allowed to migrate down on either side as the middle joint pokes through a "button hole" in the extensor hood, resulting in a hyperextension deformity of the distal joint and the typical deformity.

rheumatoid destruction, the patient should be referred to the hand surgeon for repair.

DUPUYTREN'S CONTRACTURE

This strange condition that results in a proliferative reaction occurring in the palmar fascia with resulting formation of contracting bands has no known cause. The process starts as a tiny mass in the palmar fascia that is quite tender. This is considered the "florid" stage in which early proliferation is occurring. Treatment at this point is not particularly necessary and surgical excision is contraindicated since this sometimes will provoke a massive fibrositic response with marked damage to the hand. As time goes on the mass will gradually lose its tenderness but formation of the contracting band can be seen. The involved finger is ultimately drawn into the palm with flexion contractures at the proximal and distal joints of the finger. Eighty-five percent of the contractures occur in the ring and little fingers and 15 percent in the remainder of the hand, the majority of these occurring in the region of the base of the thumb. The condition has a marked predilection for males (9 : 1 ratio) and has a strong familial tendency, though no direct hereditary features have been proven.

Most hand surgeons believe that splinting is of very little value since the contracture tends to progress at its own rate almost regardless of any type of conservative management. Most likewise do not think that the contracting bands should be excised until the patient begins to lose extension in the proximal or middle joints. If this does occur and the loss of motion has reached perhaps 10 degrees, the patient should be referred for surgical excision. Contracture should not be allowed to progress to a marked deformity since in these instances joint contractures accompany the contracting band and are difficult to correct by any type of surgery. In the case of the florid nodule small dose of x-ray therapy (600 or 800 rads) usually stop the pain and swelling and perhaps inhibit growth. Likewise, systemic steroid administration over 3 weeks in gradual diminishing oral dosage will often curtail the acute inflammatory response in these small nodules. Other types of medication are considered of little value in the treatment of either the acute florid or the later contracting stages.

STENOSING TENOSYNOVITIS

Stenosing tenosynovitis in the flexor canals usually has a predilection for the thumb and the middle or ring fingers and is usually related to the formation of a nodule in the flexor tendon with a reactive band forming in the flexor canal. The mass then becomes caught behind the stenotic band, resulting in locking of the finger. In the fingers, locking usually occurs from a stenosis at the A1 pulley level. Likewise, in locking of the thumb the stenotic band usually occurs at the base of the thumb in the region of the A1 pulley. In instances of tenosynovitis involving the digits, injections of steroids into the canal early (before locking occurs), will many times reduce the progress of the disease and the patient may be able to get by for some time on conservative management. If, however, incapacitating, locking has occurred, the patient should be referred to the hand surgeon for section of the tendon sheath and resection of the stenotic band, usually including the A1 pulley.

A variant of the stenosing tenosynovitis in the hand occurs in de Quervain's canal at the radial styloid. This small fibroosseous canal contains the tendon of the extensor pollicis brevis and the abductor pollicis longus. The abductor tendon quite often is duplicated several times: as many as three or four long abductors may lie in the canal along with the single extensor brevis tendon (which is usually not reduplicated). The symptoms are usually rather nondescript but the pain can be quite severe at times and is located over the radial styloid area. The pathognomonic indication is Finkelstein's test, which consists of holding the thumb in the clinched fist with the fingers so that it is acutely flexed (see Fig. 10-6). In this position the hand is suddenly forceably deviated to the ulnar side, thus pulling the abductor and extensor tendons through de Quervain's canal. If the inflammatory reaction exists in this canal with binding of the tendon the patient will experience an acute pain. Absence of this pain on Finkelstein's test almost eliminates the possibility of pain related to a de Quervain's stenosing tenosynovitis.

Early treatment consists of injection of methylprednisolone into the canal, usually 40 mg diluted in a small amount of local anesthetic (see Ch. 17). This, accompanied by splinting, application of heat, and nonsteroidal anti-inflammatory agents orally, will sometimes give indefinite relief. For those who do not respond to this treatment, or who respond but then relapse in a relatively short period of time, surgical unroofing of de Quervain's canal is indicated and the patient should be referred to the hand surgeon for consideration of surgery.

MEDIAN NERVE COMPRESSION: CARPAL TUNNEL SYNDROME

Median nerve compression in the wrist, or the so-called carpal tunnel syndrome, is a relatively common condition wherein the median nerve becomes compressed in the volar canal at the wrist to create symptoms of motor or sensory deficit or both. Other symptoms are usually pain the the area and sometimes hypesthesia over the distribution of the median nerve. It is the author's opinion that carpal tunnel syndrome is probably a misnomer, since the compression will almost invariably be found to occur at the level of the transverse palmar ligament, which either occurs as a separate structure distal to the volar carpal ligament or certainly occurs at its distalmost margin.

The condition occurs often in pregnancy due to swelling in the volar canal. In other instances, it is related to any condition that increases the volume of the canal with compression of the nerve. Rheumatoid disease, chronic mechanical irritation of the flexor tendons from overuse, and various other causes can be seen.

The patient will quite often have a positive Tinel's sign over the volar canal, which can be elicited by thumping the area with the middle finger. Tinel's sign is most likely to be in the base of the palm at the distal portion of the canal or up above the flexion crease of the wrist, above the upper margin of the volar carpal ligament. Various amounts of diminution of sensory acuity may be seen by pinprick and there is quite often weakness in the thenar musculature. Occasionally atrophy will be quite pronounced in these cases, usually on the radial side of the thenar mass at the location of the abductor pollicis brevis. Phalen's test, which is elicited by allowing the wrist to fall limply into acute flexion and holding it in this position for 1 minute to reproduce the symptoms of numbness and tingling in the fingers, will often be positive but is by no means pathognomonic of median nerve compression at the wrist.

Nonoperative treatment consists of injection of steroids into the volar canal, usually 40 mg diluted in a quantity of local anesthetic solution. Caution must be exercised to avoid injecting the steroid directly into the nerve. Oral anti-inflammatory medication may be given. A volar splint to maintain immobilization of the wrist and the application of heat will be of some benefit. If the patient does not respond to conservative management or response is later followed by exacerbation of the symptoms, surgical decompression of the nerve in the volar canal should be considered and the patient be referred to the hand surgeon. The results of surgery, even in long-standing cases with some apparent nerve damage, are excellent. The patient can be expected to be relieved of a considerable amount of his pain and most likely experience a prompt return of sensibility in the touch pads of the fingers and thumb.

MASSES

Masses in the hand are not common. When they do occur they usually represent manifestations of a relatively small number of conditions.

Synovial (Ganglion) Cysts

Synovial cysts on the dorsum of the wrist are extremely common and are evidence of cystic degeneration of the dorsal wrist joint capsule with maturation of the cyst and communication of the cyst with the wrist joint. These cysts are characterized by rapid growth in some occasions only to be followed by sudden diminution in size without known cause. These usually represent the leakage of joint fluid in and out of the associated wrist joint through the pedicle stalk by which they are ordinarily connected.

Multilocular cysts depend upon the simultaneous maturation of multiple small capsular cysts and denote a greater amount of capsular disease that may require a more extensive operative procedure than simple excision.

If synovial cysts are to be removed surgically the procedure should be done in the operating room under tourniquet control of bleeding. Regional anesthesia with an axillary block will suffice though general anesthetic is quite satisfactory. If the procedure is done under tourniquet control, one should be able to follow a pedicle down to the joint capsule so that a segment of capsule may be removed at the point of attachment of the pedicle. The capsular defect should then be prepared and the wrist held in a volar splint postoperatively to maintain a mild extension for up to 6 weeks, depending upon circumstances. Since these cysts are not harmful and are not likely to cause any damage to the joint, surgical excision is left to the discretion of the patient in most instances. Surgical resection is recommended only if the cyst grows large enough to become unsightly or causes pain of any magnitude.

Synovial cysts also occur quite frequently on the volar side of the wrist and in these instances usually arise either from the synovium of the tendon sheath of the flexor carpi radialis tendon or from the underlying carpal joint capsule. These cysts are quite intimately involved with and often adherent to the radial artery that passes in the region. Though these cysts are relatively small they are apt to be quite painful and are usually excised.

The decision to excise or not is usually left up to the patient. If cysts are to be excised, this should be done in the operating room under tourniquet control. Excision should only be attempted by one well versed in the anatomy of the area since damage to the radial artery can easily occur because of the close proximity.

Synovial cysts often occur in the flexor tendon sheath at the base of the fingers. These are very tiny, not much larger than a "BB" shot. They are quite hard and are often seen on either side of the volar base of the finger, so digital nerve compression or irritation may cause some of the painful symptoms. Even though they are extremely small, they are apt to be quite painful because of their location. The patient tends to put pressure on them by using the hand.

For this reason surgical excision is often indicated. It should be done in the operating room under a general or a regional anesthetic and removal should be attempted only by one experienced in surgery of this region. It will most likely be necessary to dissect out the digital nerve on this side and hold it out of harm's way while the cyst is removed along with a small plug of the flexor pulley from which it arises. Ordinarily, recovery is almost certain and quite rapid.

Giant Cell Tumor

Other types of tumors are seen with some frequency in the hand but probably the next most common tumor is the giant cell tumor of tendon sheath origin or the so-called xanthoma. These tumors are usually hard, may be multilocular, and usually occur only on the digits and much more frequently on the flexor than the extensor side of the finger. Diagnosis is ordinarily made by the pathologist after excision, but the lesion is often suspected because of the location. These tumors may become quite large, making excision difficult. Excision, when it is done, should be accomplished in the operating room under aseptic conditions and with tourniquet control of bleeding. Either regional or general anesthetic is required. The procedure should be done only by one experienced in surgery of this area.

Malignant Tumors

Malignant tumors of the hand are uncommon but when they do occur they are usually quite dramatic, with a gradually increasing mass that is very painful and often demonstrates inflammatory signs.

It is not within the scope of this chapter to discuss all of the possible tumors that can be seen. If there is any doubt about the identity of the tumor, the patient should be referred for evaluation and treatment by the hand surgeon.

INFECTIONS

Infections of the hand occur as localized entities or may result in widespread extension though synovial-lined cysts and along recognized pathways.

Paronychia

The most common infection in the hand is most likely the "run around" or paronychia (Fig. 11-16). These infections occur around the margin of the nail and involve the ungual fold. They should be treated rather aggressively since delay can cause rapid extension of the abscess to surround the nail margin completely and often damage to the matrix can occur with permanent damage to the nail formation. Other than antibiotics and general supportive measures, treatment consists of surgically incising the area of pus formation. If it has become quite extensive and seems to lie underneath the ungual margin and nail, radical excision of the nail is mandatory. The abscess in the area of the matrix should be opened with packing to allow for subsequent healing. If treated early and aggressively, these infections can be brought under control quite readily.

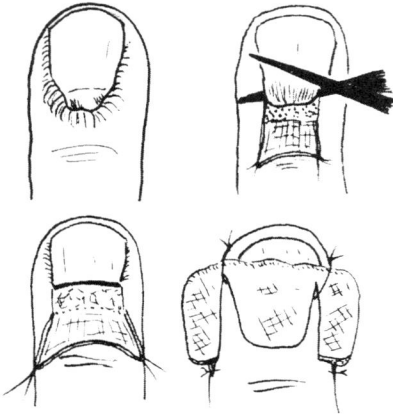

Fig. 11-16. Draining an extensive paronychia usually must include excision of the proximal portion of the nail. A skin flap is created to allow for debridement of infected material, and then the skin margins are sutured back over a pack that is left in to maintain drainage. The nail matrix is exposed but will usually form a new nail if not destroyed by the infectious process itself. (Lewis RC, Jr: Infections of the hand. Symposium on Treatment of Hand Emergencies. Emergency Medicine Clinics of North America 3(2):263, 1985. Reprinted with permission from W. B. Saunders Co.)

Closed Space Infection

Another type of specialized infection is the anterior closed space infection or "bone felon" (Fig. 11-17). These infections occur in the pulp of the finger and are particularly resistant to treatment because they are in the area occupied by multiple small fibrous tissue septa that extend from the volar aspect of the distal phalanx out to the skin. These septa contain fatty material. Once an infection occurs within them a closed space infection occurs and pain can be extreme because of the build-up of pressure. The pressure will result in loss of blood supply to the area and destruction of bone from this pressure may be seen in untreated cases.

Surgical drainage of closed space infections should be done by incision through the lateral margins of the touchpad up near the margin of the nail. The so-called fish mouth incision is unnecessary and results in a considerable amount of residual scarring and loss of sensation. Simple drainage through a lateral incision is usually all that is necessary, provided the incision includes all the fibrous tissue septa so that evacuation of the closed space infections may occur when the drainage is established. Packing of the wound with subsequent changes of pack and filling in by granulation usually results in a permanent cure without significant residual disability.

Tendon Sheath Infections

Tendon sheath infections may become quite severe. They usually are initiated by a puncture wound, though they may occur without known cause. The infection rapidly travels down the synovial-lined sheaths, which have very little inherent resistance to infection and will rapidly extend the entire length of the

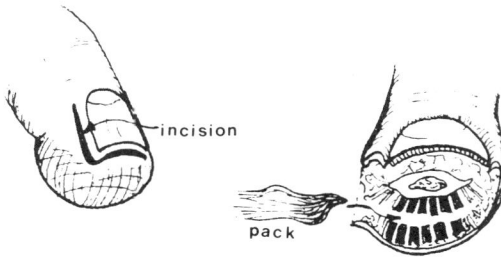

Fig. 11-17. Incision necessary for drainage of an anterior closed infection (the bone felon). The incision must extend across all of the fibrous tissue septa present in the pulp of the finger in order to secure adequate drainage. The "hockey stick" incision shown is much preferable to the old "fish mouth" incision. (Lewis RC, Jr: Infections of the hand. Symposium on Treatment of Hand Emergencies. Emergency Medicine Clinics of North America 3(2):263, 1985. Reprinted with permission from W. B. Saunders Co.)

finger. From this point they may extend down into the midpalmar or thenar spaces in the central portion of the hand where they will result in abscess formation even in the face of massive antibiotic therapy (Figs. 11-18 and 11-19). When the acute suppurative tenosynovitis is suspected, the patient should be promptly referred to the hand surgeon for expert care since surgery of these

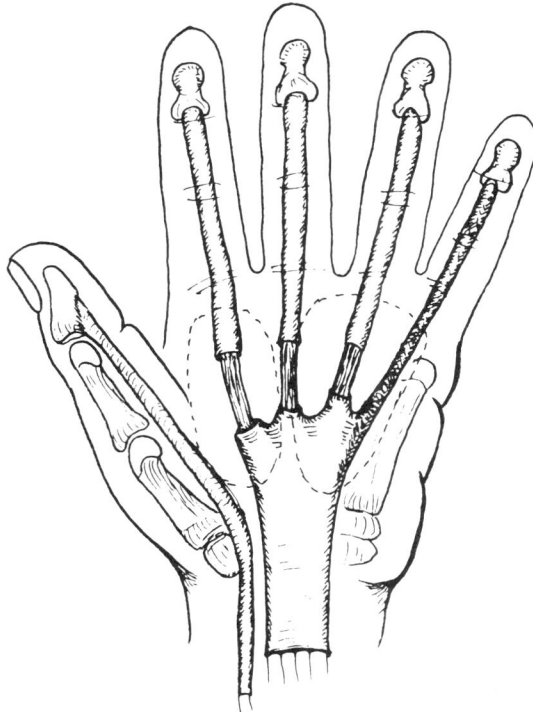

Fig. 11-18. The tendon sheaths and their extensions are shown, indicating that the sheath of the flexor pollicis is not connected to the midpalmar sheath. Flexor sheaths of the index, middle, and ring fingers stop at the base of the finger, whereas the sheath of the little finger extends down into the volar canal. (Lewis RC, Jr: Infections of the hand. Symposium on Treatment of Hand Emergencies. Emergency Medicine Clinics of North America 3(2):263, 1985. Reprinted with permission from W. B. Saunders Co.)

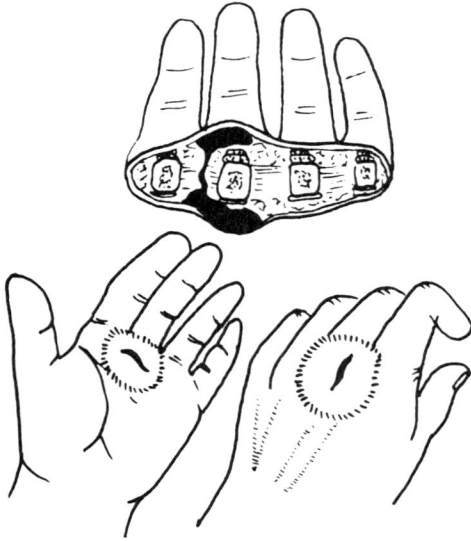

Fig. 11-19. Infections on either the volar or dorsal aspect of the hand extend through the hand and create the so-called collar button abscess. (Lewis RC, Jr: Infections of the hand. Symposium on Treatment of Hand Emergencies. Emergency Medicine Clinics of North America 3(2):263, 1985. Reprinted with permission from W. B. Saunders Co.)

conditions may be extremely complicated and difficult. Continued conservative management by the primary care physician is indicated only if the condition does not appear to be progressing and if heat, elevation, and antibiotic therapy can be seen to be effecting improvement.

Human Bite

Human bite infections constitute the particularly dangerous type of infection because of the nature of the infecting organisms. Human bites usually have a relatively high crush ratio because of the "pinching" type of injury. The devitalized tissue within the wound supplies an excellent pabulum that supports bacterial growth quite rapidly. Along with this, many of the organisms in the mouth have anaerobic characteristics. These organisms in a closed space such as a human bite with only a small puncture wound renders an excellent incubator for subsequent growth of bacteria and establishment of infection. Human bite infections should be left open for drainage. If a closed infection occurs, incision and drainage should be done early with debridement and packing of the wound. Treatment of the clinched fist injury of the fifth metacarpal has been discussed earlier (Fig. 11-11).

ARTHRITIS

Arthritis of the hand occurs with great frequency and is related to either the wearing out of joints with development of degenerative joint disease or the joint manifestations accompanying rheumatoid disease. The joints of predilection with degenerative disease are those at the first metacarpal–trapezium articulation and usually involvement of the distal joints is seen with about the same frequency. The middle joints of the finger are involved with somewhat less frequency while the proximal joints are seldom involved.

The disease is slowly progressive. Particularly at the carpometacarpal joint at the base of the thumb, gradual subluxation of the joint may occur from disruption of the restraining ligament and pull of the abductor muscle on the base of the metacarpal. The changes seen in the distal joints are first manifestations of osteophyte formation with the creation of Heberden's nodules. Ultimately complete destruction of the joint surface may occur, with angular deformities being common.

Injection of these joints with methylprednisolone has little place in treatment. For the most part, these patients are treated with supportive measures and systemic nonsteroidal anti-inflammatory medication. A great amount of relief of extensive degenerative changes in the hands can be obtained by paraffin baths. While they are possible at home, they are hazardous since the temperature cannot be well controlled. Unless absolutely necessary homemade paraffin baths are not recommended. Surgical supply houses in most locations, rent thermostatically controlled paraffin baths. The bath is usually set at 127°F and is quite safe if maintained at this level. Paraffin baths consist of the repeated dipping of the entire hand in the hot paraffin with withdrawal to allow the paraffin to solidify and form a "glove." By dipping the hand repeatedly eight or ten times a glove of perhaps one-fourth inch in thickness can be formed. Once this has been done the hand can be wrapped in a towel and allowed to stay in the solidified paraffin for 10 or 15 minutes. The paraffin can then be peeled off and dropped back into the bath to remelt. The hand will then seem to be quite red, soft, and pliable and most of the stiff joints can be stretched quite readily to improve motion. Though these units can be rented, patients with significant and widespread changes in the hand do well to consider purchase of these units for long term use since they are relatively inexpensive and quite effective.

Rheumatoid arthritis has a completely different appearance in the hand with involvement of the proximal joints and middle joints of the fingers. Involvement of the distal interphalangeal joint being relatively uncommon. Involvement of the first metacarpal–trapezium joint of the thumb is extremely common and subluxation occurs relatively early in rheumatoid disease. Likewise, involvement of the proximal joint of the thumb is common with the resulting loss of stability and the so-called "90–90" deformity is characteristic of the rheumatoid involvement of the thumb. In this deformity the proximal joint is flexed to near 90 degrees with a 90 degree hyperextension deformity of the distal joint. These deformities become quite fixed and, of course, the thumb is relatively useless with this type of deformity.

The characteristic changes in the hand in rheumatoid disease are swelling and gradual volar subluxation of the proximal joints of the fingers and gradual ulnar drift as the extensor tendons migrate over into the ulnar groove. This results in a loss of active extension of the proximal joints and adds greatly to the amount of functional disability in the hand. Changes in the wrist are often seen in association with the hand changes and destruction of the wrist may be a very significant part of the ultimate deformity.

The reader is referred to textbooks dealing with this subject exclusively for more detailed description of the deformities and treatment possibilities (see Suggested Readings). Splinting will be appropriate and helpful during the course of the disease but it must be expertly done. If there is any question, the patient should be referred to the hand surgeon relatively early in the course of the disease so that treatment may be started early and perhaps some of the deformity prevented. Injections of hydrocortisone into the rheumatoid joints are usually not indicated except in very acute exacerbations of the disease in a single joint. The steroid will cause a cessation of the acute reaction but will generally have no long-term effects. The general supportive measures used in all types of joint disease are equally applicable in the joints involved with rheumatoid disease.

12

THE HIP

GENERAL FEATURES

While the hip is one of the most stable joints in the body, being basically a complete ball and socket-type joint, its mechanical integrity depends upon an adequate fit of the ball within the socket. (Fig. 12-1) Since the weight-bearing surface is uniquely small, the hip joint is the site of many mechanical difficulties.

The weight-bearing line through the femur from the knee is relatively straight underneath the hip joint. The skeletal arrangement is such that the femur extends upward and inward slightly through the base of the neck, which usually subtends an angle of near 127 to 130 degrees as it extends medially and transfers the load-bearing of the skeleton over to the relatively small femoral head. This results in the need for tremendous load-bearing for a relatively small square area of joint space.

Articulation between the superior aspect of the head and the roof of the acetabulum usually takes up not more than 4 cm^2. When one considers that in each step the entire body weight is transmitted through this relatively small area, one can see that the mechanical stresses on the hip joint are tremendous. Nevertheless, it is surprising that the hip joint works extremely well and that it experiences difficulty only in relatively rare cases.

Conditions affecting the hip joint will be classified here into those occurring during childhood and those involving adults. The common conditions that often are perplexing from the standpoint of both recognition and management, rather than the many rare conditions involving the hip, will be discussed.

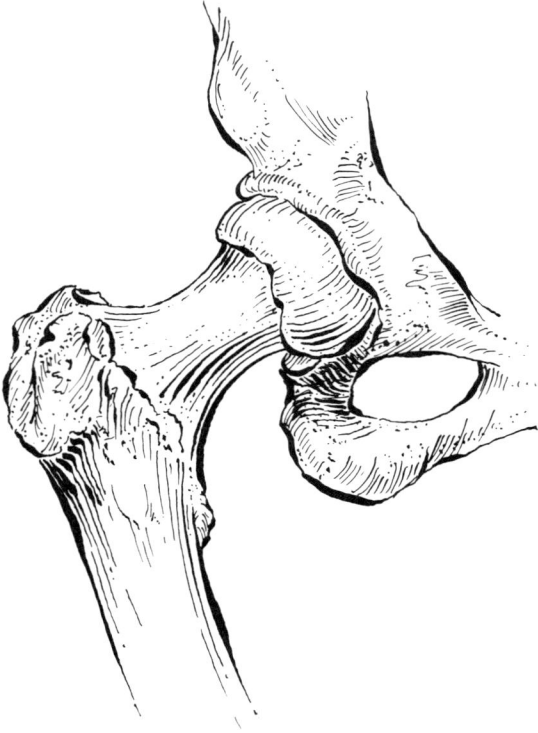

Fig. 12-1. Basic configuration of the hip joint.

CHILDHOOD DISORDERS

The developing hip joint may progress completely through maturation and ossification of the various incorporated bones without difficulty (Fig. 12-2). However, in some instances a deficiency in development occurs and in others the early development is normal but diseases of the synovium of the joint, affectations of the epiphysis itself, or sometimes complete separation and dislocation of the capital femoral epiphysis occurs. These are the concern of the primary care physician.

Congenital Hip Dysplasia

Congenital hip dysplasia is much more common than has been previously suspected principally because many of the early cases were not identified, particularly when the dysplasia was not great. Since the primary care physician is likely to deliver these children and proceed to examine them, it is his responsibility to recognize faulty development of the hip joint in the newborn.

The newborn should be examined as soon as practical after birth. As part of the examination of the skeleton the baby should be placed on its back with the hips and knees both flexed at 90 degrees and an attempt made to abduct widely the two legs simultaneously. In the newborn one can often approximate the

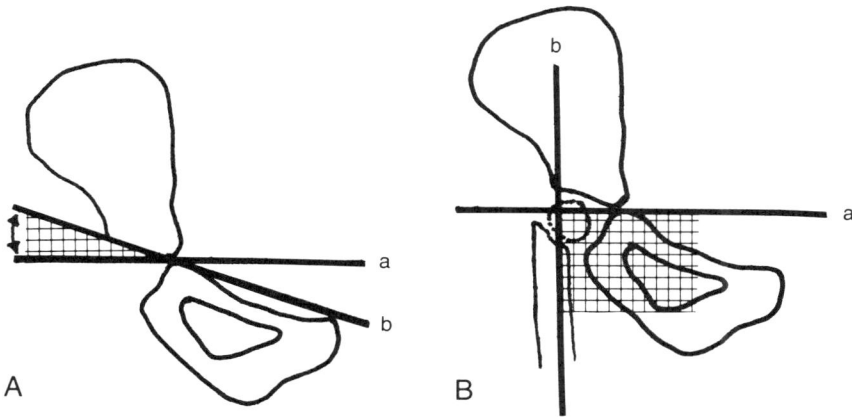

Fig. 12-2. (A) The method of measuring the acetabular index. Line *a* is drawn horizontal to the "Y" cartilage on both sides, usually resting upon the innominate portion of the stem of the "Y" cartilage. The second line (*b*) is then drawn along the roof of the acetabulum to cross the horizontal line at the "Y" cartilage stem. The angle thus created is measured and expressed in degrees. **(B)** The same horizontal line is drawn as described in (*a*) and a second line is drawn directly perpendicular to it from the lateral lip of the acetabulum. The majority of the femoral head epiphysis must then lie in the inner lower quadrant. If it lies elsewhere, abnormal hip positions should be suspected. If the epiphysis for the femoral head has not yet calcified its position should be visualized and perhaps drawn out on the x-ray film with the same implications as above.

lower extremities on either side with the top of the examining table. In other instances the hip may be slightly tight but in all cases the abduction should be near complete on both sides.

Marked loss of capacity for abduction on one side should be immediately evident, and the asymmetry if nothing else should catch the examiner's eye. Identification is much more difficult when there is a bilateral dysplasia since the lack of abduction is likely to be equal bilaterally. The asymmetry is therefore not present so that the symmetrical loss of abduction is taken to be normal. If there is a possible loss of abduction, either unilateral or bilateral, the evaluation should include x-ray examination. The hip that is completely dislocated will usually not pose as many problems as the simple dysplastic hip. The dislocated hip will have a pistoning effect when the infant is examined lying flat on the back with the hip and leg in abduction. When intermittent traction and compression are applied to the hip one can feel the hip dislocating in and out of the acetabulum. These individuals, however, still have markedly limited abduction and this is probably the most reliable sign.

The other sign that is of some value in the unilaterally dysplastic hip is unequal or asymmetrical gluteal creases visible when the infant is lying prone on the examining table. While some normal individuals have asymmetrical gluteal creases, this asymmetry in the newborn should raise considerable suspicion as to the integrity of the hips. It should at least warrant further evaluation, probably an x-ray examination, to be certain that its acetabular development is normal.

While many other signs have been described for detecting dysplasia and dislocation of the hip in the newborn, those listed here will most often identify the child with faulty hip development. Most likely, failure to examine the child's hips is responsible for the failure to diagnose a dysplastic hip.

X-ray examination requires two films. One film should be taken in the anteroposterior (AP) view with the legs completely straightened down from the trunk and patellae as near forward as possible. The second is the so-called frog-leg view, in which the hips and knees are both flexed at 90 degrees with the child lying on its back; the hips are then abducted as far as possible. This gives a relatively clear view on the lateral architecture on the neck of the hip and of its relationship to the long axis of the shaft of the femur.

For the primary care physician who must interpret his own films the most reliable information probably can be obtained from the first view of the pelvis in the AP plane with the legs straight down from the trunk. It is necessary on this film to determine the acetabular index in order to determine the integrity of the acetabular roof. To do this a horizontal line is first drawn through the "Y" cartilage. It will probably be easier to use as a landmark on either side—the superior extension of the ischium in the underside of the defect for the acetabular cartilage. This is easily indentifiable and usually does not vary much with varying degrees of difference in position. A second line is then drawn to correspond with the inclination of the acetabular roof. The landmarks here are the prominences at the acetabular rim and at the intermost aspect of the acetabulum. A line connecting these two points will then transect the horizontal line and create an angle that can be measured: the "acetabular index" (Fig. 12-2A.) In a newborn the acetabular index should not be greater than 30 degrees and in most instances it will be found to be actually between 25 and 30 degrees. If the index is greater than 30 degrees, the hip can be considered dysplastic and treatment should be given.

As the child grows, the acetabular index normally decreases slightly. In an infant between 3 and 6 months an acetabular index over 25 to 28 degrees should be considered excessive.

X-ray evidence of complete dislocation is easy to identify when it is unilateral because of the obvious asymmetry. When the dislocation is bilateral it is somewhat harder to identify. One should visualize the approximate location of the normal femoral head (which is not seen on the x-ray of the newborn since it is still cartilaginous) and in most instances it may even be better to trace the outline of the position of the head with a wax pencil. This will help the examiner to decide whether or not this head is situated under the acetabular roof.

A third line can be drawn along with the two used to measure the acetabular index, which may help identify locations without a great amount of displacement. It should be exactly perpendicular to the horizontal line and drawn through the acetabular rim. This creates four quadrants in relationship with the horizontal and vertical lines. The visualized femoral head outlined in wax pencil is found to lie, for the most part, in the inner lower quadrant and one can be reasonably sure that the hip is reduced. If the visualized head lies, for the most part, outside this inner lower quadrant, one should strongly suspect a subluxated or perhaps a frankly dislocated hip (Fig. 12-2B).

It is probably not wise for the average primary care physician to treat the severely dysplastic, subluxated, or truly dislocated hip in the newborn since this often requires follow-up care utilizing judgement gained only through specialty training. However, very mildly dysplastic hips can often be very satisfactorily treated and probably should be treated by the family practitioner. These cases of dysplasia should be treated by any method that mechanically holds the hips in an abducted and flexed position.

This usually takes the form of some sort of padding to be applied between the legs to hold them in this position. It is not often adequate merely to apply extra diapers, as is so often recommended, since this does not constitute a strong enough mechanical force to hold the hips in abduction. Though it may ultimately improve the amount of dysplasia, it certainly will not be adequate in more severe amounts of dysplasia and should not be used at all. Instead of this, a "pillow" splint should be made by the mother or the local bracemaker and can very adequately mechanically hold these hips in the abducted or "frog-leg" position.

The Frejka splint usually requires a pillow of some sturdy material, preferably felt or something similar, that can be inserted into a garment for use 24 hours a day. The pad should be wide enough to extend between the popliteal creases on each knee with the legs as widely abducted as possible. It should be wide enough to extend from the lower abdomen anteriorly to a point up above the buttocks posteriorly. The garment to contain the pillow can be fashioned as overalls, with a bib in front connecting to straps in the back that pass through the garment near the waist line. This can allow for a small pocket into which the pad can be inserted. The pocket, of course, should be made of some water-resistant material to prevent soiling of the pad. Several of these garments should be made utilizing the same pad, which can be changed when the garments become soiled.

Radiographs in the AP plane should be taken during the treatment period. If the practitioner is not certain that improvement is occurring, the infant should be referred to an orthopedic specialist for evaluation.

The importance of diagnosing dysplasia or dislocation of the hip initially in the newborn cannot be overemphasized. Several degrees of dysplasia and occasionally even mild subluxations can be very satisfactorily treated by conservative means with excellent results if they are discovered early.

If, however, the dysplasia or subluxation is not discovered until the infant has begun to walk or is several months old, the treatment is much more difficult and prolonged. It would follow then that the responsibility usually lies with the physician who does the original examination. In instances in which dislocations have not been discovered until the child begins to walk or until several months have passed, general anesthesia with closed reduction and casting are often required. Occasionally even closed reduction is not possible; skeletal traction and open reduction may be necessary to secure good reduction of the hip. It goes without saying that results in these instances are not nearly as good and certainly good results are not nearly as reliable when treatment is started this late in life as they are when the treatment is instituted soon after birth.

Legg-Perthe's Disease

Legg Perthe's disease involves the capital femoral epiphysis in young children. It is much more common in boys than girls and usually occurs around the 7th to the 10th year. The age of occurrence may vary greatly with geographic distribution; most investigators in European countries describe this condition occurring at a much earlier age.

The onset of symptoms is usually insidious; the parents notice that the child begins to limp. Most of the time the pain is not severe enough to warrant much spontaneous complaint but the limp is usually antalgic, indicating that some pain does occur when the child bears weight on the hip. When pain does occur, it usually radiates into the region of the knee on the same side and may often be mistaken a condition in the knee. On occasions the symptoms will occur immediately following injury, so that the cause of the pain is mistakenly related to this injury. Occasionally the pain becomes quite severe, particularly at night, and these instances may be the reason for consulting the physician.

Examination usually reveals the antalgic gait but otherwise there are no outward signs. Examination with the patient lying on the examining table reveals limitations of motion usually in all directions with some pain experienced, usually at the extremes of motion. There is usually no outward sign of swelling or other indications of inflammatory reaction and the child otherwise appears healthy with normal joints. These patients should undergo complete laboratory investigation to rule out any of the infectious or inflammatory diseases of joints and, of course, x-ray studies should be done.

When all laboratory studies and x-ray results are within normal limits, the assumption is that the youngster has a nonspecific synovitis of the hip. This is a poorly understood and rather obscure condition that affects the hip joints, particularly in young children. It has no demonstrated cause in most instances and is characterized by negative laboratory and x-ray findings in the face of a painful, somewhat stiff, hip. The diagnosis is mostly that of exclusion. One must be on guard lest the patient have an early Legg-Perthe's disease that has not yet shown objective signs. In these instances the youngster is usually placed on restricted activities with hot tub baths once or twice a day and moderate doses of silicylates. If the symptoms clear up readily, reexamination by x-ray should be done periodically for several months to be certain that changes are not developing in the capital femoral epiphysis. If changes do not develop in 3 or 4 months, one can begin to allow resumption of normal activities. If symptoms recur upon resumption of activities, treatment should be reinstituted until the patient becomes asymptomatic. When symptoms resolve relatively rapidly on conservative management, continued periodic x-rays should be obtained over a period of time, as in the case of the congenital hip.

Early diagnosis and institution of treatment are imperative if one is to obtain a good final result. When x-ray examination does reveal some changes in the epiphysis, these usually involve fragmentation of capital femoral epiphysis itself. This may vary in degree depending upon the duration between the onset of symptoms and the time the radiograph is taken. One hopes that the radiograph has been taken early enough that actual architectural distortion of the head has not occurred.

The watchword in treatment of Legg-Perthe's disease, once the diagnosis has been established, is *non-weight-bearing*. It has been repeatedly proven that the changes in the capital femoral epiphysis with Legg-Perthe's disease are reversible, though considerable time may be necessary for these changes to revert to a normal epiphysis. Therefore, though the fragmentation early in the course of surveillance may gradually increase in severity and magnitude, these fragments will gradually coalesce so that the architecture of the head will be restored. If, during this time of fragmentation and active changes in the femoral head, weight-bearing is allowed, femoral distortion will occur usually in the form of flattening of the head at the point of weight-bearing. When this does occur, ultimate healing of the fragments in the head still occurs, but with a misshapened head that results in incongruity at the ball and socket joint with the obvious resulting degenerative changes. It would follow, then, that if the diagnosis can be made early and the child placed on a non-weight-bearing program during this time until healing has occurred, an essentially normal hip may often be expected.

How best to maintain the non-weight-bearing status in this often uncooperative youngster? There have been volumes written on the various methods of protecting the hip joint from weight-bearing, from rest in bed over many months down to the use of very complicated braces that hold the leg not only in the weight-bearing position but in other positions.

The treatment of choice of the average physician is a relatively simple mechanism to maintain the non-weight-bearing status. The old Perthe's strap consisted of a small strap around the ankle with a chain attaching it to a similar strap around the waist, thereby, holding the hip and the knee flexed so that weight-bearing was impossible. It has several drawbacks. During the time that this is worn, the youngster must walk on crutches and unless the apparatus is made quite secure it is very easy for the chain holding the ankle strap to the waist strap to be detached so that periods of surreptitious weight-bearing occur.

Most observers find that failure of treatment mechanisms based on non-weight-bearing is usually related to lack of cooperation on the part of the patient and illegal weight-bearing is the cause of the ultimate distortion of the head. The Perthe's strap also has the disadvantage of allowing considerable atrophy of the extremity. Holding the leg with the knee rather acutely flexed over a long period of time likewise results in some changes in the knee joint capsule.

For this reason the author prefers the so-called Perthe's brace, which has an ischial weight-bearing ring, a markedly elevated foot on the other side to balance, and thus allows no possible weight-bearing. Since, the treatment of Legg-Perthe's disease requires expert judgement in management. It can best be treated by those specialized in treating these conditions. Probably the primary care physician should do nothing further than to assist in the management. The parents should be warned, however, that it often takes as much as 3 years of total non-weight-bearing treatment for the femoral head to be restored so that they will be prepared for this extended period of inconvenience.

A

B

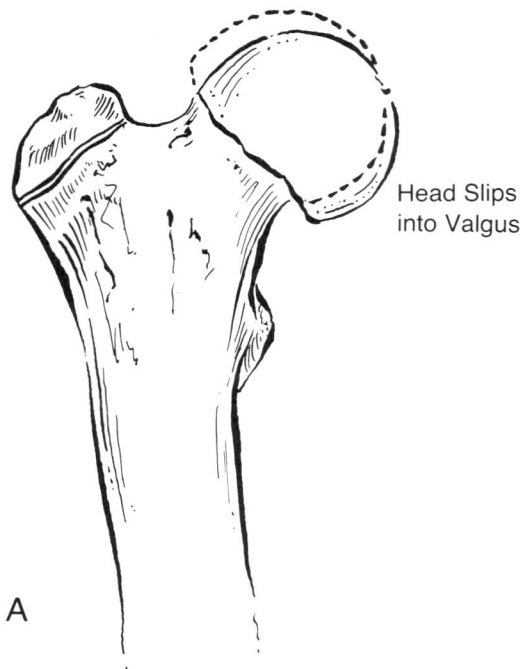

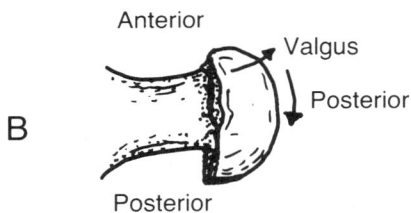

Fig. 12-3. **(A)** Anteroposterior view shows the position of the femoral head with the slipped capital femoral epiphysis. It has rotated downward. **(B)** On the lateral view it has rotated posteriorly.

Slipped Capital Femoral Epiphysis

Slipping of the capital femoral epiphysis in the adolescent can occur either insidiously or as a sudden, acute, major shift in the position of the femoral head epiphysis with relationship to the neck (Fig. 12-3A). In cases of the gradual slip the diagnosis is often hard to make since the patient's complaint is basically pain on weight-bearing and particularly with excess activity. Even then the pain may not be in the hip area, but in the knee. This is extremely important since many missed diagnoses of slipped capital femoral epiphysis have occurred because the patient was treated over long periods of time for a painful knee. If the teenager presents with painful knee but no physical findings in the knee (swelling, tenderness, or other evidences of localizing disease), a radiograph of the hip should always be taken to determine whether this may be referred pain from the hip. The acute slip may occur spontaneously as the presenting symptom or it may result from the gradual slipping. Minimal symptoms then suddenly become extremely acute as the epiphysis slips entirely off of the neck or at least into an extremely poor position. The diagnosis in these instances, of course, is easy to make.

The typical youngster with a slipping of the femoral epiphysis is an early to midteenager, usually male, and overweight. The typical patient has Fröhlich's syndrome: reasonably tall but with feminine distribution of fat, very wide hips, and poorly developed musculature. Though postpubertal, the Fröhlich's syndrome individual often has infantile genitalia and pubic hair is slow to appear and sparse. When a boy with Fröhlich's syndrome appearance begins to develop symptoms referable to his hip or knee, the index of suspicion is extremely high. There are, of course less classic variations in which the youngster is merely chubby but even in these instances there is usually some delay in the appearance of sexual characteristics.

On observation of the individual with an early, gradually developing, slip one notices an externally rotated extremity during gait. On physical examination there is limited motion, particulary in rotation, and attempts to rotate the hip, when it is flexed particularly, cause pain.

There is seldom any real shortening until the gradual slipping has become quite marked but since the hip tends to be held abducted, this often is not noticed. Patients with the sudden slip tend to lie with the hip shortened, slightly flexed, and in external rotation. These patient are ordinarily in acute pain and usually have sustained some type of injury, such as a fall.

Proper x-ray examination is imperative if the diagnosis is to be made early. A spot AP film of the hip may not show the earlier stages since the initial slip tends to be posterior. For this reason, however, it is quite easy to identify even the early changes in position on a true lateral film. As a general rule the "frog-leg" type lateral is not sufficient and a true "across the table" lateral is necessary for diagnosis. This lateral projection is taken with the patient supine with the tube on the contralateral side and the contralateral extremity flexed up to allow a straight shot of the x-ray beam through the lateral projection. The x-ray film is then held lateral to the involved hip at an angle parallel with the neck of the involved femor and of course at right angles to the x-ray beams. The early stages of migration of the hip posteriorly can be seen and if there is any question as to the diagnosis the opposite hip should be documented for comparison (Fig. 12-3B). One should remember, however that there is often bilateral involvement but usually the opposite hip, if involved, will present symptoms that make it suspicious. As the migration continues over a period of time the posterior slippage is accompanied by some development of varus deformity which, of course, can be seen easily on the AP film later in the course of the migration.

Most orthopedic surgeons believe that the patient with an early slip should have operative fixation of the epiphysis to prevent further slippage. Even with non-weight-bearing on crutches there is still some likelihood of an acute slip, in which case the hip can probably not be restored to normal. In the cases of early slippage, adequate internal fixation by pins will usually stop the progress of the migration but in even those instances the patient will be required to remain non-weight-bearing until the epiphyseal line has closed. Therefore, any case of slipping of the capital femoral epiphysis should be referred to the orthopedic surgeon for further evaluation and treatment.

DISORDERS IN ADULTS

Fractures

One of the most common conditions seen in the adult hip by the primary care physician is a fracture. As pointed out previously, poor weight-bearing exists whereby weight is shifted from the longitudinal axis of the femoral shaft along the inclination of the neck (which usually averages around 127 degrees) into the weight-bearing surface of the superior aspect of the femoral head against the acetabular fossa. This creates a severe shear force on the region of the neck of the femur and is therefore much more likely to sustain fracture when sudden loading occurs, or when the patient falls and sudden force is exerted against the trochanter. There are four basic types of position for the fracture. The location of the fracture is extremely important from the standpoint of the type of treatment that will be recommended (Fig. 12-4).

Subcapital

This fracture line extends across the neck of the femur at right angles to the longitudinal line of the femoral neck just at the point of connection of the head with the neck. It may sometimes run more obtusely or more acutely than the regular 90 degrees. This change in angle has some importance from the standpoint of the stability of the hip once it has been subjected to internal fixation. However, the displaced subcapital fracture has considerable importance because of the possibility that the blood supply to the femoral head has been destroyed by the fracture line itself. The foveolar artery that extends through the ligamentum teres supplies only a relatively small percentage of the blood to the femoral head. Most of the blood supply comes through the capsullar attachment. Since the capsule attaches around the base of the neck the blood vessels that supply the head must enter from this area and run either through the substance of the bone or on the surface of the bone into the femoral head. This rather complicated nutritional arrangement is in great jeopardy when a fracture occurs transversely across the femoral neck since the normal blood supply to the femoral head is largely disrupted. If, of course, the fracture remains largely nondisplaced (so-called "compacted" fracture) the blood supply will occasionally remain intact and the prognosis is much better.

Completely displaced fractures of the subcapital region, however, carry a relatively high risk of avascular necrosis of the femoral head. That risk is obviously greater in older persons because of the greater fragility of the blood vessel walls. For this reason the patient who is past 70 with a subcapital fracture should usually undergo excision of the femoral head and replacement with a prosthesis of some type. This, of course, obviates the need for any type of blood supply to the area and the patient will most certainly get along quite well.

On the other hand, the patient between 60 and 70 is considered marginal;

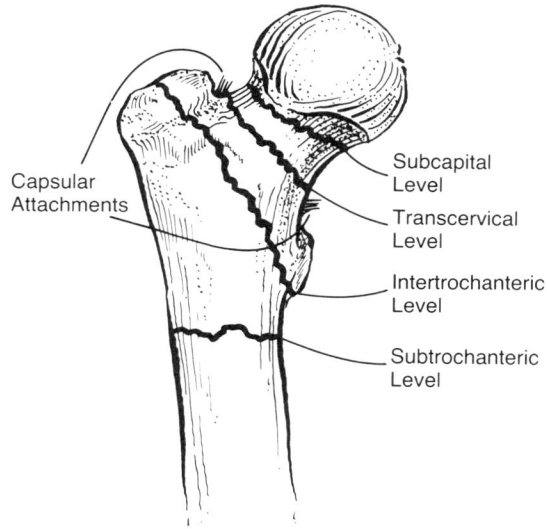

Fig. 12-4. Location of various fractures of the hip. The subcapital and transcervical fractures lie within the joint capsule and, therefore, are much more likely to interrupt the circulation by tearing the vessels that lie in the periosteum extending into the head. Note the extracapsular location of intertrochanteric and subtrochanteric fractures. The obliquity of the intertrochanteric fracture allows for considerable shortening in this type of fracture.

depending upon the circumstances and the appearance of the fracture some orthopedic surgeons will insert a femoral head prosthesis while others will resort to pinning the fracture in its compacted position following fracture. Generally the pinning technique in this type of fracture uses a long threaded pin drilled up into the head to give some further impaction but it is never driven across the fracture line such as with a large Smith-Peterson type nail since this might further disrupt the already precarious blood supply. Many types of threaded pins are generally used for fixation.

It is unfortunate that there is no good way to tell whether the femoral head is going to survive once pinning has been done until changes of avascular necrosis begin to show up on the x-ray films. Some of the more recent techniques using the radioactive bone scan and other imaging techniques identify the avascular necrosis earlier. However, for the most part, a period of watchful waiting is necessary following pinning of a subcapital fracture before one can determine the success of the procedure from the standpoint of healing and maintenance of good blood supply to the head.

If the patient goes ahead to a frank nonunion and/or avascular necrosis of the femoral head, the head must be removed and replaced with a femoral head prosthesis. An additional advantage of inserting the femoral head prosthesis in the older patient is that early weight-bearing can be allowed, which is often of great benefit to the more elderly patient. On the other hand, following pinning of the fracture, non-weight-bearing with crutches must be maintained over a good many months before healing can be expected.

In the patient under 60 years of age the chances of healing are much greater. The chances of avascular necrosis are much less, so most orthopedic surgeons will consider pinning in this age group unless there is a definite contra-indication in the patient or the type of fracture sustained.

Subcapital fractures are occasionally hard to see on the original radiographs. This type of fracture can occasionally be missed and the patient is allowed to walk on the hip until the fracture becomes disimpacted and completely separates. A true lateral film is of paramount importance in determining the presence or absence of a fracture in this area. Most of the time a questionable line across the subcapital region can either be confirmed or completely ruled out on the lateral film. In instances in which it is still not possible to diagnose fracture with complete certainty, but in which symptoms that lead the physician to believe that there is truly a fracture persist clinically, the best course of action is to put the patient on non-weight-bearing with crutches for several weeks and then to x-ray the hip again. If a fracture does exist, the demineralization that occurs along the margins of the fracture line during the first few weeks following injury will make the line immediately obvious on these delayed films.

Transcervical

Transcervical fractures are, as the name implies, "across the neck." They are located within the neck of the femur between the subcapital location and the base of the neck near the intertrochanteric line. These fractures have many of the characteristics of the subcapital fracture and are often treated similarly. As the level of the fracture, however, approaches the base of the neck, treatment is more likely to resemble that of the intertrochanteric fracture rather than the subcapital since the mechanical forces are more similar to those in the intertrochanteric area.

Intertrochanteric

Intertrochanteric fractures occur at the base of the neck, roughly following the intertrochanteric line of the femur. These are often comminuted but since they occur in an area comprised of cancellous bone they tend to heal quite well. Nonunions of intertrochanteric fractures are not common. This type of fracture is usually seen in older persons, particularly when there is rather marked demineralization of bone. The comminution may be so extreme that the greater trochanter may itself be isolated as a separate fragment, but the lesser trochanter is almost invariably a separate fragment since it is usually pulled off by the insertion of the iliopsoas muscle. Whereas the fractures of the neck or the subcapital region are "intracapsular" and seldom bleed to any great extent, the great amount of cancellous bone and the great amount of comminution in trochanteric fractures lead to a considerable amount of bleeding. A large hematoma often forms in the area of the fracture. Likewise, while the patient with a subcapital fracture may not have any obvious deformity of the lower extremity, intertrochanteric fractures are identifiable by the marked shortening, abduction, and external rotation of the lower extremity.

Treatment requires that a pin be inserted up into the neck and head of the femur and then connected to a plate that can be attached to the shaft of the femur with screws. The angle created by the nail and plate can be varied to restore the normal relationship between the shaft and the head of the femur.

Various types of apparatus include both those with the pin and the plate made as a single unit and those with two separate pieces that are later connected. The mechanism is the same, however, and any mechanism for reattaching the neck and head fragment to the shaft fragment of the femur is satisfactory. Following pinning of these fractures, weight-bearing is ordinarily is not allowed until healing has occurred and can be demonstrated on the radiograph.

Subtrochanteric

Subtrochanteric fractures occur in the upper part of the shaft of the femur and lie in the region of the level of the lesser trochanter or sometimes extend down into the shaft of the femur for a short distance. These fractures are ordinarily quite comminuted and require a considerably greater force to sustain. These fractures, like the intertrochanteric, require internal fixation by some mechanism that can grasp the neck and head fragment and attach to the shaft fragment at approximately the normal 127 degree angle of a hip. Again, as in the intertrochanteric fracture, unaided weight-bearing is not allowed on these fractures until bony union has occurred regardless of the presence of the fixation device since it is not strong enough to withstand the stresses of weight-bearing.

Arthritis

Arthritis of the hip joint is common and is particularly symptomatic because it occurs in a weight-bearing joint. Various types of rare conditions give rise to arthritic changes in the hip but the usual two types of arthritic involvement of the hip are degenerative joint diseases and arthritis related to rheumatoid disease.

Degenerative Joint Disease

Degenerative joint disease in the hip joint is common and usually related to overuse, such as in the obese patient; posttraumatic changes in the joint that lead it to be incongruent; or variations in the architecture related to congenital dysplasia. When one considers the relatively small surface area of the hip joint and that each step requires the entire body weight to be placed on this highly constrained joint, one can easily see why it so easily becomes the site of wear and tear in degenerative joint disease. Add to this the small cartilaginous and subcartilaginous injuries that occur from sudden trauma such as jumping or other sudden impact and it is easy to see why this joint, even with normal architecture becomes the site of wear. If the architecture is abnormal, such as is seen from posttraumatic distortions, it is easy to see why the joint wears out rather rapidly in some individuals. Since there is a high degree of constraint between the acetabulum and the femoral head, abnormalities in the shape of the head or of the acetabulum result in the incongruity that rapidly increases the wear of the covering articular surface of the joint. Finally, in instances of insufficient support from a very shallow acetabular cup, seen in untreated or poorly treated congenital dysplasia of the hip, a lack of stability allows for abnormal motion during weight-bearing, and abnormal shifting of the weight as the hip joint tries to subluxate on weight-bearing, resulting in a rapid loss of articular surface.

The greatest number of patients seen in the usual primary care practice have hip joint disease related to obesity: the hip joint is asked to carry greater loads than it is mechanically capable of carrying. Even when distortions of the normal architecture occur from trauma or congenital abnormalities, the overweight patient is much more likely to have a rapid progression of the wearing out of his hip than the individual of more normal weight. The stresses and strains seen in the acrobat, on the other hand, probably do not contribute a great amount to the degenerative changes as long as they do not compromise the ligamentous stability of the joint.

Another factor contributing to degenerative disease in some cases is muscular paralysis or weakness, particularly of the abductor group. The poorly stabilizing mechanism offered by weak musculature results in abnormal stresses and shifting the weight in the joint during weight-bearing, which wears out the joint surface. The person with abnormal abductor musculature who is forced to walk with a Trendelenberg limp or with shifting of the pelvic weight over the hip with each step (forcing it into marked abduction) expends a considerable amount of motion between the joint surfaces for the same amount of distance covered, resulting in a greater amount of wear and tear.

Nonoperative treatment of degenerative joint disease of the hip includes the following measures.

Stress on the joint should be limited by weight reduction and by minimizing the amount of activity that requires weight-bearing on the joint. A more sedentary life style that does not include prolonged or excessive weight-bearing on the hip will often result in a dramatic improvement of symptoms, as will the reduction of weight to optimal levels.

Additional support may be gained by use of a cane. Many patients are reluctant to use a cane because of the psychological stigma. However, proper use of a cane (in the hand opposite to the involved extremity) will quite often markedly relieve symptoms in the hip. Use of a cane along with measures for reducing the weight borne on the hip, will often allow the patient to go for some time with a reasonable degree of comfort.

Exercises used in degenerative hip joint disease include measures to stretch the joint out gently to keep as full a range of motion as possible, to stretch out flexion contractures that may occur in the joint, and to improve the strength of the supporting abductor musculature. The details of an adequate physical therapy program are not within the scope of this chapter, but these three measures should be considered when asking the therapist to outline a program for home use.

Heat and other supportive measures usually have already been tried by the patient when first seen by the physician, but are nevertheless effective and should be encouraged.

Anti-inflammatory medications tend to have a dramatic effect on degenerative joint disease of the hip. While salicylates alone are adequate in many cases, the physician will want to try other nonsteroidal anti-inflammatory agents which often will bring about a dramatic relief, particularly when accompanied by the other measures described.

The occasional injection into the hip of intra-articular steroids is probably justified during an acute episode of pain. However, this is not proper treatment over the long term for any joint involved with arthritic changes.

If the changes have progressed to the point that the patient cannot be kept comfortable using these nonoperative measures, consideration should be given to surgical treatment and the patient referred to the orthopedic surgeon for evaluation. In the past the medial displacement osteotomy popularized by Coventry often proved effective and some surgeons prefer this in the earlier stages. For the most part, however, the surgical treatment of degenerative joint disease of the hip that has failed to respond to other forms of treatment is total joint replacement. While the use of methyl methacrylate cement first made the hip joint replacement procedure possible, it also became one of the major hazards of the procedure and was the one feature that made one hesitate to recommend total hip joint replacement until the patient had no other choice. However, the newer porous-coated metals seem to have great promise and may obviate one of the restraining factors. The procedure may well become not only highly successful in relieving symptoms but also much safer.

Rheumatoid Disease

The hip joint is, of course, one of the joints most often involved with rheumatoid disease and since it is a weight-bearing joint the symptoms of rheumatoid involvement of the hip joint are often disabling. The same measures described above for the treatment of degenerative joint disease are often somewhat effective in the patient with rheumatoid hip disease. Unless the systemic disease is brought under control by medication, there is likely to be a progression of the hip joint disease.

Patients with significant involvement of the hip joint, however, should receive the nonoperative measures described previously, particularly the exercise program to strengthen the abductor musculature, and should be very cautious about the development of flexion contracture of the hip joint. This occurs quite often in rheumatoid disease because of the painful day-and-night synovitis in the hip joint. Total joint replacement is quite satisfactory in the rheumatoid patient and some of the most dramatic results are obtained in these patients.

13

THE KNEE

ANATOMY AND FUNCTION

The knee joint is unique for several reasons. To start with, there are actually two joints in the knee joint itself; that between the femur and upper tibia and that between the femur and the patella. The primary knee joint is weight-bearing and bears the entire body weight on a relatively small surface area each time a step is taken. The second important characteristic is that the ligamentous structures are far from strong enough to hold the joint were it not for the supporting musculature, particularly the quadriceps. The supporting muscula-ture posteriorly has neither the excursion nor the mechanical advantage that the quadriceps does and is merely the interweaving of the tendinous insertions of the gastrocnemius—soleus group to the lower femur and the attachment of the hamstring musculature to the tibia medially. This, along with a strong posterior cruciate ligament and a strong posterior knee joint capsule, affords a consider-able amount of static stability to the posterior knee joint. It is therefore possible to stand with the knee fully extended bearing full weight of the body without much supporting mechanism as long as the knee is kept extended against the posterior restraining structure so that it will not go into recurvatum. On the other hand, the knee is quite instable anteriorly so that if the knee is flexed only a few degrees while carrying full body weight, it would immediately collapse were it not for the strength of the quadriceps mechanism. By pulling through the patella and its insertion into the tibial tubercle, this affords a strong mechanism to maintain the extended position. When the knee is flexed for a few degrees it becomes the responsibility of the quadriceps mechanism to maintain that stability in all degrees of flexion with weight-bearing. The knee flexed in weight-bearing at 45 degrees depends almost entirely upon the quadriceps strength for its stability. The collateral ligaments merely keep the joint surfaces intact and the anterior cruciate prevents the forward excursion of the tibia on the femur in the flexed position. The knee joint depends not only on *strength* in the quadriceps muscle but also on a certain amount of *intrinsic tone* in that muscle to maintain normal stability. A muscle that has become atrophic, even if there is good active strength in extension, will have a certain amount of instability because of lack of muscle bulk and tone.

It would then follow that one of the most important features in rehabilitation of the knee is regaining strength and tone in the quadriceps musculature. This is true after injury or surgery and in the knee diseased with arthritis to the extent that the supporting musculature has become atrophic and gradually decreasing stability aggravates the already existing joint disease. Even in these individuals a rigorous program to rehabilitate the knee by vigorous quadriceps

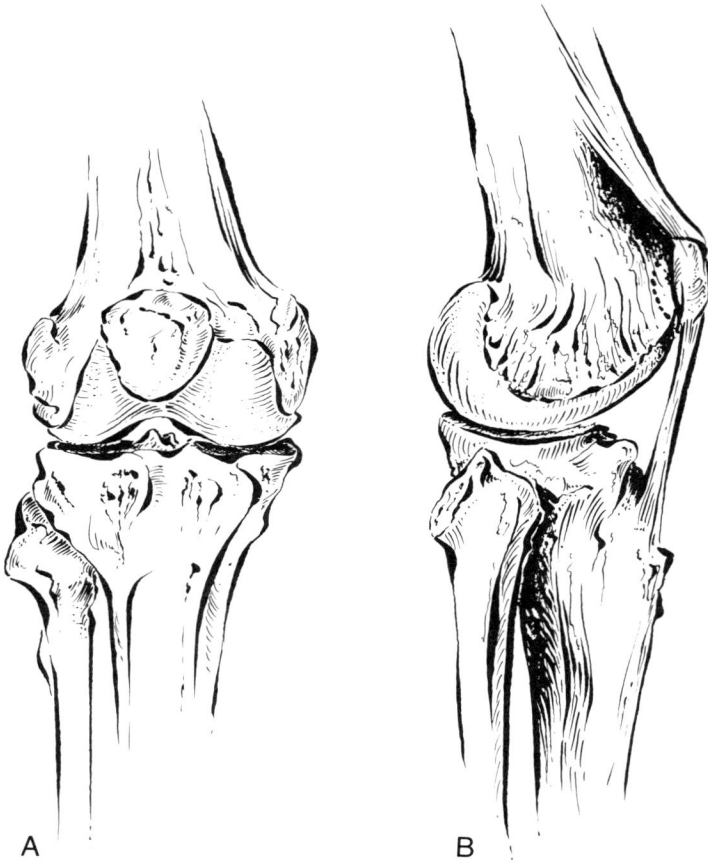

Fig. 13-1. (A) AP and **(B)** lateral anatomic views of the knee.

exercise greatly improves the symptoms in the knee, primarily by affording a greater amount of stability. Of course, it goes without saying that the less total body weight the knee joint is required to carry, the less support it requires to maintain its stability. Maintaining optimal body weight is therefore extremely important.

The knee joint proper consists of the articulation of the two condyles of the femur against appropriate depressions in the upper tibia or in the tibial plateaus (Fig. 13-1). The medial condyle is somewhat larger than the lateral and has a larger weight-bearing surface. With the normal knee in the completely extended position in full weight-bearing, 75 percent of the body weight is carried on the medial compartment of the joint, whereas only 25 percent is carried on the lateral compartment. As degenerative disease causes a wearing out of the articular cartilage on the medial side, a certain amount of genu varus develops. This increases the amount of weight-bearing on the medial compartment from 75 percent upward, which, in turn, aggravates the wearing out of the joint. This constitutes a vicious cycle. It is on this premise that the upper tibial osteotomy was formulated many years ago to redistribute body weight across the knee joint in an effort to prevent the progressive increase in wearing out of the medial compartment in ordinary individuals.

Since the upper surface of the tibia is relatively flat with only small depressions for articulation with the femur, two structures in the knee joint serve to deepen the recess in which the femoral condyle articulates and to create more of a cupping of the upper tibia. These are called the menisci and occur on both the medial and lateral sides, with somewhat different characteristics.

On the medial side, as would be expected, the cartilage is a larger and somewhat broader structure with a "wider open" C-curve. The lateral cartilage is smaller, thinner, and has a relatively closed C-shaped configuration. These cartilages are both attached anteriorly and posteriorly and along their peripheral surfaces. Neither cartilage is attached underneath to the tibia. Injuries that result in a tearing loose of the cartilage from its peripheral attachment result in a hypermobility of the cartilage. The resulting effect is that the cartilage may become caught in between the articulating surfaces of the femur and tibia, resulting in various degrees of cartilage damage and symptoms of internal derangement or locking.

The collateral ligaments exist on either side and, as previously mentioned, serve to hold the knee joint intact and maintain the normal stability of the joint. (Fig. 13-2). These ligaments are thickenings in the capsule of the joint and are not strong enough to maintain the stability of the knee were it not for the supporting musculature. Since the majority of the weight-bearing is on the medial compartment, the medial collateral ligament is obviously stronger, thicker, and more resistant to stretch or tear than the lateral collateral ligament.

The other two ligaments within the knee joint are the cruciate ligaments. The posterior cruciate ligament supports the knee in extension and prevents recurvatum of the joint normally. The anterior cruciate attaches to the femur posteriorly and the tibia anteriorly to prevent the excursion of the tibia anteriorly on the femur with the knee flexed. Testing of the anterior cruciate ligament is

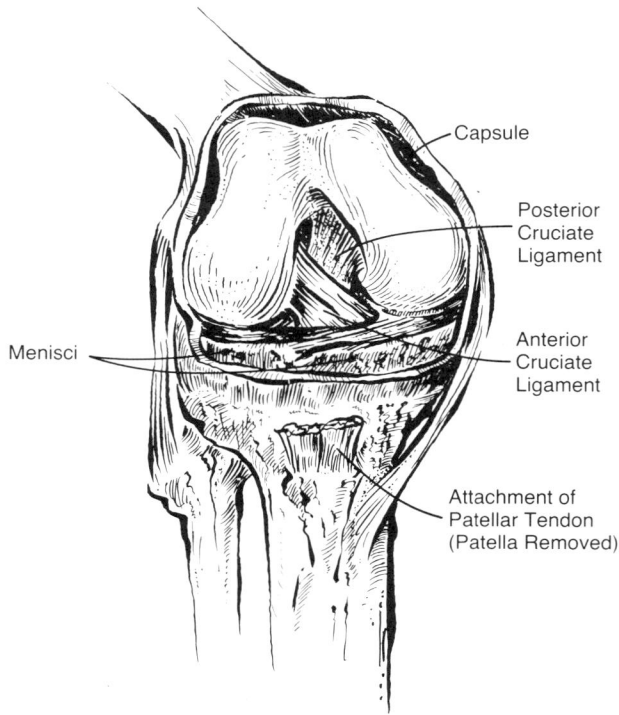

Fig. 13-2. AP view of the knee with the femur flexed on the tibia and the patella removed. Note the extension of the capsule around the entire femoral condyle anteriorly, and the attachment of the anterior and posterior cruciate to the region of the tibial spines. The anterior cruciate is attached to the intracondylar notch on the medial side of the lateral condyle, with the posterior cruciate attached to the superior aspect of the notch. Note the location of the menisci, extension of the sartorius tendon medially into the pes anserinus, and the collateral ligament attachments.

done with the patient seated with the knee flexed. While the knee is trapped between the examiner's knees, as he sits on a stool, the tibia is drawn forward on the femur in this 90 degree flexed position. If the tibia has a considerable amount of laxity so that it can be pulled forward on the femur, this is a positive "drawer" sign and represents anterior cruciate instability.

The knee joint synovial sac is rather voluminous and extends up a variable distance above the superior pole of the patella in the structure commonly known as the suprapatellar pouch. When the joint is filled with effusion this pouch becomes distended and can be easily palpated above the patella, since it extends across the entire breadth of the femur and often 2 cm above the upper pole of the patella.

Posteriorly, the synovium and capsule are likewise somewhat redundant, extending from an attachment above the superior margin of the joint surface down to the margin of the joint surface on the upper tibia (Fig. 13-3). The knee joint with effusion or interarticular bleeding may hold an enormous amount of fluid and become quite distended usually with blood and increased joint fluid after injury. If the capsule is distended the knee usually cannot be flexed past 90

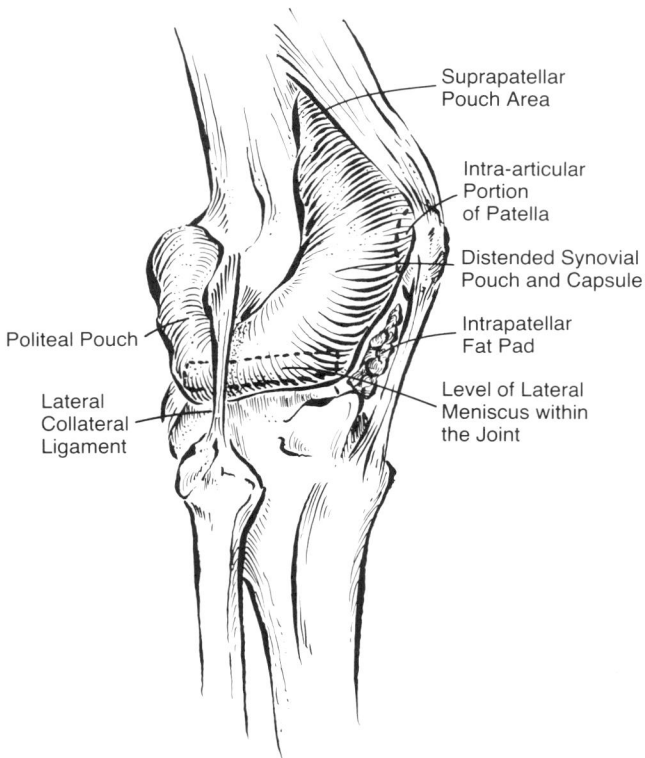

Fig. 13-3. Anteriolateral view of the knee showing the extent of the synovial pouch and capsule of the knee joint. It extends superiorly for some distance anteriorly, creating the suprapatellar pouch. The inclusion of the articular surface is on the under side of the patella in the joint space. Note the level of the meniscus on the lateral side within the joint space and the extension of the capsule and synovium in the popliteal area above the joint surface of the condyles.

degrees because of pressure on the suprapatellar pouch area. It cannot be extended past about 15 degrees because of the pressure on the posterior capsule as it is stretched during complete extension of the knee. The injured knee found to have loss of complete extension cannot be thoroughly evaluated until the fluid has been aspirated. Lack of extension may represent a tear of the meniscus with locking of the knee, or may merely be due to the effusion present with stretching of the capsule. This cannot be determined until the knee joint has been aspirated; many times, it will be found that the knee joint will go completely straight once pressure has been relieved.

X-RAY EXAMINATION

X-ray studies should be made of any knee presented for examination. Four views should be taken in the usual case: anteroposterior (AP), lateral, "notch" view with the knee flexed and the tube pointed to take a picture of the intercondylar notch area of the femur, and the tangential patellar or "skyline" view. This is taken with the knee flexed and is shot along the long axis of the patella so that the condition of the patellofemoral joint can be evaluated and the relative position of the patella ascertained with respect to the femoral condyles. If the knee if flexed either from excess fluid or from locking with a torn cartilage it may be necessary to take two AP views: one for a true AP of the lower femur and one for a true AP of the upper tibia. Also, as mentioned above, the knee should be aspirated if a great amount of effusion exists so that if the loss of extension is from capsular pressure, full extension may be obtained before the radiograph is taken.

In many instances of internal derangement of the knee joint an arthrogram is of significant value in determining the condition of the menisci and other structures. This procedure should be done by a radiologist experienced in the technique and evaluation of the results. Occasionally, computerized tomography of the joint is indicated but this depends entirely upon the circumstances; this particular test should not be ordered indiscriminately because of its considerable cost.

SPECIFIC PROBLEMS IN CHILDREN

Several specific injuries seen in the knee in childhood bear special mentioning because of their unique clinical characteristics and treatment.

Osgood-Schlatter's Disease

This is probably a misnomer since the usual case of Osgood-Schlatter's "disease" is a "condition" that occurs because of the unique attachment of the patellar tendon to the upper tibial epiphysis. If one looks at a lateral radiograph of a 10-year-old, the epiphyseal plate of the distal femur is a transverse structure extending across the entire breadth of the femur in a uniform manner. The upper tibial epiphyseal plate extends transversely across the upper tibia except anteriorly where it curves downward and extends down to include the tibial tubercle. This arrangement makes it necessary for the quadriceps tendon to attach to the epiphysis of the upper tibia; because of this unusual stresses to the tibial tubercle may occur. Repeated trauma to this small anterior extension of the upper tibial epiphysis often results in an inflammatory reaction is seen as fragmentation of the epiphysis on the radiograph.

The clinical symptoms are swelling, tenderness, and sometimes even an increased local temperature. The area becomes exquisitely tender and since this is the area that strikes the ground first when a child falls on his knee the condition becomes quite painful and is considerably disabling to an active child. On occasion the inflammatory reaction may be severe enough that the child even has some difficulty in walking. It is often bilateral.

Various treatments have been used but none with any permanent effectiveness. The extremity may be immobilized in a cylinder cast with the knee in complete extension to prevent the child from falling on the inflamed epiphyseal center and also prevent the pull of the patellar tendon on the epiphysis. The child almost invariably becomes asymptomatic and is much improved until the cast is removed; it then usually takes only a relatively short time before the clinical manifestations recur. Likewise, injections of methylprednisolone into the area will result in a short period of remission but these almost invariably recur with time.

The only effective treatment is reassurance of the patient and his parents that the condition is self-limited and will heal in most instances as soon as the epiphysis has closed. Occasionally a detached ossicle remains even after the remainder of the epiphysis is closed. The patient and his parents should be informed that if this occurs and if symptoms are severe enough, surgical excision of the small ossicle can be done. Otherwise, the parents can be assured that as soon as growth has been completed and the epiphysis has closed, the child will no longer be symptomatic. An additional problem, particularly in girls, occurs when the epiphysis heals but with considerable enlargement. The anterior prominence seen at the tibial tubercle area, many times, is unsightly. If this occurs to the extent that the mass creates cosmetic problems, consideration may be given to diminishing the size of the mass surgically. The patient must decide whether the presence of the mass is worth going through an operative procedure which will, of course, leave a scar even without the mass. In most instances, if it is explained in this manner, the patient will elect to tolerate the mass and not undergo surgery.

During the acute stages of the disease the pain can sometimes be improved by heat and aspirin as needed. Youngsters intent on engaging in athletics in spite of the condition often benefit from a soft sponge rubber pad that can be sewn into an elastic knee support to give some padding across the knee and make it somewhat less painful when he falls on the knee. The child and his parents should be instructed that he be allowed to engage in all types of activities including football as long as he is willing to do this without complaining continuously about the pain. Some children use this as a method of gaining sympathy or perhaps even complain subconsciously to their parents to keep them in a constant state of concern. If this is true then the child should be prohibited from playing athletics because his symptoms will certainly improve when he reduces the trauma to the inflamed epiphyseal center.

For the most part, however, careful, sympathetic counseling of the child and his parents will suffice for treatment and nothing will be necessary other than the few supportive measures previously described. Referral to an orthopedic surgeon is seldom necessary unless some unusual condition is seen or the physician feels that some reinforcement of his opinion about the condition is necessary to gain acceptance from the patient and his family.

Osteochondritis Dissecans

The cause of osteochondritis dissecans is unknown though the patholophysiology appears to be some condition resulting in the disruption of blood supply in the subchondral bone, resulting in detachment of a segment of articular cartilage. The condition will occasionally be seen in the elbow or the ankle but the most characteristic and frequently observed location is in the articular surface of the medial condyle adjacent to the intercondylar notch. This unique location may in some way be related to the unknown causative factor, though this has not been established.

The symptoms are usually pain and recurring effusion in the joint. Locking only occurs if the devitalized segment of cartilage becomes detached and floats loose in the joint. When the symptoms first occur the ossicle usually is still situated in its normal location and can be seen on the radiograph. Often, because of its location near the intercondylar notch, the lesion can be seen only on the so-called notch view described previously. This is another instance in which the full group of projections should be obtained if an x-ray examination of the knee is made.

If osteochondritis dissecans is discovered in a joint, the patient should be referred to the orthopedic surgeon. In most instances if the ossicle has not become detached the patient may be treated by non-weight bearing either with crutches or with a long leg brace adjusted to block extension to 25 or 30 degrees. (This of course results in the inability to bear weight over the articular surface of the femur where the lesion is located.) In many instances, however, progression of the condition is documented by serial radiologic examination to the extent that excision of the detached cartilage will be necessary. Drilling of the base promotes fibrocartilaginous replacement and saucerization of margins of the defect in the normal cartilage to minimize the roughness of that cartilage. These decisions, however, of course are left up to the operating surgeon since he has the responsibility of achieving a good knee joint in these cases. Most of the time the prognosis is good, however. Though these patients are likely to develop degenerative joint disease earlier than others, the immediate symptoms usually subside with treatment and the patient is able to resume normal activities once the lesion has been treated and has healed.

Fractures

Fractures about the knee in children are unique because of the presence of epiphyseal centers in both the lower femur and upper tibia. Fractures in this area often involve the epiphysis. One of the characteristic configurations of injury to the lower femur is a dislocation of the distal femoral epiphysis with inclusion of a segment of the diathesis. This so-called "Salter type II" fracture requires special attention and a very accurate reduction to prevent alteration in epiphyseal growth. All of these cases should be referred to the orthopedic surgeon since the chance of developing joint disturbances with epiphyseal involvement is present.

ATHLETIC INJURIES

Considering the poor mechanical situation of the knee joint and the severe stresses to which it is subjected, it is not surprising that knee injury is one of the most frequent disabilities seen in athletes. This is particularly true in football, where one of the objectives is to knock the other person off of his feet by "blocking" against his leg. Similarly, the sudden "cutting," which amounts to a sudden change in direction accompanied by a pivoting on a single outstretched lower extremity, results in a tremendous amount of strain both to the supporting structures and to the menisci within the knee joint. Combinations of these various injuries run the gamut from simple sprains or strains of the capsular support of the joint to severe ligamentous damage with marked instability and cartilage tear.

Capsular Injuries

The most frequent injury to the knee is a sprain that results from stretching the capsule and the associated ligamentous attachments beyond their normal length. The common mechanism of injury is a sudden blow to the side of the leg at about the level of the knee. When administered from the outside, this forces the knee into a sudden valgus strain, causing a severe stress on the supporting capsule and ligamentous structures. Similarly, when the patient is struck from in front there is a marked tendency to hyperextension of the knee, resulting in possible damage to the supporting structure including the posterior capsule and posterior cruciate ligaments. In cases where actual disruption of fibers does not occur, the patient may have sudden severe pain with point tenderness over the joint margin and ligamentous attachments, but examination fails to reveal evidence of ligamentous instability and the instrinsic stability of the knee is not lost. These should be considered serious injuries, however, and should be treated by rest with non-weight-bearing and possibly immobilization during the 6 weeks required for healing. The application of a cylinder cast gives excellent support for healing but also results in a considerable loss of strength and tone in the quadriceps muscle, so it is advisable only in more severe cases. Patients with less severe cases should be restricted from running and from contact sports during the healing period but may be allowed to bear guarded weight during this time. If possible the patient should receive physical therapy in the form of whirlpool or hot soaks twice daily plus a rigorous program of quadriceps exercises to strengthen the supporting musculature. The patient should not be allowed to return to contact sports, however, for 6 weeks.

Ligamentous Tears

Ligamentous tears are a step further in severity of the capsular and ligamentous injuries. The fibers are actually torn in the body of the ligament or the bony attachments of the ligaments are torn loose. These allow for loss of stability. The patient should be tested for ligamentous instability as soon as he can be examined since it is usually much easier to determine before swelling and soreness occur. During this first short period after injury, the knee can be checked for instability on the lateral or medial side by stressing it with your hands. If instability is found, it should be confirmed by stress radiographs. Since the posterior capsule affords a considerable amount of stability to the knee even in the lateral position, the collateral ligaments can be tested only with the knee slightly flexed to relax the posterior capsule. In cases, of course, in which the capsule is torn along with the collateral ligament, this is not important since the knee can be placed into valgus or varus strain with separation of the joint line in either position.

If the patient is examined the day after the injury instability will be difficult to determine because of pain. In this instance, if there is a strong suspicion of ligamentous instability, the area should be anesthetized or the patient given an intravenous narcotic so that stress radiographs can be done adequately to determine the stability. Unfortunately, testing the anterior cruciate ligament is difficult; there is not much of a way that stress radiographs can be taken to confirm an injury to the anterior cruciate. The loss of stability in this ligament must be determined by examination, as previously described.

If the patient can be shown to have even slight loss of stability in the knee compared to the opposite side, he should be referred to the orthopedic surgeon for evaluation and treatment. Many times if the instability is not great the patient will be treated merely by immobilization in plaster to see whether repair will occur with immobilization alone. However, acute ligament tears with loss of stability require prompt surgical repair.

If the knee is not examined by the physician until after the acute state and ligamentous instability is discovered after some healing has occurred, the patient should be referred to the orthopedic surgeon for consideration of a reconstructive procedure to restore ligamentous stability. If in doubt, the best policy is to refer the patient to the orthopedic surgeon for a more thorough evaluation and to leave the responsibility for the decision-making to be the specialist.

Meniscus Tears

Tears of the meniscus probably are the most common major injuries to the internal structures of the knee without ligamentous tear (Fig. 13-4). As mentioned above, the menisci are attached both anteriorly and posteriorly at their extremities and along the peripheral margin. The undersurface and the inner surface are not attached, so the meniscus more or less swings free within the joint. The meniscus also has a peculiar configuration on cross-section: it is wider at the periphery where it is attached to the capsule and slopes down to a knife edge at its inner portion. Tears of the peripheral attachment allow the cartilage to become hypermobile, so it may be dislocated far enough into the articular surface that it becomes pinched by the femoral condyle as it glides through its tract in the upper tibia. Similarly, some injuries are of such an acute nature that a tear occurs within the substance of the cartilage itself. The body of the cartilage may become displaced into the intercondylar notch with the peripheral attachment still intact. This resembles vaguely a bucket with a handle on it; these are often called "bucket handle tears." These generally result in complete locking of the joint. Unless the cartilage is reducible by manipulation the knee is usually irretrievably locked in flexion until the cartilage is surgically removed.

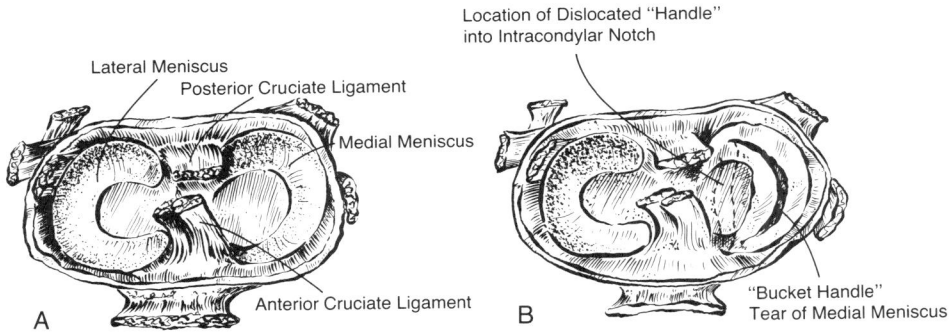

Fig. 13-4. (**A**) View of the tibial plateau area from above. The attachments of the cruciate ligaments are in the central portion of the tibia near the spines. Note the ligamentous and tendinous relationship peripherally and the intact medial and lateral menisci. (**B**) Longitudinal "bucket handle tear" of the medial meniscus. The torn bucket handle portion of the cartilage is now attached only anteriorly and posteriorly, but no longer medially, so that it can dislocate over into the intracondylar notch, as shown by the dotted lines.

The medial cartilage is torn much more frequently than the lateral since it is the larger of the two, it has the wider configuration or the more open curve, and it lies on the medial side of the joint where most of the weight of the body is borne. Lateral menisci may likewise be torn but this is not nearly as common. Tears of the meniscus with dislocation of the major portion of cartilage into the interconcylar notch result in locking of the knee with the loss of the last 30 degrees of extension. Remember that an accumulation of fluid and blood in the joint will distend the capsule and the knee will be unable to be extended because of tightness of the posterior capsule. If the knee is distended and a cartilage tear is suspected, the knee should be aspirated to remove the excess fluid and then examined to determine if extension can be achieved once the joint has been emptied.

Arthrograms may be helpful in establishing a diagnosis of cartilage tears since they are usually quite distinctive in their appearance. In this age of internal examination by arthroscopy, a diagnosis can be established rather simply with a procedure of no great magnitude; this should be done where the tear of the cartilage is strongly suspected. These patients with suspected cartilage tears of course should be referred to the orthopedic surgeon for evaluation and appropriate treatment. If the knee joint is normal except for the torn cartilage, arthroscopic removal can be accomplished quite simply and the patient can be restored to full activities in an amazingly short time.

Dislocation of the Patella

Dislocation of the patella may occur in the young athlete but also in any adolescent with the appropriate predisposing factors. The major cause of dislocation of the patella is the lateral displacement of the attachment of the patellar tendon to the tibial tubercle. This usually occurs in an individual with considerable genu valgus; the valgus deformity plus the lateral attachment of the insertion of the patellar tendon result in a subluxation of the patella laterally as the knee is completely extended. Many times the patella can be felt to progress back and forth across the femoral condyles as the knee is flexed and extended. Many of these individuals develop changes in the undersurface of the patella relatively early because of this abnormal movement. Many of these individuals are overweight, which adds to the poor mechanics of the knee joint and to the likelihood of recurring dislocation of the patella. Even if dislocation does not occur, they develop patellofemoral arthritis relatively early, indicating that some form of stabilization of the patella surgically should be considered. The patient should be referred to the orthopedic surgeon for this evaluation.

The other patient with an acutely dislocated patella has an immediate problem since there will be severe pain and inability to extend the knee. The patient should be given some type of intraveneous medication so that he can tolerate a small amount of pain and the patella can be reduced quite simply by merely extending the knee, which allows it to fall back into its normal relationship. The knee should be immobilized in a walking cylinder cast in complete extension for 6 weeks after dislocation, but the patient should be warned of the strong possibility of recurring dislocation of the patella unless surgical stabilization is done.

Strengthening the quadriceps mechanisms helps to "take the slack out" of the extensor mechanism and minimize the possibility of recurring dislocations, but the mechanical deficit responsible for the subluxation usually must be treated before the patient can become completely comfortable. Treatment by the orthopedic surgeon usually will amount to a translocation of the tibial tubercle medially and somewhat distally to realign the extensor mechanism and give a better line of pull. This procedure (known as the Houser procedure) has many variations, including release of the lateral capsule and embrication of the medial capsule. Whichever procedure is used, however, the patient can generally be expected to obtain an excellent functional result with complete relief of the symptoms referable to the patellofemoral joint and of the tendency to recurring dislocation.

FRACTURES

Fractures of the knee joint may occur in any of the three associated bones and may be associated with other fractures or occur alone. Fractures that occur into the joint ordinarily cause sudden bleeding into the joint with severe distention of the joint capsule that requires aspiration and drainage to relieve the pressure. When blood is withdrawn from an injured knee joint in which a fracture is suspected it should be placed in a pan and observed for the appearance of fat droplets on the surface. If a fracture communicates with the joint, and if the bleeding is occurring from that fracture, many small droplets of marrow fat will be floating on the surface of the blood. These can be easily identified and help to substantiate the diagnosis. Of course, radiographs should be taken before a final opinion is made.

Patella

Patellar fractures usually occur from a direct blow. Fractures may result either in a transection of the patella, which usually results in an immediate separation due to the pull of the quadriceps on the upper pole, or may be stellate in nature, which refers to extreme comminution that will often occur to a surprising degree in this largely cancellous bone. If the patella has been transected in its central portion and the two ends separated, the defect can usually be palpated at the time of the examination. It will likewise be found that the patient cannot actively extend the knee due to loss of continuity of the extensor mechanism. Of course, transections through the upper or lower pole have different variations on these findings. Again, confirmation can only be made by x-ray examination.

Fractures that are nondisplaced and have no great deformity of the joint surface may be treated by simple immobilization in a cylinder-type cast. This may be true of nondisplaced fractures through the central portion of the patella (which are usually incomplete) or of fractures in the upper or lower poles that do not involve the joint surface and are not markedly separated because of the effect of the lateral expansion of the capsule. These fractures require 6 to 8 weeks for healing. The patient should be started on isometric contractions of the quadriceps mechanism with straight-leg raising many times per day as soon as possible. These should be continued until the cast is removed so that quadriceps atrophy is kept at a minimum.

If there is marked deformity of the articular cartilage, such as is seen in a stellate fracture, or if there is separation of the fragments, the patient should be referred to the orthopedic surgeon for consideration of surgery. If the joint surface can be reestablished the surgeon will probably merely do an open reduction and internal fixation. However, if there is marked damage and destruction to the articular surface a complete patellectomy may be necessary.

Tibial Plateau

Tibial plateau fractures usually occur with a severe stress into either valgus or varus that results in a pressing of the femoral condyle down into the upper tibia with a depression of the plateau. These are sometimes severe enough to fracture through the entire plateau and depress it on the involved side. Other times there may merely be a defect in the tibial plateau that is depressed but that will alter the joint surface considerably. All tibial plateau fractures, except those with very minimal displacement, should be referred to the orthopedic surgeon for consideration of surgical reduction. On some occasions there is a stress on the cruciate ligament attachments that results in a fracture of the tibial spine rather than a rupture of the ligament. In these instances radiographs will show what amounts to an avulsion of the spine. Usually, when there is not a great amount of displacement, these fractures can be treated by immobilization in the appropriate position, usually full extension. Since this is cancellous bone, healing usually occurs in 6 weeks and the patient can then be started on gentle exercises.

Exercises to maintain quadriceps tone and strength should be instituted early. If there is any question about the degree of displacement of the tibial spine fracture, the patient should be referred for evaluation by the orthopedic surgeon.

Distal Femur

Fractures of the distal femur usually result in a fracture through the intercondylar notch with loss of continuity of a condyle on the side in which the maximum stress has occurred. These usually are caused by sudden severe valgus or varus strain and result in marked displacement of the condylar fracture fragment. On occasion a "T" fracture may exist: a fracture across the femur in the condylar area with extension down into the intercondylar notch so that three fragments are present. All of these cases, of course, require open operation and should be referred to the orthopedic surgeon for treatment.

Fractures of the femoral shaft likewise require referral to the orthopedic surgeon. Often with femoral fractures a tremendous amount of soft tissue bleeding occurs so that the patient may become hypovolemic and shock may occur during the period of transfer. For this reason, patients with fractures of the femur should always have intravenous fluids started and the fracture should be stabilized as well as possible prior to transfer.

ARTHRITIS

The knee is one of the most common joints in the body to be involved with arthritis. Because of its small size and relative mechanical instability the joint is prone to early development of wear and tear changes. These usually occur in the medial compartment because of the greater amount of weight-bearing on this side. The loss of joint surface in the medial compartment results in an increasing amount of varus deformity, which further increases the weight-bearing load on this side and exaggerates or accelerates the development of degenerative changes. Similarly, in individuals with a lateral insertion of the tibial tubercle and a lateral subluxation of the patella, degenerative changes in the patellofemoral joint may occur . These changes may become quite severe and may constitute the major focus of arthritic changes in the joint.

The patients seen for the first time with mild to moderate degenerative changes should be placed on a conservative management program. The stress of weight-bearing should be diminished. This requires weight reduction in the overweight patient and abstinence from activities that require prolonged and stressful weight-bearing on the knee. These features alone may considerably improve the symptoms. External support should be used, including nonrigid elastic support that gives some compression to the joint and helps to limit effusion in the joint. In the more severe cases actual support with various types of knee cage braces may be indicated. The use of a cane during an acute episode will markedly diminish the amount of weight borne on the joint and this should be encouraged. The use of a cane or a single crutch in the opposite hand will decrease weight-bearing stress. Properly used, the cane and the involved extremity are used simultaneously (thereby sharing the weight) and then the good leg is used as the involved leg and the cane are brought forward again. This may markedly improve the patient's symptoms and should be used at least during the acute episode.

The building up of intrinsic support is the keystone of treatment of the knee damaged by arthritic process. The patient should be shown a quadriceps exercise program, preferably using a sandbag in the following manner. The patient should sit on the side of a table or stable platform so that his legs swing free over the side, and the knees are flexed to 90 degrees. The sandbag, usually weighing approximately 4 lb, is attached to the foot. The patient then gradually extends the foot and the weight out to 0 degrees of extension, holds the extended position for a few seconds, and then gradually releases it back down to the 90 degree flexed position. This should be done in sets of 25 and the patient should strive to complete six sets (150 times). This can be done twice daily without difficulty. If the knee is very painful it may be necessary to start out with a smaller weight, but it should be possible to get up to 4 lb as a plateau. Probably no other single form of treatment will do as much to improve the pain of a knee involved with degenerative arthritis or rheumatoid arthritis.

Injection with methylprednisolone is thought to be undesirable in most cases. During an acute episode, with acute fluid formation and severe pain, the knee should be aspirated. If it has not been recently injected with steroids, a small dose (40 to 80 mg) may be instilled into the joint in an effort to reduce the acute synovial reaction. This injection, however, should not be repeated for many months since it has been well documented that repeated injections of hydrocortisone into the joint may result in neurotrophic changes and joint destruction with a Charcot-type picture. For this reason the injection of steroids should be only an emergency procedure for the acutely inflamed and swollen joint. When the patient does have a joint injection for an acute episode he should be immediately started on all the procedures as described previously and should be told that another injection will not be done in the near future.

Anti-inflammatory steroids give a considerable amount of improvement in many patients. Some patients do not tolerate these medications and some patients do not respond to them so they are far from 100 percent successful. It should usually be tried, however, using the medication the practitioner is most familiar with. If no results are achieved or if sensitivity develops the patient should be treated accordingly.

Finally, the use of heat in all forms usually improves the joint symptoms. Hydrotherapy seems to be quite soothing, but the use of various heat-producing medications at bedtime with the leg wrapped in a towel usually provides a considerable amount of relief, particularly from morning stiffness. The patient should be cautioned to prevent hyperreactivity of the skin.

As the patient progresses to the point where conservative management is no longer successful, he should be referred to the orthopedic surgeon for consideration of surgical intervention. The use of the upper tibial osteotomy to correct the weight-bearing line has been described previously and is still used, particularly in younger patients. Total knee joint replacement has become quite popular in recent years and is generally extremely successful. It is not within the scope of this chapter to discuss the various facets of the total joint replacement; the patient should be referred to the orthopedic surgeon if it is a consideration.

RHEUMATOID DISEASE

Rheumatoid disease often involves the knee joint and results in a severe synovial reaction during the earlier stages. It ultimately will become much more boggy, with varying amounts of joint effusion. The joint is much more likely to be hot and tender to pressure, which occurs in the degenerative joint only during the acute exacerbations.

Treatment of the knee involved with rheumatoid disease is not much different in the early stages from that described for conservative management of degenerative joint disease. This, of course, should be individualized and the patient should be on appropriate medication for the rheumatoid disease. The one difference in treatment in the earlier stages is that a knee that develops a chronic synovial reaction, and is continuously swollen with varying amounts of fluid, should be considered a candidate for synovectomy before joint destruction has occurred. Synovectomy of the knee joint is extremely successful early in the course of rheumatoid involvement of this joint and often will cause a long remission. Immediately following the resection of the synovium the patient should be started on vigorous exercise programs and be restored to the conservative management program described.

When joint destruction has become severe and the patient has developed irretrievable damage to the joint, he should be referred to the orthopedic surgeon for consideration of total joint replacement. This is an extremely gratifying operation in most cases.

14

THE ANKLE

General Observations	**Sprains**
Anatomy and Function	**Fractures**
X-Ray Examination	**Arthritis**

GENERAL OBSERVATIONS

The ankle is unique in the musculoskeletal system for several reasons. It is a weight-bearing joint with a relatively small area of weight-bearing surface: when each step is taken the entire body weight is placed on a relatively small articular surface area between the talus and the lower end of the tibia (Fig. 14-2). This results in a considerable amount of pressure per square inch and allows for wear, particularly if the joint has been injured and has incongruous surfaces. The ankle joint has no muscular support like that of the knee or hip joint and relies instead entirely upon its mechanical structure and ligamentous support for stability. The joint is, in fact, very tightly constrained. Superiorly, it is an inverted "U" structure comprised of the inferior surface of the talus along with the medial and lateral malleoli. Into this inverted "U" the talus fits, with articular surfaces on both the superior and lateral surfaces (Fig. 14-2). Thus the ankle joint has only motion in extension and flexion and no lateral motion whatsoever; this is prevented by the constraining features of the two malleoli. Since the inverted "U"-shaped superior joint surface is comprised of two separate bones, an additional chance for instability occurs with disruption of the supporting ligamentous structures that hold the tibia and fibula together.

ANATOMY AND FUNCTION

This joint is enclosed by a very stout capsule that envelops the entire joint and has enough laxity both anteriorly and posteriorly to allow considerable flexion and extension of the joint. The joint is supported on either side by ligamentous structures. On the medial side the basic ligamentous structure is the deltoid ligament, which attaches from the tip of the medial malleolus to the underlying talus. This short, thick ligament is so strong that it seldom ruptures as

219

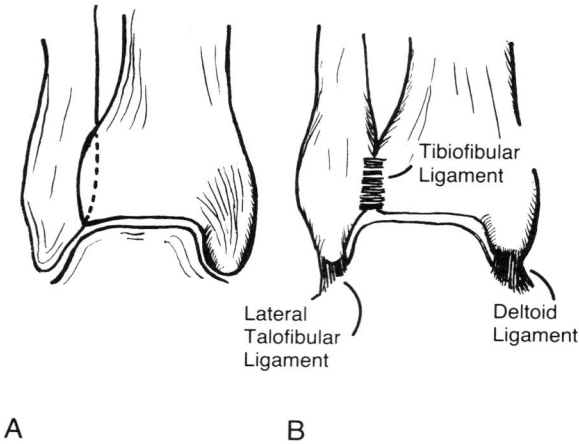

Lateral
Talofibular
Ligament

Tibiofibular
Ligament

Deltoid
Ligament

A   B

Fig. 14-1. (A) The true AP view of the ankle joint, indicating that there is some overlap of the fibula by the tibia, since the latter lies somewhat behind. **(B)** With the AP view taken in 15 degrees of internal rotation, the true ankle mortise can be seen as well as the integrity of the tibiofibular ligament holding the distal tibia and fibula together.

an isolated feature. Rupture can, in fact, only occur if the support on the opposite side of the ankle is disrupted, such as with a complete tear of the lateral collateral ligament or a fracture of the fibula in the joint line. For the most part, however, the deltoid is quite strong; since the foot is usually injured more by inversion forces the deltoid ligament is seldom the site of injury.

The lateral collateral ligament is more often torn, resulting in instability of the ankle joint. There are two separate ligamentous systems on the lateral aspect of the ankle. The collateral ligament attaching from the tip of the lateral malleolus to the talus forms the true lateral supporting structure of the ankle. Along with this accessory ligaments occur anteriorly (Fig. 14-1). These are often torn in the usual sprain of the ankle that occurs with the foot in plantar flexion. Even though these ligaments are the ones usually injured in the average "sprain," this does not result in a loss of instability of the ankle joint.

The third set of important ligamentous structures stabilize the articulation between the distal fibula and the talus. These very strong ligamentous structures are quite short and are torn only with difficulty. However, when tear does occur with loss of stability, a separation of the fibula and tibia occurs, resulting in widening of the ankle "mortise." Loss of stability and severe alteration of the ankle joint mechanisms follow. Long-standing widening of ankle mortise with hypermobility of the talus within the mortise usually results in degenerative changes in the joint.

The other important structures around the ankle joint are the tendinous structures. Medial stability is aided by the posterior tibial tendon and the peroneals provide additional stability laterally. These structures provide stability of the body when balanced on the foot when standing or walking. They also give a certain amount of additional support to the ankle joint. The very strong tendo Achilles posteriorly prevents dislocation of the ankle joint in acute dorsiflexion of the foot by its restraining nature posteriorly. The tibialis anterior tendon,

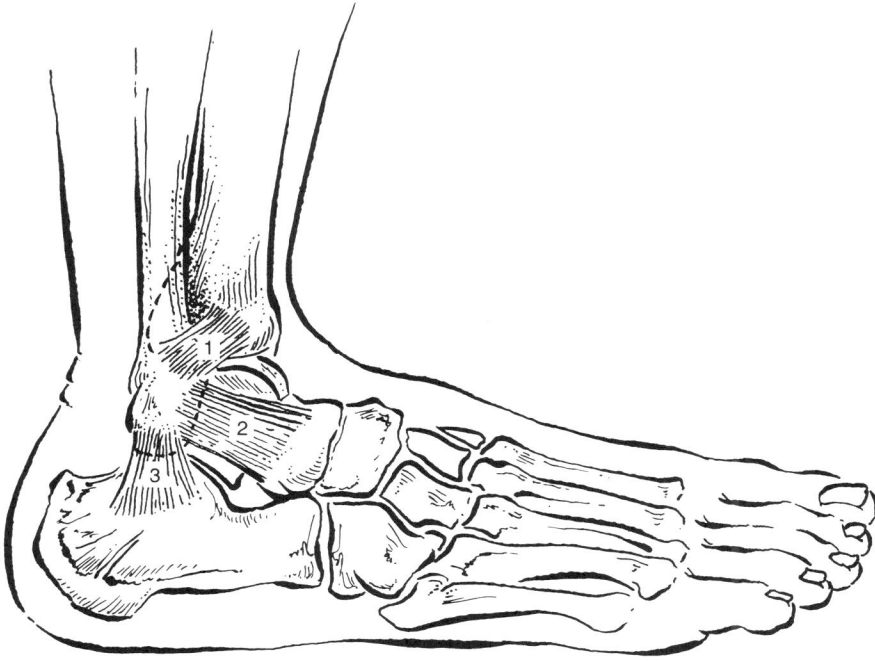

Fig. 14-2. Lateral view of the ankle shows the various ligamentous structures that may be injured in an ankle "sprain." These consist of the (1) tibiofibular, (2) talofibular, and (3) the calcaneofibular ligaments.

along with the long toe extensors, provide the same restraining effect anteriorly when the foot is placed into forced equinus.

X-RAY EXAMINATION

X-ray examination should always be done in at least the following three positions.

1. An anteroposterior (AP) view with the foot straight.
2. An AP view in approximately 15 degrees of internal rotation so that the fibula, which ordinarily lies lateral and somewhat posterior to the lateral aspect of the tibia, can be rotated exactly parallel to the tibia. Only in this way can the integrity of the distal tibiofibular joint be ascertained and the status of the ankle mortise be determined. As demonstrated in Figure 14-2, the ankle mortise is created by the inverted "U"-shaped structure of the superior joint surface of the ankle which includes the two malleoli. The articular surface of the talus, with its superior and two lateral surfaces, must articulate precisely within this inverted "U." If the "U" is widened by a loss of stability of either the lateral or medial constraining malleoli, or by a separation of the tibia and fibula at the distal tibiofibular joint, the talus does not fit properly and there will be additional space

between the lateral articular margin of the talus and the corresponding malleolus. This indicates a loss of stability and the need for prompt reduction and probably internal fixation.

3. A lateral view will demonstrate the relationship between the superior joint surface of the talus and that of the distal tibia. The width of the joint surface can be ascertained as well as the relationship between these two bones. At that time other structures, such as the subastragalar joint, can be visualized and their integrity evaluated.

The important point on x-ray examination is that a single AP and a lateral view of the ankle are not sufficient; the additional AP view in 15 degrees of internal rotation must be taken to determine adequately the true mechanical status of the ankle joint.

SPRAINS

Since, as indicated previously, the ankle relies almost entirely upon ligamentous structures for its support and stability one would expect injuries to these structures to occur frequently. Sprains of the deltoid ligament, as indicated, seldom occur because the usual injury to the foot occurs with the foot in marked inversion. Injuries to this ligament occur only with the loss of the supporting structures laterally so that the entire foot can be slid laterally with respect to the joint mortise. Sprains of the lateral ligaments occur most frequently and require careful analysis and treatment. As shown in Figure 14-3, there is usually point tenderness over the ligamentous structure that is most acutely injured, even though the entire lateral aspect of the foot and ankle may be quite swollen. If one is careful to apply direct pressure over a relatively small area one can differentiate between acute tenderness over the lateral malleolus, the lateral collateral ligament, or the anterior ligaments of the lateral aspect of the joint. In the individual with an acute sprain with marked swelling over the entire area, this differentiation may be very important in the early stages because the type of treatment to be used depends on the maintenance of stability. If the patient feels exquisite tenderness below the tip of the malleolus at the point shown on Figure 14-3 (location C), one should suspect a complete tear of the lateral collateral ligament. Treat the ankle with immobilization in a plaster cast for at least 6 weeks to heal this supporting structure. If, however, the tenderness is present over the anterior ligamentous structures on the lateral aspect of the ankle (location B), one can be more certain that the sprain involves only the anterior ligaments, which are not important from a structural standpoint. Treatment may be directed more towards control of symptoms and diminution of swelling rather than towards maintaining lateral stability of the ankle.

When one is sure that the injury has occurred only in the anterior ligamentous structures simple treatment with a heavy cotton compressive dressing for a few days will give support and allow the swelling to subside. Early weight-bearing using only an elastic ankle support can be allowed once the swelling and soreness are reduced. During these first few days, even with a severe ligamen-

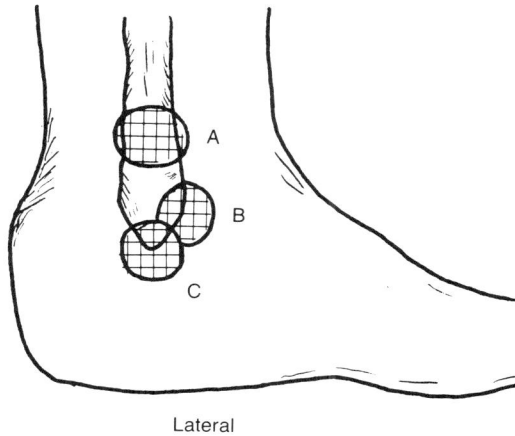

Fig. 14-3. The three diagnostic areas of acute pain to palpation. Location A represents the likelihood of a fracture of the distal fibula, location B represents the area overlying the anterior ligaments and capsule, and location C represents the lateral collateral ligament per se.

Lateral

tous strain, the patient should not bear weight on the ankle. If it is more convenient for the patient to have some weight-bearing instead of using crutches, a walking cast can be applied even though there does not appear to be any compromise in the lateral stability of the ankle. In these instances the cast need only be worn for 3 or 4 weeks instead of the 6 weeks required for complete ligamentous healing.

Treatment of the usual ankle sprain depends entirely upon the presence or absence of lateral stability. If one can determine that the ankle is stable, it is proper to allow early ambulation and to treat the ankle sprain more or less subjectively: non-weight-bearing for a few days in a compressive dressing followed by hot soaks and gradually increased ambulation with an elastic anklet. The usual elastic anklet can be purchased from the drug store but should have an enclosed heel, since this allows for greater comfort and probably gives better stability. The toe of the elastic anklet may be open but the anklet should extend several inches above the malleoli to help control swelling. Twice-daily treatments with hot soaks and/or hot packs will help diminish the swelling and soreness. If the maximum tenderness is at location A (Fig. 14-3) one should suspect a fracture of the fibula.

For repeated or chronic sprains of the lateral aspect of the ankle joint, one should allow the swelling and soreness to subside and then do stress radiographs of the ankle joint. These films are made by holding the lower leg at approximately 15 degrees of internal rotation. While supporting the lower leg with one hand, marked inversion force is placed on the foot to force it into maximum inversion. These radiographs, if normal, should show no change in the relationship of the talus inside of the inverted "U" of the superior ankle joint surface.

If the integrity of the lateral collateral ligament has been lost, the relationship between the talus and the inverted "U" of the ankle joint surface will be lost: the talus will drop out of this close relationship. Chronic ligamentous instability of the lateral aspect of the ankle requires surgical reconstruction by the orthopedic surgeon. This relatively simple operation uses the tendinous structures on the lateral aspect of the ankle and requires approximately 6 weeks of immobilization in a plaster cast postoperatively. These types of operation are ordinarily successful and one can expect to have almost complete restoration of normal function following successful surgery.

Tears of the ligamentous support between the distal fibula and the tibia occur ordinarily with other ligamentous damage or with fractures and result in a loss of the tight fit of the "U"-shaped superior joint surface and the talus. With a separation of the fibula and tibia, this "U"-shaped structure widens so that the stability of the fit of the talus within the structure is lost. A lateral instability of the talus will then occur that can be demonstrated by sliding it back and forth between the two malleoli. When tears of this ligament are demonstrated clinically, surgical repair by metallic fixation across this joint is mandatory. Since tears of this ligamentous support almost invariably are associated with other injuries, the entire ligamentous integrity of the ankle should be restored surgically at the same time.

FRACTURES

Fractures in the ankle joint are usually limited to the lateral or medial malleoli or, less commonly, to compression-type fractures to the superior joint surface or fractures of the talus (Fig. 14-4).

Fractures of the medial malleolus may occur in three basic locations; the location of the fracture determines the treatment.

Fractures at location E in Figure 14-4 occur at the tip of the malleolus. They result from avulsion of the attachment of the deltoid ligament or a small fracture through the bone that occurs when the ligament is stronger and resists tear. These fractures are quite stable. If they are not displaced, they may be treated by immobilization in a short-leg plaster cast with weight-bearing by means of a heel or cast shoe for approximately 6 weeks.

Fractures at location D through the base of the malleolus result in a loss of integrity of the medial aspect of the ankle joint, since the talus along with the medial malleolus can slide medially. This results in loss of integrity of the inverted "U"-shaped superior articular surface. These fractures are extremely unstable. Even when they heal without internal fixation, healing time is prolonged and nonunion is common. For this reason, internal fixation is usually recommended. The operative procedure required in open reduction and internal fixation using a single screw is relatively simple, healing occurs quite promptly (usually in 8 weeks), and almost invariably healing *does* occur with solid bony union. For this reason, almost all of these fractures should be treated by open reduction and internal fixation with a screw.

Fractures at location C occur in the distal tibia and often involve the weight-bearing portion of the articular surface of the distal tibia. Some that are not displaced and have no disruption of the joint surface may be treated by immobilization alone. However, if any separation at the fracture site has occurred and if

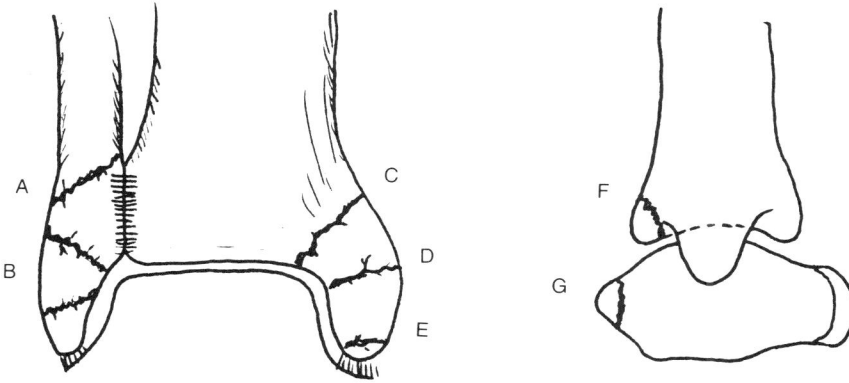

Fig. 14-4. Fractures of the ankle classified on the lateral side as to whether they lie above the tibiofibular synchondrosis (A) or below (B). On the medial malleolus location, C represents a fracture occurring up into the body of the tibia itself with entrance into the joint space past the angle in the joint surface, at the base of the medial malleolus. Location D represents a true medial malleolar fracture, which occurs usually at the base. Location E represents a small avulsion fracture in which the deltoid ligament attachment has been avulsed. On the lateral view, location F represents a fracture of the "posterior malleolus" with avulsion of the capsular attachment of the posterior tibia. Location G represents a "red herring" in which an os astragulare is often mistaken for a fracture of the posterior aspect of the astragulus or talus.

there is any disruption of the common contour of the weight-bearing surface of the superior ankle surface, open reduction should be done to restore it and ensure healing. These fractures have large surfaces and occur in cancellous bone, so healing is usually prompt.

Fractures of the lateral malleolus have similar implications for treatment. Fractures just at the tip (location B) are uncommon since the ligamentous structure usually tears rather the bone fracturing. However, when it does occur and the reduction is good, treatment by immobilization alone will usually result in solid bony union. When, however, the fracture occurs up in the fibula (location A) with involvement of the integrity of the lateral malleolus, consideration should be given to open reduction and internal fixation. Leaving an offset or widening of the lateral malleolus results in widening of the ankle mortise and the instability described previously. Since fractures of the lateral malleolus are ordinarily oblique or spiral, one must be careful to recognize offsets and widening of the ankle mortise. This fracture is usually oblique in the sagittal plane so it is often better evaluated on the lateral view. If this is seen to occur an open reduction is mandatory.

Fractures of the distal fibula that occur above the joint line can often be treated nonoperatively by immobilization in a plaster cast. Since these do not involve the integrity of the joint mortise, complete anatomical reduction is not required.

The rule of thumb, then, as in the other structures around the ankle should be that fractures resulting in loss of stability of the lateral aspect of the ankle joint should be reduced and internal fixation used. Fractures that do not result in a loss of the integrity of the lateral aspect of the ankle joint may be treated by closed reduction and immobilization in a plaster cast alone.

In the lateral view, fractures of the "posterior malleolus" (location F) are seen usually with hyperextension injuries of the ankle and may be associated with fractures of the lateral and medial malleoli, the so-called trimalleolar fracture. Fractures of the posterior malleolus reduce spontaneously when the foot is brought into dorsiflexion and seldom need internal fixation. Apparent fractures at location G usually represent an anatomical variation called the os astragulare and need no treatment.

ARTHRITIS

Arthritis of the ankle joint occurs relatively frequently in the form of both degenerative joint disease and rheumatoid disease. The ankle is frequently involved with rheumatoid disease and since it is a weight-bearing joint with poor supporting structures and with a relatively small weight-bearing surface, marked involvement of the ankle can be quite disabling. In the early stages, a synovectomy can sometimes be done to remove the diseased synovium and stop the progression of the rheumatoid granulation tissue, which actually destroys joint cartilage. In later stages of the disease, however, with complete joint destruction, either an arthrodesis of the joint may be necessary or consideration given to total joint replacement. Arthrodesis of the ankle joint, contrary to popular belief, is not a greatly disabling procedure since it removes only ankle joint motion. If the patient has a good subastragalar joint, flexibility of the foot is not greatly disturbed. The patient usually does quite well with restoration of complete stability to the ankle and complete relief of pain. Solid arthrodesis of the ankle, however, does require some months to achieve after surgery and prolonged immobilization in plaster is often necessary.

Total joint replacement, on the other hand, is usually quite successful in the ankle joint. A number of different prostheses have been developed. For the most part they consist of restoration of one joint surface with high-density polyethylene and the other with stainless steel. Both components are cemented in place with methyl methacrylate. The clinical results following total joint replacement have generally been quite good.

Degenerative joint disease occurs less frequently than would be imagined considering the poor mechanical design of the ankle joint. When degenerative disease does occur in the ankle it is often associated with alterations of joint congruity following trauma, or in grossly overweight patients. The general supportive treatment consists of elastic support, heat, medication, and weight reduction. These will suffice most of the time. If the patient is severely disabled, consideration may be given to either arthrodesis or a total joint replacement as described previously.

15

THE FOOT

ANATOMY AND FUNCTION

The foot has the unusual duty of serving not only as the end point of weight-bearing of the body but also as the primary propelling mechanism in gait. When one stands erect with the feet evenly spaced, a weight-bearing line is created down through the tibia, talus, and calcaneous to the floor. The foot creates two lever arms working through the ankle joint. The posterior limb extends from the central weight-bearing line to the tip of the os calcis; the anterior lever arm extends from the weight-bearing arm to the metatarsal heads (Fig. 15-1). The most powerful mover of the foot is the group of muscles ending in the attachment of the tendo Achilles to the calcaneous. This powerful motor group acts to pull the heel proximally and creates the mechanical advantage of a lever arm working through the fulcrum at the ankle joint. Even though this lever arm is shorter than the anterior, the very strong powerful gastrocnemius—soleus group acting through the tendo Achilles is able to force the foot into the equinus position, even bearing the entire weight of the body. This mechanism is essential in normal gait and in propulsion of the body but creates a tremendous tension force at the point of attachment of the tendo Achilles to the os calcis. It also creates a tremendous pressure point across the metatarsal head arch as the foot is forced into plantarflexion or equinus, bearing the weight of the body.

The anterior lever arm extending from the fulcrum of the ankle joint out to

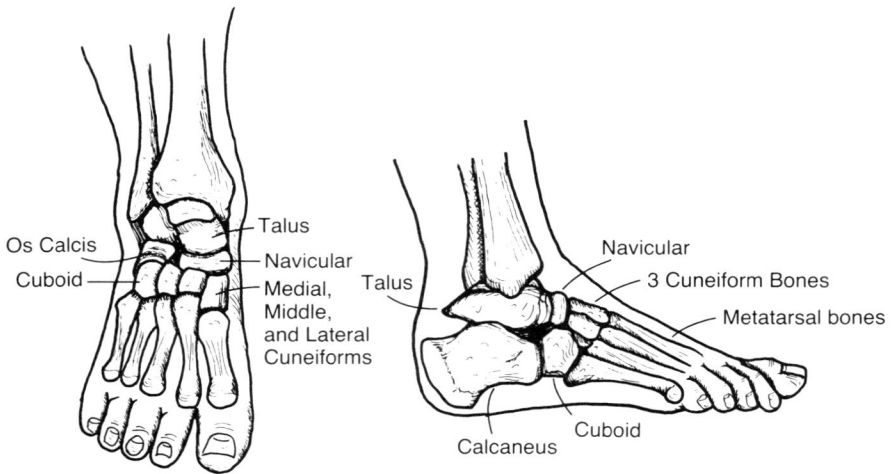

Fig. 15-1. Normal skeletal relationships in the foot and ankle.

the metatarsal head arch is involved basically with dorsiflexion or extension of the foot. This is achieved not by a single muscle, as the posterior motivating force is, but by a combination of muscles acting each in its various way to create a composite force to pull the foot in a balanced direction proximally with the rotation at the ankle joint. Whereas the motivating force posteriorly acts at the very end of the lever arm, the motivating forces anteriorly act partially through pull activated through the end of the lever arm at the metatarsal heads and partially through the function of the tibialis anterior, which attaches not at the end of the lever arm but approximately half way out to the end. Since the tibialis anterior is the strongest of the muscle groups, it loses much of its power by inserting proximal to the end of lever arm. It also loses a considerable amount of its power by attaching far medially on the foot so that it becomes a foot inverter as well as a foot dorsiflexor. The long extensors of the toes, which form the other part of the extensor mechanism of the ankle, do attach near the end of the lever arm at the metatarsal head area but extend through the area to the distal phalanges of the toes without a firm attachment at the metatarsal head area.

As long as the balance of the foot is proper between flexors and extensors of the toes, and as long as the foot extensors are capable of doing their job without difficulty, these toe extensors (both long and short) function quite well in their action as foot elevators or extensors. However, any disruption of this finely adjusted mechanism results in abnormal pull through the toes with resulting deformity. As an example, the loss of power in the dorsiflexing mechanism ordinarily results in an acute flexion deformity of the toes as the toe extensors attempt to pull through against mechanical disadvantage. By overpulling, a turned up position of the toe results from attempting to dorsiflex the foot. This is probably one of the most common causes of hammer toe formation.

One of the most common attitudes of the foot with dorsiflexor weakness in the tibialis anterior group is the so-called claw foot: all five toes become acutely flexed as the toe extensors attempt to add additional force to their effort at dorsiflexion. This force is transmitted through the tendon out to the distal phalanx so that an acute hammer toe deformity occurs. This constitutes the basis of the tendon transfers in poliomyelitis residuals known as the Hibb's-Jones transfers: the extensor of the great toe is translocated into the neck of the first metatarsal bone while the long toe extensors of the other four toes are translocated en masse into the dorsum of the foot. By this means the strength of these muscles is markedly improved since extension of the toes is removed from their action. At the same time the toes are no longer pulled into this clawing deformity since the long extensors are not pulling through them in an effort to dorsiflex the foot.

Another important feature in the general function of the foot is the unique function of the subtalar or subastragalar joint. This joint is comprised of two different sections but has as its single function the movement of the foot from lateral to medial in the coronal plane. Other than some yielding to stress, there is virtually no other motion in the subastragalar joint. The ankle joint then provides, by its hingelike movement, the flexion and extension of the foot without regard to lateral motion. The subastragular joint supplies lateral motion in both directions without regard for flexion and extension. This allows the considerable amount of flexibility that remain in the foot following fusion of the ankle joint. It also is the reason why the foot can still flex and extend through the ankle joint even with a subastragalar fusion. However, the patient does lose a considerable amount of flexibility of the foot so that he is no longer able to walk comfortably on uneven ground, even though his locomotion and normal function in walking remain unchanged. Since weight-bearing occurs through the metatarsal head area, the toes may be used in a completely extended position and not alter their flexion in propulsion as long as the metatarsal phalangeal joint is still functional. This composite function of plantarflexion of the foot caused by the gastrocnemius, with the additional power created by flexion of the toes, provides propulsion of the foot in locomotion.

A final word concerning balance. Since the foot is not nearly a large enough foundation to support the body were it not for the effects of the supporting musculature, it follows that the interplay between the anterior and posterior muscle groups provides the "guy wire" effect necessary to support the perpendicular skeleton on the relatively small foot. In the normal individual this balance between the foot extensors and dorsiflexors is adequate in any position to maintain a good solid foundation and prevent collapse of the foot. If there is any change in this delicate balance, various alterations in stability and gait will occur.

In addition to the anterior and posterior stability in the sagittal plane, the foot must be supported medially since by its very design the foot is arranged to act as a weight-bearing surface from the heel along the lateral margins of the foot curving around onto the metatarsal heads. This supporting mechanism is furnished by the tibialis posterior muscle with a small amount of help from the flexor hallucis longus. The posterior tibial muscle, by its point of insertion, acts as a "ridge pole" through the longitudinal arch of the foot, holding up the central part of the foot and allowing weight-bearing on the heel and metatarsal heads. It would immediately follow, then, that this muscle is important in maintaining the integrity of the longitudinal arch and preventing flexible flat foot deformities. It would also follow that in instances of pes planus, seen with eversion of the entire foot toward the lateral side, measures to strengthen or tighten the posterior tibial muscle constitute the foundation of treatment. Exercises that strengthen the posterior tibial muscle will often considerably improve the flat foot, particularly in the youngster. Even though the foot is not improved cosmetically there is invariably symptomatic improvement in the individual who has pain in the foot because of pes planus. These exercises will be discussed in greater detail in the section on flat foot.

CONGENITAL DEFORMITIES

Webbed Toes

Ordinarily there is no functional loss from webbing of the toes and no treatment is necessary. Many parents will confront the family physician with demands that the foot be operated on and the toes separated. They should be counseled that the toes can be surgically separated but that the operative procedure does not warrant the end result since the toes will most likely not cause any problem. On the other hand, they should be told that as growth occurs there may sometimes be an inequal amount of growth in the toes that are webbed. There then occurs a rotatory deformity from one toe outgrowing the opposite one in the syndactyly. In this instance treatment will be necessary and the patient should be referred to an orthopedic surgeon for treatment. Even in this instance, the toes will usually not be separated but the elongated toe will be shortened back to match its companion and the deformity eradicated. There are other types of malformations of toes and many of these assume somewhat greater proportion than is acceptable. These instances, however, require expert opinion and the patient should be referred to an orthopedic surgeon for appropriate treatment.

Calcaneovalgus Deformity

The calcaneovalgus deformity, in which the foot is acutely dorsiflexed and lies anterior to the tibia, is relatively common. Many youngsters are born with varied amounts of calcaneovalgus deformity since, as the foot is brought up into acute dorsiflexion, a certain amount of valgus accommodates the change in position of the ankle. Most of mild calcaneovalgus deformities do not require treatment other than by stretching by the mother two or three times daily. She can be taught the simple measures of stretching the foot into equinus and varus. If she does this faithfully approximately ten times, twice daily, most such children will recover without difficulty.

In the cases that are more refractive to treatment or that seem to be severe enough that manually stretching alone will not suffice, the application of Dennis-Browne splints early in the youngster's life will usually correct the deformity without much difficulty. The Dennis-Browne splints should be attached to small

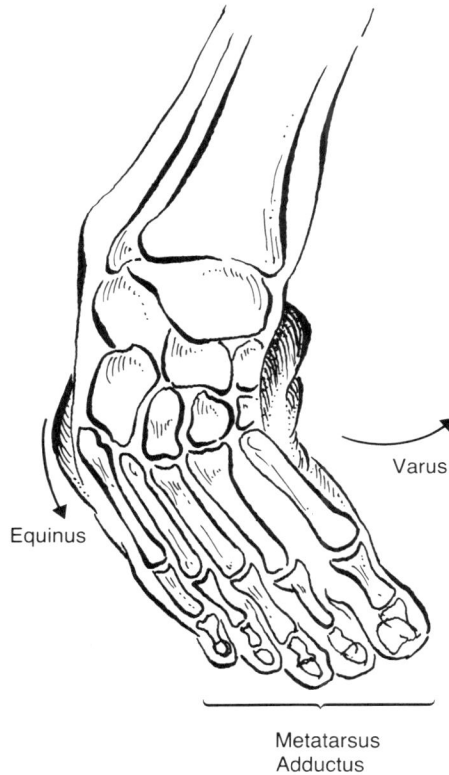

Fig. 15-2. Typical club foot has three major components: equinus deformity with the toes pointing down; varus deformity with the entire foot being inverted, or rolled inward; and metatarsus adductus, in which all of the metatarsal bones are deviated medially.

shoes so that the feet can be well attached. Care must be taken to avoid having the brace bar too long, since the feet will tend to slip out of the shoes rather easily. The average length of the bar in a newborn or young infant will be 8 inches or less. The bar should be bent very slightly so that the foot is in a minimal amount of varus to help compensate for the tendency to valgus associated with the severe calcaneal foot. If the foot does not respond promptly to stretching and/or the application of Dennis-Browne splints, the child should be referred to an orthopedic surgeon for further evaluation. Some cases of severe calcaneovalgus foot may include bands of abnormal tarsal coalition that will preclude response to these stretching procedures. The vast majority of cases of calcaneovalgus foot deformity in the newborn, however, have a benign problem that responds very well to the treatment described.

Club Foot

The typical equino varus club foot has three primary components (Fig. 15-2). Each is present to a greater or lesser degree, but in the severe club foot deformity all three of the deformities are profound. First, the foot is held in a marked equinus so that the ankle cannot be brought up to anywhere near a neutral position. Second, there is a marked varus so that the foot curls inward and often the deformity may be so severe that the sole of the foot is actually pointing cephalad. The third part of the deformity is a metatarsus adductus. The typical picture in a severe club foot deformity includes a tiny foot extended with the toes pointing downward and rolled so as to form a C-shaped deformity. The majority of the hindfoot is present in the severe varus deformity and the forefoot adductus continues the deformity by creating the anterior part of the "C." Along with these features the child with a club foot will have a prominent smallness of calf on the involved side. This is, of course, not of great importance in the bilateral deformity since the calves will be equal though small. However, in the unilateral involvement the smallness of the calf may constitute a considerable cosmetic deformity as the child grows older even though the club foot is completely corrected.

The pathology involved is basically severe soft tissue contracture on the medial aspect of the foot along with an extremely tight heel cord. However, intrauterine growth occurring in face of this soft tissue deformity causes accommodation of the bones of the foot so that the newborn has both bony and soft tissue deformity.

The time to begin treatment of the club foot deformity is soon after birth. Most orthopedic surgeons will want to wait a week or so until the skin has stabilized in its new nonaqueous environment. A cast should be applied as soon as the skin appears to be stable to withstand its application. The treatment of club foot deformities is a very specialized procedure and these patients should be referred to the orthopedic surgeon as soon as the club foot deformity is discovered at birth. A very high percentage of these will respond to periodic casting; most of the time at least the varus and the equinus deformity can be corrected by this mechanism. Occasionally the metatarsus adductus will persist despite casting, though when the casting is begun early and done properly the majority of youngsters respond well to nonoperative correction of the deformity. Later on, if the varus deformity is persistent, if a totally uncorrectable equinus deformity occurs, or if the foot becomes corrected in plaster but the deformity recurs after the plaster is removed, surgical intervention may be necessary. This, of course, will depend upon the judgement of the treating surgeon. The family may be reassured, however, that in most instances the foot deformity can be completely corrected so that an essentially normal foot can be achieved. The problem of the smallness of the calf, however, should be discussed early and the parents made aware of this persistent deformity.

STATIC CONDITIONS OF VARIOUS ETIOLOGIES
Longitudinal Arch Problems

A longitudinal arch is not mandatory for a good, stable, comfortable foot. Lack of a good longitudinal arch is a characteristic of many races and most members of these groups go through life without any serious foot problems (Fig. 15-3). However, when the loss of a longitudinal arch is associated with the

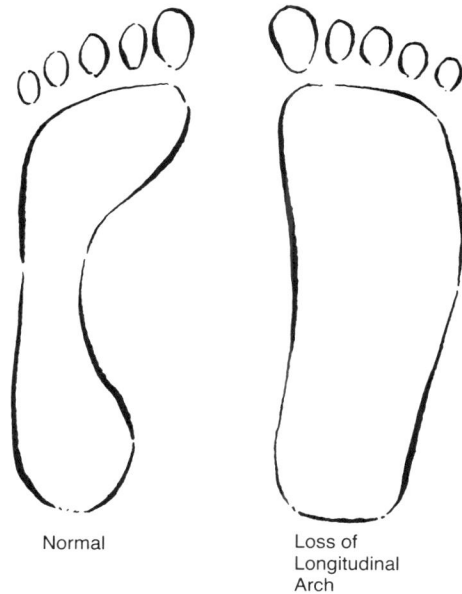

Fig. 15-3. Imprint of the weight-bearing foot shws a loss of the longitudinal arch but no specific indication as to the eversion of the foot. This is a "flat foot" but does not give any indication of the relative position of the hind foot.

Normal

Loss of Longitudinal Arch

tendency of the foot to evert, the foot becomes structurally unsound and the likelihood of painful symptoms is much greater (Fig. 15-4).

All infants are born without a visible longitudinal arch and for the most part do not develop an arch that can be seen until about the fourth year. Until that time parents need to be reassured that their child has otherwise essentially normal foot development as long as the foot is structurally normal. The arch begins to develop as do the supporting structures of the longitudinal arch: the plantar fascia and, of greater importance, the supporting effect of the tibialis posterior muscle. If the longitudinal arch then does develop in a normal manner the foot assumes a two point base of support: the tuberosity of the os calcis at the heel and the transverse metatarsal head arch anteriorly. It is upon these structures that the entire weight is carried (Fig. 15-5A).

Patients without a longitudinal arch do not necessarily develop symptoms, as mentioned above. However, the addition of even small increments of eversion of the foot are likely to result in gradually increasing symptoms due to instability. Since many people do develop this additional foot eversion, many people with pes planus (flat foot) experience painful symptoms. Many types of treatment have been devised in the past, most of which are at least somewhat effective. The basic treatment, of course, is support of the foot with a longitudinal arch support (Fig. 15-5B). These are commonly called "oval pads" and are either made of very firm sponge rubber or some type of piano felt. The support is fitted so that the medial aspect fits against the side of the shoe and then the pad is shaved off around its margin so that it feathers out into the normal insole of the shoe. Oval pads of this type should be cemented into place or added to a properly shaped

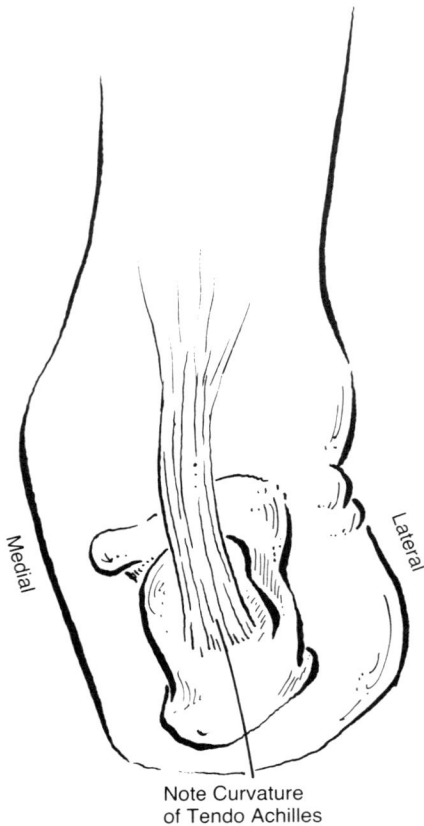

Medial

Lateral

Note Curvature
of Tendo Achilles

Fig. 15-4. Posterior view of the weight-bearing foot shows eversion. This may give a weight-bearing imprint, as seen in Figure 15-3, since the additional mechanical instability occurs because of the abnormal weight-bearing line.

insert so that the pad will be in the proper position each time the shoe is worn. If the painful foot syndrome is associated also with metatarsalgia or pain over the weight-bearing metatarsal head, addition of an anterior so-called Morton's pad to the complex will place the weight-bearing somewhat behind the metatarsal heads and allow greater comfort. (Fig. 15-5C). The combination of oval pads with anterior Morton's pads has been combined into a single pad known as the "Dixon and Dively inlay" (D & D inlay) (Fig. 15-5D). Again, these pads should be cemented into the shoe permanently or fashioned into an inner sole that correctly fits the shoe heel so that the pad is always in the proper position in the shoe. Otherwise, it may not only be ineffective but also uncomfortable to wear.

Along with the static "propping up" of the flat foot, additional dynamic exercises may be done to give intrinsic support. An exercise program to support the longitudinal arch of the foot often relieves symptoms of the painful flat foot without changing the outward appearance of the foot. Two exercises seem to be most effective and should be done twice daily with each foot. The first exercise strengthens the tibialis posterior muscle. The foot is placed in a position of some equinus with rather marked inversion and held in this position for five counts. The position can be imitated passively by pressing on the base of the little toe, inward and downward, and then actively holding the foot in this position with

Cross-Sectional View of Pads

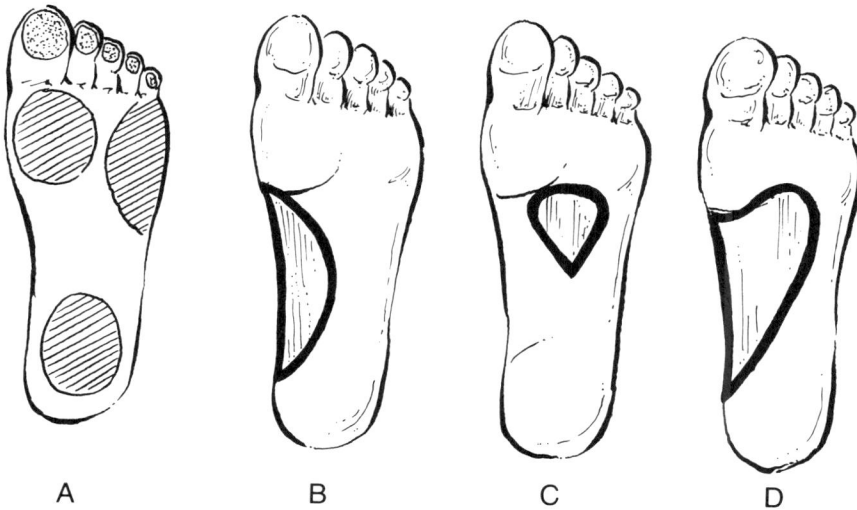

Fig. 15-5. (A) Weight-bearing areas of the foot, the greatest of which are seen to be in the heel, first and fifth metatarsal head areas, with a lesser degree on the touchpads of the toes. **(B)** Simple longitudinal pad that supports the longitudinal arch only, as shown by the silhouette of the cross-section. **(C)** Morton pad applies pressure behind the metatarsal heads and is used primarily for metatarsalgia, whether due to pressure over the metatarsal heads or to a plantar neuroma. **(D)** D & D inlay is a combination of the longitudinal pad and the Mortons pad made into a single appliance to give protection to the whole foot.

the posterior tibialis tendon. Even patients as young as 4 years of age can be taught to contract this particular muscle actively in this manner.

The other exercise is to strengthen the tibialis anterior that, though acting as a primary dorsiflexor of the foot, still provides some medial support. From the equinus and inverted position previously described, the foot is brought into a dorsiflexed and inverted position and held there for five counts. Care must be taken in both the posterior and anterior tibial exercises to refrain from contracting the toe flexors or extensors; to be effective, the exercises must isolate the single function of either of the tibial muscles. These two exercises are done for 10 repetitions for each foot, twice daily. It is sometimes impossible to teach younger children both exercises but the more important tibialis posterior exercise is relatively easy for even these youngsters. The importance of this exercise program cannot be overemphasized: it will sometimes completely obviate the symptoms of a painful flat foot even more than the addition of support to the shoe. Proper treatment, however, should include both the passive support of the foot with the pads and the active strengthening of the foot with exercises.

The "painful heel syndrome" that is seen relatively frequently in adults is thought to be due to plantar fasciitis related to the lack of support in the longitudinal arch of the foot. Whereas the plantar fascia attaches to a broad area anteriorly (attaching to all five of the metatarsal head areas), it attaches to a relatively small area posteriorly, just at the margin of the tuberosity of the oscalcis. When repeated stress is placed on the longitudinal arch of the foot the plantar fascia tends to act as a bowstring and increased pressure is placed upon both ends of its attachment. The broader-based anterior attachment seldom gives rise to symptoms. However, the attachment to the os calcis can become extremely painful and often times people with the "painful heel syndrome" are relatively disabled with pain in this area. Treatment of this type of plantar fasciitis depends again, upon strengthening the active support of the foot. The anterior and posterior tibial exercises described previously are the cornerstone of this treatment. The addition of a relatively thin "horseshoe" pad that rings the circumference of the heel but leaves the area of tenderness over the midportion of the heel without pressure on it usually gives considerable symptomatic relief.

Finally, nonsteroidal anti-inflammatory medications usually give considerable relief, since this is an acute fasciitis. If the patient does not respond to the above measures over a reasonable period of time, consideration should be given to the injection of methylprednisolone into this area of attachment of the plantar fascia to the os calcis. Since this is such an extremely painful area and since the injection should be in the form of a "needling" with multiple repeated injections through the area to distribute the steroid evenly, it is extremely difficult to do this under a local anesthesia. A more preferable and more frequently successful method is to ask the anesthesiologist to administer a very short pentothal anesthesia so that the heel can be adequately injected as described above. This can, of course, be done as an outpatient procedure with safety. It makes possible a much more adequate injection than is possible with the almost always incomplete anesthesia obtained from the local anesthetic agent. As mentioned, repetitive puncturing of the attachment of the fascia to the oscalcis is mandatory if one is to distribute the steroid through the inflamed area.

If the patient continues to have severe symptoms of painful heels even after all of these measures, then one should consider surgical sectioning of the plantar fascia. It should be noted that it is not necessary to attack the point of the attachment of the fascia to the oscalcis even though this is the point of symptoms. Instead, a small curved longitudinal incision made in the non-weight-bearing portion of the concavity of the arch will expose the extremely tight plantar fascia. This fascia can be sectioned in its entirety with perhaps a small segment being actually removed. This, in effect, "lengthens" the plantar fascia and releases the extreme tension on the two ends of its attachment. The procedure should be done under a general or regional anesthesia and a convalescent period of 6 to 8 weeks should be anticipated. However, the procedure can be expected to yield almost 100 percent successful results if done properly.

Spastic or Peroneal Flat Foot

In the flexible flat foot (even when painful), the foot may be restored to a normal anatomical position passively when non-weight-bearing. In the case of the spastic flat foot, even in the non-weight-bearing (relaxed) condition the foot cannot be restored to its normal position because of spasm of the peroneal musculature. This has been found to be due to a condition known as "coalition foot," in which a congenital bridge occurs between various of the tarsal bones that alters the basic flexibility of the foot. This then leads to acute peroneal spasm that accounts for the severe symptoms these patients have. The peroneal spastic flat foot will not respond to conservative measures. If this condition is suspected, the patient should be referred to the orthopedist for appropriate radiographs to identify the coalition between the tarsal bones and surgical resection. Occasionally, even subastragalar arthrodesis may be necessary to relieve the symptoms.

Metatarsus Adductus

Metatarsus adductus was described under the section on congenital deformities as being the "front third" of the standard club foot deformity (see Fig. 15-2). However, it often occurs alone without any alteration in the anatomy of the midfoot or hindfoot. When it does occur alone, however, it is much more likely to be neglected from the standpoint of treatment since it does not appear to be as significant a deformity. While it is, in fact, not as severe as a true club foot it does constitute a significant deformity that, if left untreated, results in a considerable amount of difficulty in the adult patient. Radiographs taken with the foot flat on the x-ray plate reveal a marked deviation of all five metatarsal bones toward the medial side of the foot. This deviation apparently occurs at the tarsometatarsal junction. No other significant abnormalities are usually seen.

The foot may be completely correctable passively in the beginning but occasionally the deformity will be so severe that passive correction may not even be possible in the beginning. Early treatment in the infant consists of an application of Dennis-Browne splints. These can be ordered from bracemakers and consist of a bar between the two shoes with a ratchet at the point of attachment on either side so that the rotation of the foot may be set at the desired position with respect to the bar. The bar may, likewise, be bent slightly to alter the inversion or eversion position of the feet. The bar in the infant should be long enough that the diaper can be changed but should not be extremely wide. An average length is 8 to 10 inches and can be determined by measuring with a tape while holding the feet at the desired position. The ratchet on either side then should be set at about 45 degrees external rotation and a very slight amount of eversion. If the deformity is severe it may be better to use a straight-last shoe rather than a regular shoe on the splint. The braces should be worn almost continuously but the mother should be instructed to remove them periodically to massage the feet and to be certain that no pressure areas exist.

The mother should also be taught stretching exercises by which the forefoot is stretched into more abduction with respect to the remainder of the foot. This can be done by holding the heel and foot firmly in one hand while forcing the forefoot over into the abducted position with the opposite hand. These stretching procedures can be done eight or ten times, several times daily. In mild cases the stretching alone may be all that is necessary and the brace may not be indicated.

As the youngster begins to walk and bear weight, he should be fitted with a straight-last shoe. These are obtainable from a bracemaker or corrective shoe store. These are reasonably effective in holding the metatarsal shafts straight with respect to the foot. These shoes should be worn as long as the deformity is noticeable and the stretching procedures previously described should be continued also.

Occasionally, when a foot is completely refractive to conservative management as described, or if an older child is seen for the first time with a relatively severe deformity, consideration should be given to surgical correction and the patient referred to the orthopedic surgeon. The untreated severe metatarsus adductus deformity will result in later bunion formation: the included metatarsus primus varus will result in a hallux valgus as the patient grows older and begins wearing shoes, and the Hallux valgus will result in formation of a painful bunion.

Metatarsus adductus is often associated with internal tibial torsion, so that the child who has begun to walk shows a severe "intoeing" or "pigeon toed" gait. Internal tibial torsion associated with the metatarsus adductus must be treated as a separate entity. If it is not severe it may merely correct spontaneosly with longitudinal growth of the tibia while weight-bearing. If it is quite severe, the patient should be referred to the orthopedic surgeon for possible fitting of a corrective apparatus such as twister splints.

Cavus Foot

The opposite deformity to the flexible flat foot is the cavus foot, which is a developmental abnormality characterized by a very high longitudinal arch. The cavus foot is often a congenital or developmental abnormality but may be associated with various types of neurologic deficits, in which case it is usually associated with clawing of the toes and the characteristic "claw foot" deformity. Cavus deformity, when developmental and not associated with neurologic deficit or other foot deformities, causes symptoms related to the pressure of the binding of the shoe across the high instep. Also, this deformity will often cause pressure phenomena over the metatarsal heads because of the more acute inclination of the metatarsal shafts in the sagittal plane. Most instances of cavus foot are not severe enough to warrant treatment. However, if the symptoms are severe and do not respond to simpler methods of treatment, the patient should be referred to the orthopedic surgeon for possible midtarsal osteotomy.

Claw Foot

The claw foot consists of the cavus deformity of the foot with associated clawing of the toes. This is usually related to some type of neurologic disorder. The child with bilateral clawing of the feet should be worked up neurologically to discover whether some undiagnosed condition such as Friedreich's ataxia, Charcot-Marie-Tooth syndrome, or undiagnosed poliomyelitis might be present. Clawing of the foot often results from loss of dorsiflexor power, so the toe extensors are used to dorsiflex the foot. This results in a severe recurvatum of the metacarpolphalangeal joints of the toes with the resulting flexion deformity of the toes themselves from the countering overtightness of the flexor tendons created by the hyperextension deformities of the proximal joints.

In early instances the patient can be made considerably more comfortable by insertion of Morton's pads in the shoes. This provides pressure behind the metatarsal heads to correct at least some of the claw toe deformity. If, however, these deformities become severe referral to the orthopedic surgeon for surgical correction should be done. Again, when treating these patients with nonoperative management, the family physician must be careful to be certain that no occult neurologic deficit exists.

Metatarsalgia

Metatarsalgia is a catch-all term for conditions resulting in pain across the metatarsal head area. This is usually more severe in the region of the second metatarsal head since it is longer and accepts a greater load during normal weight-bearing. The etiologic factors may be multiple and this condition may be even related to the cavus or claw foot deformity. On the other hand, some of the more frequently causes are obesity and tight heel cords. The extremely heavy person, of course, carries a greater load on the metatarsal head area normally and frequently has symptoms referable to that area. The patient with tight heel cords has a tendency for the foot to remain in equinus. When walking, therefore, a greater amount of pressure is placed on the anterior end of the foot to force it back up into neutral or the dorsiflexed position. Unless the tight heel cords are extremely severe, they should be treated merely by stretching. If, however, the foot cannot be brought up within 15 to 20 degrees of neutral, consideration may be given to surgical heel cord lengthening.

The usual management of metatarsalgia is to provide some way of altering the amount of pressure applied to the metatarsal head. The Morton's pad can often be used. Another commonly used appliance is the transverse metatarsal bar: a strip of leather applied to the sole of the shoe transversely in a position just behind the transverse metatarsal arch. This results in a redistribution of the weight into the relatively nontender area behind the metatarsal heads and usually results in considerable relief of the symptoms. Care must be taken to watch for wearing of these bars, however, since they soon wear down to the level of the sole, in which case they become much less effective.

MISCELLANEOUS CONDITIONS

Ingrown Nails

Ingrown toenails are themselves somewhat painful but the biggest problem concerning ingrown nails is the periodic infections that develop as a result of the trapping of bacteria in the interval between the nail grown into the soft tissue and the soft tissue bed itself (Fig. 15-6A). These bacteria begin to multiply and an infection develops which sometimes is very difficult to treat on a local basis. During the period of infection the nail should be debrided as much as possible so

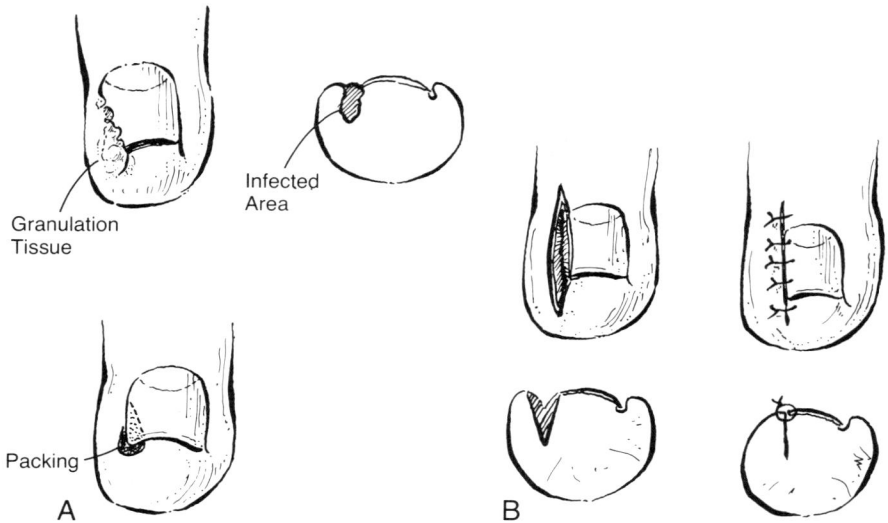

Fig. 15-6. (**A**) A typical ingrown nail with the granulation tissue likely to occur at the point of infection. The cross-sectional view shows the area of the infection in the "gutter." (**B**) Steps in the "gutter" operation for removal of the margin of the nail for total cure of the ingrown nail and the healed foot with absence of the gutter on the involved side.

that the soft tissue elements are removed from over the nail. The tip of the nail then can be very satisfactorily elevated with a small pledget of cotton passed underneath using a small blade or one side of a small forcep (Fig. 15-6A). This cotton soaked in alcohol usually will act as a drying agent and trains the nail to grow out straight, preventing the recurrence of nail ingrowth into the soft tissue. If the infection is quite severe, it may be necessary to resect this protruding part of the nail with the idea of surgically excising the nail later.

Recurrent infections of the nail are usually a cause for resecting the nail margin and the associated gutter. The ingrown nail is considered a "problem of the gutter." Excision of the nail as it extends down into the ungual fold will usually result in a permanent cure (Fig. 15-6B). The surgical procedure for removal of the gutter can be done under local anesthetic if desired. However, complete anesthesia must be present in the toe if the operation is to be done satisfactorily. The skin incision should include the area shown in the lower left of Figure 15-6B which demonstrates the inclusion of the nail fold along with the curved part of the nail. When this defect is closed, as shown on the right in Figure 15-6B, the nail merely comes to a margin that meets the margin of the skin and no "gutter" is present. The incision should be long enough so that you are certain that all nail matrix is removed in the area to be closed. If any matrix cells are left, a spiked remnant of nail is likely to grow out at the base and cause considerable difficulty. If no active infection is present, the healing time is relatively short (10 to 14 days). It is usually recommended that this procedure be done only after the acute infection has subsided so that a primary closure can be accomplished. If the opening is packed, a considerable amount of time is required for healing and often a scar is left that can become painful. Excision of the gutter can be done on both sides of the same nail simultaneously if both sides are involved. It is not necessary to remove a great amount of the body of the nail, but merely that portion that curves over into the ingual gutter.

Onychogryphosis

Badly thickened and deformed nails are characteristically seen in older people and are related to an ungual infection with fungus. This nail will often form the "stag-horn" type of deformity in which the tip of the nail becomes a mere point and rises up so high that it presses on the shoe and causes considerable discomfort. Removing the nail will effect only a relatively short term cure; the nail that grows back soon becomes involved with the same fungus and results in the same deformity, usually within a period of some months. There is no satisfactory treatment of the fungus infection of the nail per se since most of the fungicides do not seem to be effective.

When the nail has become painful and causes a mechanical problem with the toe, total excision of the nail, nail bed, nail base, and a portion of the distal phalanx with closure of the defect with a plantar flap is usually the procedure of choice. This procedure is known as the "terminal Syme" procedure and is shown in Figure 15-7. The procedure can be done on an outpatient basis, but it usually requires an anesthetic that is profound enough in the great toe to allow for the removal of a portion of the phalanx as well as the other material. If care if taken, the flap closure can be very smooth and even quite acceptable cosmeti-

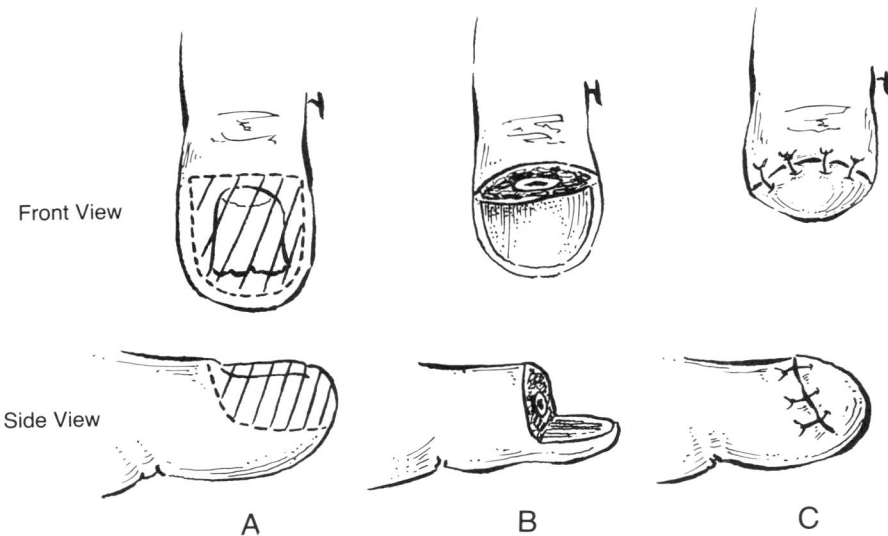

Fig. 15-7. Terminal Syme procedure for chronic deformities of the great toe nail. (**A**) The toe nail along with the matrix is removed and then (**B**) a portion of the distal phalanx is removed so that a flap of plantar skin can be folded over and sutured, (**C**), thereby completely obliterating the nail and creating a smooth great toe.

cally. It is a mistake to leave a large bulbus flap with a wide scar at its point of healing since the scar per se will sometimes rub and cause a pressure callus.

Corns and Calluses

Formation of a corn or a hard clavus, is usually the result of one or more of three factors acting on the area (Fig. 15-8): perspiration, friction, or, pressure.

Perspiration

Excess perspiration of the feet is present in many individuals and it is thought that the repeated cycle of the skin becoming soggy with perspiration and then drying out that creates callus. In individuals with this type of sweating mechanism, callus may be quite extensive and difficult to care for. Most of the time, the callus related to perspiration has some pressure area which allows it to form and, therefore, the relief of the callus is related not only to control of perspiration but also to removing or padding the offending pressure area.

Calluses in themselves are the primary cause of pain. When a callus is present, even over an area of some pressure phenomenon, the pain can be considerably removed by nothing more than removal of the callus itself. This can be shaved away in small layers using a #15 Bard-Parker blade. It can also be removed by the patient to a great extent using the coarse side of a regular emery board. Usually the callus is more responsive to being ground away with an emery board when it is somewhat moistened, such as after being soaked.

The use of a pumice stone has been recommended but it has not been found to be quite as effective as the emery board since it is not as rough. Care must be taken both in the shaving and the filing with the emery board to prevent intrusion upon normal skin that underlies the callus. This skin is often altered in its appearance and microscopic characteristics by the presence of the callus. Once it has been allowed to resume its normal function following removal of the callus, it usually will toughen up quite readily. The use of various solutions, most of which contain salicylic acid, to remove corns is generally inadvisable since these quite often will lead to an acute secondary infection.

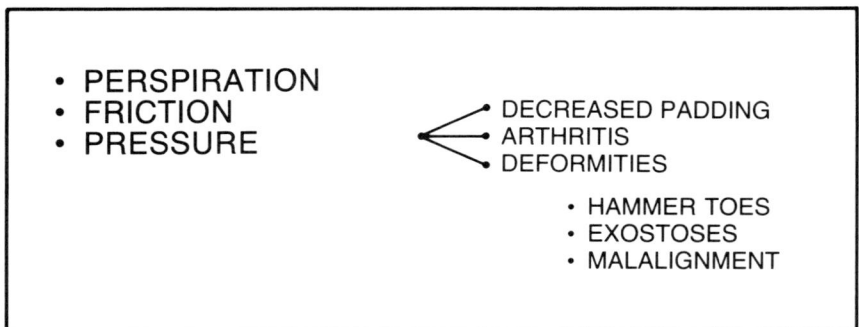

- PERSPIRATION
- FRICTION
- PRESSURE ← DECREASED PADDING / ARTHRITIS / DEFORMITIES
  - HAMMER TOES
  - EXOSTOSES
  - MALALIGNMENT

Fig. 15-8. Factors related to "corn" formation.

The problem with perspiration has often been helped considerably by the use of powdered alum, which can be dusted into the socks or shoes daily. Alum seems to have an astringent effect and results in a considerable decrease in the amount of sweating. Frequent changes of socks and foot gear also seem to help alleviate the problems related to perspiration.

Friction

Calluses caused by friction are usually obviated only by the alleviation of the friction point. The skin in the area can be covered with moleskin, which will absorb the friction and prevent some of the callus formation. Often, however, it is necessary to alter the foot gear to relieve the situation.

Pressure

The pressure phenomena are usually the most common and are related to (1) decreased padding, (2) arthritic changes with marginal lipping of the joints or (3) deformities such as hammer toes, exostosis, or malalignment. It is often necessary to relieve the pressure area surgically by removing the offending exostosis or correcting the deformity. For the most part, patients with static deformities of any extent should be referred to the orthopedic surgeon for possible corrective surgical procedures.

Plantar Wart

An additional type of callus should be discussed since it occasionally is seen: This type of callus occurs in a "plantar wart." It is amazing that many of the calluses seen on the foot are thought to be caused by "plantar warts" and in reality are related only to pressure phenomena or one of the factors mentioned previously. If, when the callus is shaved away, a warty lesion can be seen in the central portion of the callus, this can be considered to be a true plantar wart. However, it is impossible to diagnose a plantar wart until the callus has been removed. Treatment of choice is probably fulguration with an electrocoagulation unit. Care should be taken to avoid deep burns in the foot. If there is any question as to the depth or the extent of the warty lesion, the patient should probably be referred to a specialist for appropriate treatment. Injudicious coagulation or treatment of a plantar wart directly over a major pressure area of the foot will often lead to a painful scar that is just as bad as the wart was prior to its removal. Likewise, if a wart recurs several times consideration should be given to surgical excision. This procedure is not universally successful, so probably the responsibility of removing this recurrent wart should be left up to the orthopedic surgeon.

Hammer Toe

As shown in Figure 15-9, the hammer toe usually creates three pressure areas: (1) under the metatarsal head, (2) over the distal end of the proximal phalanx, and (3) over the tip of the toe. If the toe is not badly deformed, the

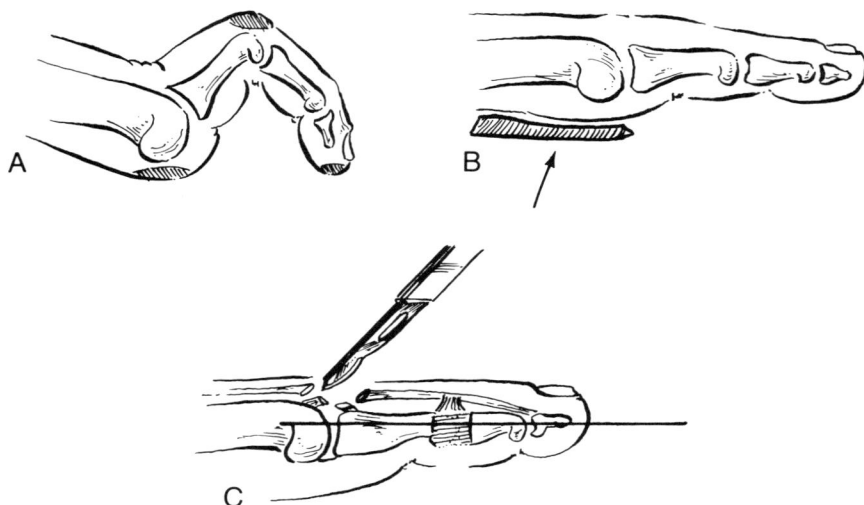

Fig. 15-9. Typical hammer toe deformity. (**A**) Three pressure points in a common hammer toe and the hyperextension of the proximal joint with hyperflexion of the middle joint. (**B**) Correction by pressure with the pad under the metatarsal head results in shortening of the flexor to pull the toe out straight. (**C**) Surgical correction of a hammer toe includes arthrodesis of the middle joint with fixation by means of intermedullary Kirschner wire associated with a dorsal capsulotomy of the proximal joint and sectioning of the long extensor tendons.

addition of a Morton's pad or a pad just behind the metatarsal area will usually result in a stretching of the flexor tendon, which will allow the toe to become straight. If it is not possible to correct a hammer toe by padding surgical correction usually consists of sectioning the dorsal capsule of the proximal joint and usually an arthrodesis of the middle joint of the toe in a position of 0 degrees extension using fixation with a single, longitudinally placed Kirschner wire.

Plantar Neuroma (Morton's Neuroma)

The anatomical arrangement of the plantar nerves causes a condition conducive to the formation of a neuroma between the third and fourth toes. In the interspaces between the first and second, second and third, and fourth and fifth toes there occurs a branch of the respective lateral or medial plantar nerve, with resulting common digital nerve that makes a "Y-type" division into two branches, serving the adjacent sides of the web spaces.

The medial plantar nerve serves the entire great toe, second toe, and third toe. But in the interspace between the third and fourth toe it is joined for a short distance by the corresponding branch from the lateral plantar nerve to create a common digital nerve that then soon divides to serve the adjacent sides of the web space between the third and fourth toes. The connection of these nerves for only a very short distance that results in continued stretching, with the resulting creating of a small neuroma. These neuromas are usually not much larger than a small pea, but once they become large they allow for trapping of the neuroma

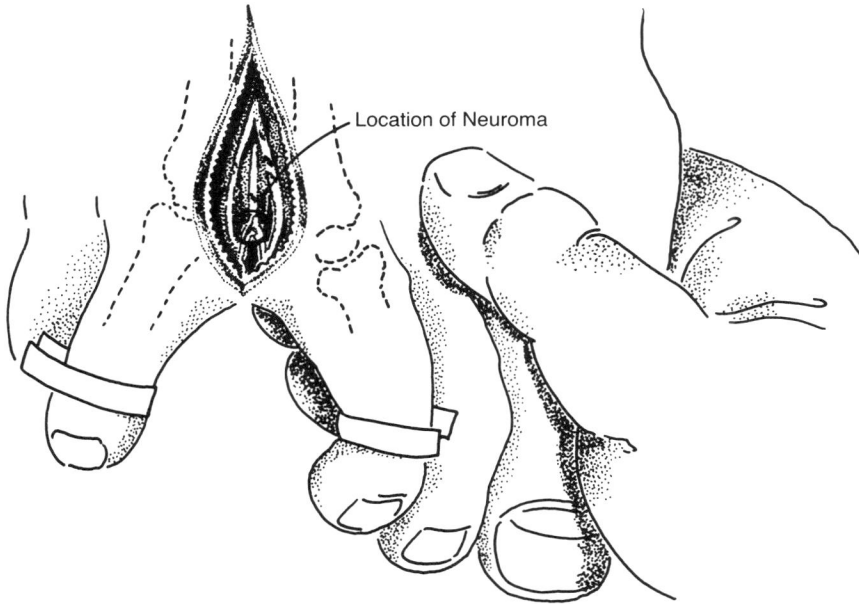

Fig. 15-10. Typical location of a plantar neuroma at the time of surgery. Note the dorsal incision and the rather easy accessibility of the nerve through the dorsal approach.

between the third and fourth metatarsal heads with sometimes exquisite pain.

The symptoms that the patient describes can often afford a diagnosis merely by listening since they are rather characteristic. The patient states that he seldom has pain when walking barefoot but with any shoe on, particularly a tight fitting one, the patient experiences a sudden severe pain with tingling out into the toes. Often, the third and fourth toes cannot be identified specifically but patients will almost always relate that the tingling is in the toes on the lateral side of the foot. The patient will further relate that if he sits down and pulls the shoe off and gently manipulates the lateral side of his foot, the pain suddenly stops. He can then put his shoe back on and walk again until the pain recurs after a variable length of time.

Smaller neuromas can often be successfully treated with the Morton's pad, as previously described. This pad will allow pressure to be exerted behind the metatarsal heads that are separated enough that the small nerve tumor does not become entrapped. However, once the pads will no longer afford good relief, surgical excision should be done. Figure 15-10 shows the small dorsal incision that is made, usually under a general or regional anesthesia. The small neuroma is seen encircled in the depths of the incision and occurs at the Y-shaped division of the common digital nerve. Simple excision leaves some anesthesia in the interspace between the third and fourth toes for a period of time, but this usually is not long-lasting and is no real problem. The symptoms are immediately improved in the patient's foot, however, as soon as he begings to walk in a few days and usually the result is quite gratifying.

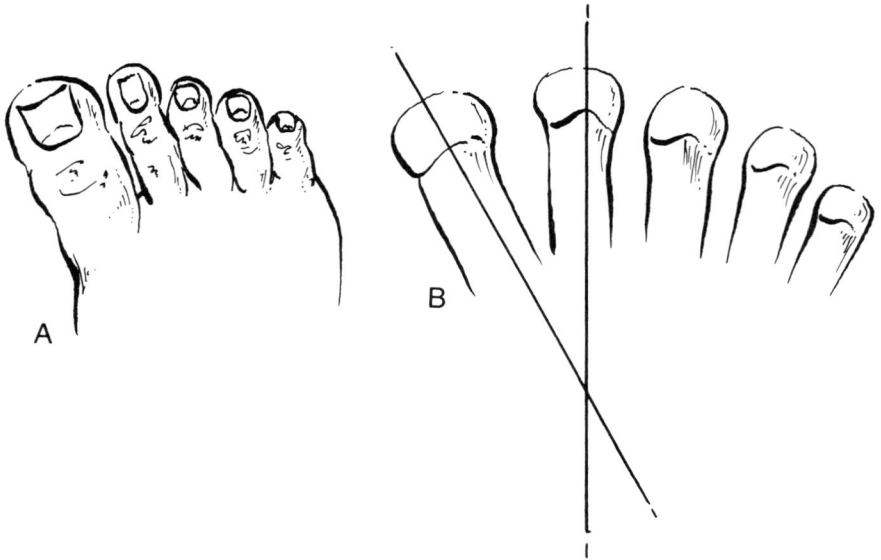

Fig. 15-11. Classical bunion development. **(A)** Metatarsus adductus including an adduction of the great toe along with the four smaller toes. **(B)** Deviation of the metatarsal bone occurring in the adult with the so-called metatarsus primus varus developing. (*Figure continued.*)

Bunion

The creation of a bunion is actually an aftermath of untreated metatarsus adductus in the child (Fig. 15-11). The splaying of the forefoot with a rather marked varus of the first metatarsal bone is part of the original mechanical defect seen in the metatarsus adductus. If the patient were to go through life without wearing shoes, the great toe would remain in varus and the deformity of a bunion would not occur. However, as the patient grows older and begins to wear shoes, the mechanical problem begins to occur. This does not imply that the shoes are ill-fitting, as may have been thought in the past. It does, however, mean that some mechanism pushes the great toe into valgus, with the apex of the angle thus created being at the medial aspect of the metatarsal head.

Metatarsus primus varus is therefore the actual cause of the development of hallux valgus. The hallux valgus therefore actually is not so much the problem, except that an exostosis invariably develops on the medial side of the metatarsal head and itself becomes what is commonly referred to as a bunion. The bony prominence is painful, particularly if the dorsal digital nerve courses over it, as it often does.

One of the other causes of pain in bunion formation is the creation of a bursa over the exostosis. The clinical picture of acute bursitis is pain, redness, swelling, and tenderness. These will be quite disabling at times. Occasionally an active bacterial infection occurs, but for the most part the acute bunion "bursitis" is due to pressure; the fluid obtained is often sterile. The hallux valgus

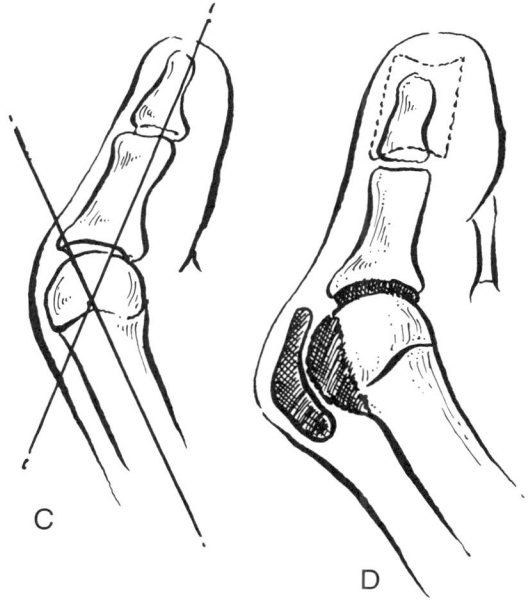

Fig. 15.11 (*Continues*). (**C**) Subsequent development of a hallux valgus caused by the overpull of the extensor tendon to pull the great toe back into the valgus position, leaving the medial side of the first metatarsal bone projecting medially. (**D**) Bunion itself comprised of the exostosis forming on the medial side of the head due to the prominence here and the ultimate bursa that forms over this bony projection, which often causes acute pain.

usually progresses so that the great toe either rides over or under the adjacent second toe. The second toe, will then often form a hammer toe deformity when it rides up over the great toe. The entire picture is of a mechanical malalignment with resulting pressure phenomena over the metatarsal head. With time, the joint that has been subluxated toward the medial side becomes the site of degenerative joint disease due to the incongruity of the joint surface in this altered position. Often the major pain a patient with hallux valgus has may be of degenerative joint disease of the proximal joint of the great toe.

Many types of bunionectomy have been suggested and some of the typical types are shown in Figure 15-12. Figure 15-12A shows the "classic" bunionectomy, in which the exostosis is merely removed and the adduction deformity of the great toe corrected by anchoring it with the flap that has been created. This is a relatively good procedure if the amount of metatarsus primus varus is not great and if the joint is good. Figure 15-12C shows the commonly used "Keller" bunionectomy, in which a new joint is created by resection of the proximal end of the proximal phalanx. This removes the joint surface articulating with the mtatarsal head. The Keller procedure allows for a cicatricial type of arthroplasty since soft tissue is brought into the intervening area by means of a pursestring in the surrounding soft tissue. A scar tissue joint is thus formed and the valgus of the great toe is again corrected with the bunion flap. More recently, Swanson has described a silicone rubber prosthesis that resurfaces the proximal end of the proximal phalanx, thereby creating a hemiarthroplasty in which the distal joint surface is made of silicone rubber. The prosthesis fits into the medullary canal by means of a stem. Variations of the original design include coating the stem with Dacron mesh so that tissue ingrowth occurs and the prosthesis is very stoutly

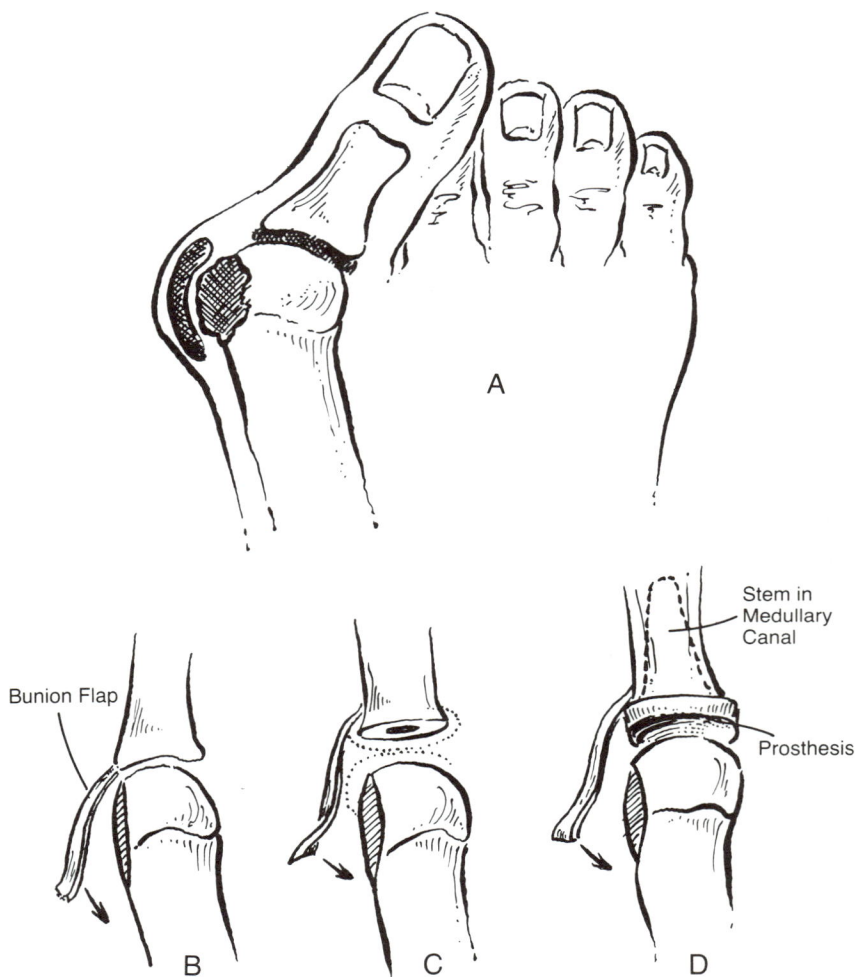

Fig. 15-12. (A) Typical bunion deformity with exostosis, hallux valgus, and bursal formation. **(B)** Classic bunionectomy in which the exostosis is removed. The joint is left intact and the bunion flap is used to correct the hallux valgus. **(C)** Typical Keller-type bunionectomy with removal of a portion of the proximal phalanx again uses the bunion flap to correct the valgus. **(D)** Bunionectomy with insertion of a silicone rubber prosthesis to create a hemiarthroplasty of the joint still uses the bunion flap.

fixed to bone. The joint surface in itself is therefore actually reestablished (Fig. 15-12D). Once again, the valgus deformity is corrected with the bunion flap.

Various other types of bunionectomies have been reported, but the author finds that one of these three usually is quite satisfactory. If a great amount of metatarsus primus varus is present, particularly in the younger individual, consideration should be given to one or another of the correctional osteotomies. An osteotomy will realign the first metatarsal bone for better mechanics. This is considered especially when the patient's life expectancy following the surgical procedure is long. The type of procedure to be used is ordinarily decided by the operating surgeon.

SHOE PADS

One is often in a quandary over what type of padding to use in a shoe. Selection of shoe pads depends upon the condition to be treated. When one looks at the plantar surface of the foot, one sees three major points of pressure with secondary points presented over the touchpads of each toe (see Fig. 15-5). The use of pads is primarily designed to relieve pressure over these areas and three basic types of pads are ordinarily used.

The pads are usually made of very firm sponge rubber or felt which the corrective shoe store can buy as blanks and alter to the individual needs. Figure 15-5 shows the three types of pads along with their cross-sectional silhouette. Type "A" is the so-called longitudinal pad or "oval" pad, which is primarily for an arch support itself. As you can see from the cross-sectional version, a slanting type of pad feathers out to the edge anteriorly, laterally, and posteriorly. It merely holds up the longitudinal arch, thereby relieving strain on the foot and stretching of the plantar fascia. Type "B" is the so-called "Morton's pad." This pad has a prominent area in the center, feathers out on both sides, has a somewhat heart-shaped design to provide support under the metatarsal heads in an area just behind these heads, and tapers off to a point posteriorly. It should be adjusted in the shoe so that the pressure point of the major prominence of the pad lies just behind the metatarsal head; pressure is taken off here and not over the metatarsal heads themselves. This type of pad is ordinarily used for metatarsalgia, painful calluses over the metatarsal heads, and plantar neuroma, as previously described. The Dixon and Dively inlay (D & D inlay), is a combination of the oval pad and the Morton's pad and provides a generalized support for the foot. It not only supports the medial arch structures but also provides support underneath the metatarsal head and gives excellent overall support for the foot. The pads should usually be glued into the shoe as in Figure 15-5A and B, so that they are in the exact location to provide support to the intended area. However, a good corrective shoe cobbler can often make an "insert" that fits the shoe exactly. The pad is then put in its proper position each time the shoe is worn. If the pad is extremely uncomfortable after a few days of "getting used to it," the pad may be set in an inappropriate location, this should be checked by the physician.

There are many other types of appliances for the foot. For the most part these are somewhat more sophisticated and probably should be left to the orthopedic surgeon. The pads, however, are quite simple and can be very easily prescribed and fitted by the family practitioner.

16

CARE OF THE FOOT IN THE DIABETIC

The Problem	**Specific Areas of Care**
Propensity to Infection	Skin
Decreased Circulation	Blisters
Neurogenic Changes	Corns and Calluses
General Cleanliness	Nails

The patient with diabetes mellitus has problems not only with his metabolic processes but also with many other physiologic functions. One of the most often neglected problems, however, concerns his feet (Fig. 16-1). Anyone familiar with patients with diabetes will recall that a surprisingly high number of them have lost portions of their lower extremities to amputation caused by ulcerations that will not heal or to frank gangrene. In some cases it is impossible to prevent certain of the serious conditions of the foot in diabetics. The following discussion will help to give the patient and his physician a better understanding of the problems and various measures aimed at preventing these many time catastrophic conditions that cause loss of the lower extremity.

THE PROBLEM

There are three primary reasons that the patient with diabetes has difficulty with his feet: propensity to infection, decreased circulation, and neurogenic change.

Propensity to Infection

It is well known that the diabetic does not have the usual tissue resistance to infection and, therefore, infection quite often is the final terminal complication that tips the balance in an otherwise controllable ulceration of the foot and makes amputation necessary. Infections in the foot occur with sudden rapidity since the feet often give many portals of entry through nail margins, cracks,

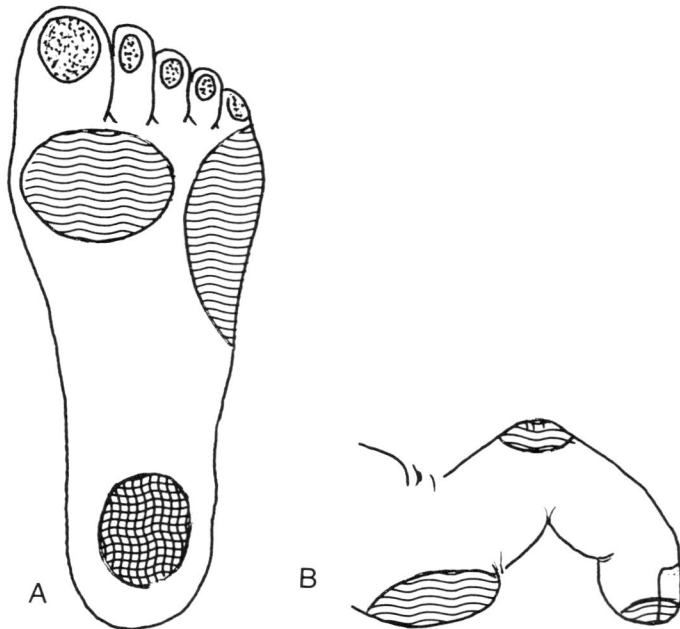

Fig. 16-1 (A) Plantar area of the foot to show the areas of weight-bearing stress. These areas are more subject to breakdown in the diabetic foot. **(B)** Lateral view of the foot showing pressure areas over the central portion of a hammer toe, and over the point of the hammer toe. Areas of pressure over the dorsum of the foot usually are due to fitting of shoes, and the same is true concerning friction blisters over the heel.

fissures, and the like. Since these areas tend to be neglected from a hygiene standpoint, particularly in the older, less active individual, the natural loss of tissue resistance in the diabetic is coupled then with a circulatory impairment. This further decreases host resistance, so that infections that might well be controlled by natural host responses in normal individuals progress to severe, life-threatening infections in the diabetic. The early and vigorous use of broad-spectrum antibiotics has decreased the ravages of infections in the diabetic foot. However, even massive treatment with antibiotics is often not enough to forestall the tremendous advantage that the organism has in an area with such markedly decreased host resistance.

The patients should be cautioned repeatedly about the importance of infection and be instructed to notify the physician even at the slightest evidence of a change in the condition of the foot that might signal infection. The cardinal signs of inflammation are heat, pain, swelling, and redness but they are often altered in the diabetic so that the classic picture of infection may not be present. Swelling and redness are the most reliable early symptoms and the patient should be instructed to watch for these and the other signs of infection. Probably most important of all is to encourage daily inspection of the feet so that an area of infection may not occur without being identified relatively early so that appropriate treatment may be started before it has become severe. Daily inspection by a patient and family who have been instructed as to the danger signs seems to be the best method for preventing serious infections in the diabetic foot.

Decreased Circulation

Many patients with diabetes develop, early in the course of the disease, an involvement of the arterial walls with atheromatus plaques; one of the cardinal signs of diabetes is a "presenile arteriosclerosis." This diminished blood supply in the foot due to arterial insufficiency constitutes one of the very important underlying forces in the diabetic foot, which renders it susceptible to infection and very resistant to healing. Added to this diminished arterial circulation is that the dependency required of the foot in ambulation allows for a greater amount of swelling with resultant capillary tamponade. The patient who develops a soft tissue defect in the foot from whatever cause will find that healing becomes almost impossible. Even small areas of ulceration in the foot are often very difficult to treat since the normal reparative forces of the diabetic foot are so low that an indolent ulcer results without any attempts at healing. Many measures can be instituted to try to help the circulation, mostly in the form of sympathetic blockage, medications to cause dilatation of peripheral vessels and measures to prevent swelling.

Even with all of these measures, however, the indolent ulcer in the diabetic foot usually will ultimately require surgical excision and either closure or grafting for final healing. The patient should be instructed in methods to improve the circulation and in the importance of frequent inspections of the foot.

Neurogenic Changes

A certain percentage of patients with diabetes develop a peripheral neuropathy that is often manifested by a loss of sensation in the foot. Decreased resistance of tissue deprived of its nerve supply is well known and this certainly creates some of the problem in the diabetic with peripheral neuropathy. More important, however, is the loss of sensibility of the foot which makes it much more susceptible to damage from friction or pressure. The protection afforded by normal sensation in the foot which warns the patient of impending trouble is absent, so a large area of ulceration or friction burn may occur before the patient realizes it. This adds a tremendous hazard in these individuals. The patient with decreased sensation in the foot must be warned to inspect his foot very often during the day to be certain that no evidence of tissue breakdown is present. Similarly, foot gear must be carefully fitted to preclude any areas of pressure or friction to the foot which will cause breakdown in an alarmingly short period of time. The loss of sensation, when superimposed on the decreased circulation and propensity to infections characteristic of many diabetic feet, often is the "final straw" that tumbles the finely balanced mechanism into decompensation, with rapidly progressive ulceration, infection, and gangrene necessitating eventual amputation.

GENERAL CLEANLINESS

Keeping the foot in as bacteria-free an environment as possible is of paramount importance in these diabetic feet for the reasons outlined above. The patient should thoroughly wash his feet, twice daily, preferably using a mildly bactericidal soap to lower bacteria count on the skin. Care must be taken in selecting the bactericidal soap since some patients have an allergic reaction to many of these stronger chemical preparations. However, the use of soaps containing hexachlorophene usually is well tolerated and will usually diminish the bacterial count of the skin tremendously when used twice daily. The foot should be gently washed in tepid water with the soap containing hexachlorophene and then thoroughly rinsed to remove all of the excess soap from the skin before being thoroughly dried. The foot should not be soaked for any length of time since this tends to cause maceration of tissue and may speed the development of infection. A thorough washing can be done in a matter of a few minutes and the foot must be thoroughly dried before shoes and socks are put on. Air drying is most appropriate after the foot has been thoroughly dried with a soft cloth. Areas that are particularly hard to dry out, such as nail gutters and fissures, may be painted with alcohol which acts as a drying agent by absorbing the water contained in these crevices and then evaporating. The socks should be changed after each washing and thoroughly laundered in water hot enough to destroy any bacteria.

SPECIFIC AREAS OF CARE

Skin

Since bacteria normally gain entrance to the skin, protection of this barrier from infection is vital in successful management of the foot in diabetes. Maceration is to be avoided at all costs since this provides multiple portals of entry in the soft soggy skin. Skin should be thoroughly dried as indicated above. If considerable sweating occurs, the socks and shoes should be removed periodically during the day to allow drying. If the skin becomes dry and scaly following drying, application of a very small amount of a lanolin-containing ointment is recommended. Care should be taken, however, to apply these preparations containing lanolin in very small amounts, to rub them well into the dry areas, and then to use a soft towel or paper tissue to wipe off all excess, so that the skin does not remain covered by an occlusive layer of ointment. Cracks and fissures can be avoided if proper care is taken to prevent long-standing maceration of the skin and to follow frequent dryings by the application of small amounts of a lanolin cream.

Fungus infections are extremely important since they tend to be insidious and often are not recognized for what they actually represent. Likewise, a blister in the skin caused by fungus lends a chance for widespread infection, since the material in the blister has a very high concentration of fungi that may be spread to other areas of the foot. When these small blisters are first recognized they should be evacuated promptly. The skin around the bleb should be thoroughly washed with antibacterial soap and then prepared with alcohol or other solutions prior to opening with any small sharp object that has been properly sterilized. The material evacuated from the cyst should be very carefully absorbed onto a cotton ball or paper tissue so that none of it is allowed to contaminate the skin around the bleb. The area around this should then be promptly treated with one of the topical fungicidal agents. A 1 percent Tolnaftate solution or one of the preparations containing undecylenic acid may be used. This medication should be reapplied twice daily until the covering of the bleb has completely dried and peeled off. Any new blebs that occur in the area should be promptly treated in the same manner.

Blisters

Blisters on the foot may be caused by either friction or fungi as indicated above. Blisters caused by friction are usually obvious because of their location. Care should be taken first to remove the object causing the friction. The biggest problem following the evacuation of blisters of any kind on the foot is the development of secondary infection. The evacuation of these blisters then should be done under strict aseptic conditions. If the bleb appears to be due to a fungal infection, treatment with the fungicidal preparation should be instituted immediately. The area should be inspected often for signs of acute inflammatory reaction that might indicate a secondary infection.

Corns and Calluses

Corns and calluses are usually caused by one of three circumstances: prolonged dampness with periodic drying; friction; or pressure. Of course, the first treatment of corns and calluses is to try to remove the offending mechanism. The treatment of dampness of the skin is discussed in detail above. The creation of calluses in an area of friction should be identified and appropriate measures taken to ensure that rubbing against shoe gear does not occur. Finally, the calluses that occur from pressure points should be very carefully guarded since this probably constitutes the most dangerous type.

If the callus does not respond to careful readjustment of pressure, the patient should be promptly referred to the orthopedist. The corns themselves should not be trimmed with a sharp instrument unless done by the physician. Patients who trim corns with a razor blade or sharp knife will almost invariably cause an open wound that may become secondarily infected and may not heal. Most corns can be kept under control by use of an emery board or pumice stone following washing with water. If the callus is somewhat softened by washing, it can be removed in layers with one of these abrasive mechanisms without fear of damage to the skin itself. Pumice stones have gained considerable favor and apparently are quite effective in abrading these calluses. However, the author's preference is for the rough side of an emery board. These boards are thin, can be shaped to fit the area to be treated, and are quite effective in removing excess callus.

Nails

Since the nails offer one of the most effective portals of entry for bacteria into the tissue of the foot special care must be taken to avoid abnormal nail conditions. Of particular importance is the ingrown nail: growth of the nail out into soft tissue results in the creation of an open wound that usually becomes secondarily infected. The patient with an ingrown nail should be seen by a physician experienced in its care so that the open area can be prevented and the foot allowed to heal. This will often require a surgical procedure to remove the margin of the nail and the associated soft tissue "gutter." This procedure should be considered particularly when the patient has experienced recurring infections in the nail. Simple avulsion of the nail by the physician usually will result only in temporary relief. The new nail that grows from the remaining matrix will usually have the same characteristics as the original nail and will be subject to the same growth patterns with the same consequences. The procedure for this "gutter excision" operation will be found in Chapter 15, The Foot.

17

THE INJECTION OF STEROIDS INTO JOINTS AND PERIARTICULAR STRUCTURES

AGENTS AND ACTION

Since the advent of steroids for clinical use in the diminution of inflammatory reactions, the relatively insoluble methylprednisolone preparations have become popular for injection directly into joints, synovial-lined cavities, and soft tissue areas in general. The very fact that these preparations are relatively insoluble constitutes the primary mode of action. These crystals are suspended in a vehicle and when injected into a joint or other soft tissue area the vehicle is rapidly absorbed leaving a deposit of slowly dissolving crystals in the soft tissue area or joint. This allows for the gradual liberation of steroids into the surrounding soft tissue as the crystals begin to dissolve slowly over a period of time. For this reason the onset of action is sometimes delayed due to the insolubility of the crystals, and the delay in beginning the absorption into the tissues. However, the action is often quite prolonged since it takes a matter of several weeks for the dose that is deposited to dissolve and be dispersed.

TECHNIQUE

The injection should be made under strictly aspectic conditions since the inoculation of microorganisms with the material injected may have devastating effects if infection develops. If microorganisms are injected in any concentration infection is likely to occur, since it is the obvious activity of the drug to diminish the body's ability to establish an inflammatory reaction, and the host resistance is markedly diminished on a local basis. It is usually better to set up a sterile table covered by a sterile towel so that the various needles, syringes, etc. may be laid out in a sterile field. The operator should wear sterile gloves. The patient's skin should be thoroughly prepared with an antiseptic solution in a wide area and allowed to dry. The area to be injected is selected, as will be discussed under each separate heading in this chapter, and the initial injection is made with the local anesthetic. It is usually better to use two syringes, one for the local anesthetic and another for the steroid. The initial injection is made with a tiny 27-gauge needle in a small area that has been anesthetized by ethyl chloride spray. This step, of course, is not mandatory but patients usually appreciate the physician doing the injection with as little pain as possible. Use a small amount of 1 percent lidocaine to raise a wheal in the skin; then the deeper injection is accomplished through this wheal.

It is not necessary to use large needles unless fluid is to be aspirated from the joint prior to injection. It is, however, possible to anesthetize the area completely with a smaller 25- or 23-gauge needle by very gently injecting the lidocaine in front of the needle as it is inserted. The almost instantaneous affect of lidocaine in anesthetizing nerve endings will allow the injection to be made with relatively little pain, if one is careful to inject the local anesthetic agent very slowly in front of the needle and then proceed with the tip of the needle through an area that has been anesthetized. This does not take a great amount of time: almost any area can be thoroughly anesthetized in only 2 or 3 minutes.

As indicated, if a large joint is to be entered for the aspiration of fluid prior to injection, a large 18-gauge needle can then be substituted on the syringe. It is then introduced through an area previously anesthetized with a smaller bore needle and, therefore, the entire procedure can be done with virtually no pain. If a joint is to be aspirated once the needle has penetrated the synovial sac, it is possible to inject several millimeters of the anesthetic agent directly into the larger joints (or relatively smaller amounts into smaller joints) so that the synovium can be anesthetized by topical application.

The dose of the steroid may vary but in larger joints it is customary to inject from 40 to 80 mg, with smaller joints receiving relatively smaller doses. By using preparations containing 80 mg/ml it is possible to place a relatively large dose of steroids into a small volume joint (such as the metacarpophalangeal joints of the hand) without over distending the joint. In the case of larger to middle-sized joints the steroid is often mixed with a small amount of the local anesthetic to give better dispersion through the joint.

Soon after injection, the joint is usually moved several times through a full range of motion to be certain that the material is evenly dispersed through the joint and comes in contact with all synovial surfaces. In soft tissue injections (such as for a lateral epicondylitis or tennis elbow), it is usually better to anesthetize the area first. The steroid is then mixed with several milliliters of local anesthetic and injected thoroughly through the area of inflammatory reaction. Again, this gives better dispersion of the crystals by the dilution method.

Once the injection is completed the needle is withdrawn and the small needle opening is covered with a spot-type adhesive bandage to prevent bleeding or expulsion of the injection fluid through the puncture wound. Other dressing than this is ordinarily not necessary.

INJECTIONS IN THE REGION OF THE SHOULDER JOINT

Four basic areas are usually injected in the region of the shoulder joint (Fig. 17-1): acromioclavicular joint, bicipital groove, rotator cuff, and shoulder joint proper (glenohumeral joint).

Acromioclavicular Joint

This small joint can be satisfactorily injected, although the joint does not have any real space and injection into the joint proper usually causes some distention of the capsule. The 80 mg/ml concentration should be used. Since it is

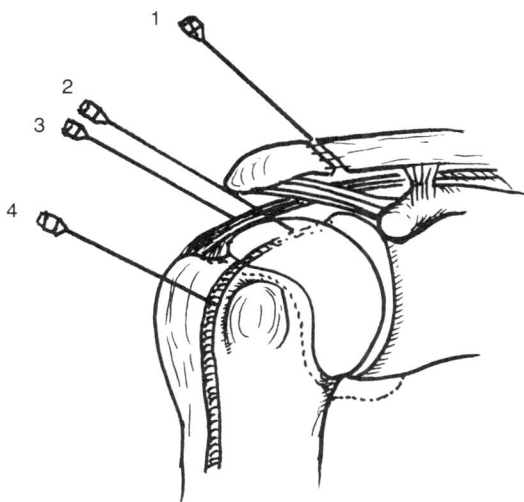

Fig. 17-1. Injection sites for the shoulder: (1) acromiclavicular joint, (2) bicipital groove, (3) rotator cuff, and (4) shoulder joint.

of such small volume, very little anesthetic can be used to dilute it. Most of the time it is possible to enter the joint with a small 25-gauge needle. After the joint has been anesthetized, a small amount of steroid can be injected but the volume will usually be quite small. The capsular structures around the joint should be carefully infiltrated with the solution since much of the pain may arise from the capsule around the joint. The steroid may be slightly diluted for this portion of the injection. It is seldom necessary to use more than 0.5 ml of a 80 mg/ml preparation.

Bicipital Groove

This groove in the humerus through which the long head of the biceps tendon courses is usually best approached anteriorly. With the patient lying down and the shoulder externally rotated so that the palm is pointing towards the ceiling, the area of the bicipital groove can be usually palpated. In obese or muscular individuals it is often impossible to feel the tendon, but in thinner individuals one can almost always feel the biceps tendon as it glides under the palpating fingers.

Using the technique previously described, the groove can usually be entered with a 23-gauge needle and if the anesthetic is administered carefully this can be done relatively painlessly. Once the area has been anesthetized the needle can be inserted until one strikes bone. By probing gently with multiple small thrusts of the needle in both directions, laterally and medially, one can feel the needle encounter the fibrous tissue covering of the bicipital groove. Once this has been palpated the needle can be felt to penetrate it and extend into the bicipital groove. It is best to inject the material into the groove between the covering and the tendon and not into the tendon itself since this may lead to attritional changes and ultimate rupture of the long head of the biceps. Once the canal has been entered it is not necessary to disperse the medication further since this is a synovial lined tunnel and material injected into the space will ordinarily travel up and down the tunnel without difficulty. Once the canal has been anesthetized, it is permissable to apply some little bit of pressure to be certain that the material has been distributed up and down the length of the canal. The patient will usually experience immediate relief of his pain after the injection, which is a good indicator that the injection has been made in the proper location.

Rotator Cuff

As you will recall from the section on shoulder anatomy, the rotator cuff extends as a hood over the humeral head, attaching to the tuberosity but extending both anteriorly and posteriorly as well as superiorly. For practical purposes the usual area of inflammatory reaction is in the superior aspect of the rotator cuff (supraspinatus portion) due to impingement between the humerus and the acromion. Likewise, it is often necessary to include the anteriosuperior aspect of the hood since this is the portion that impinges under the acromioclavicular ligament with the arm in the abducted and forward flexed position (the position of usual functional activity of the upper extremity).

The injection is made from directly lateral: attempt to palpate the acromion process and slip the needle into the space underneath the underside of the acromion. In this position one will penetrate first the deltoid muscle and then probably go through the subdeltoid bursa without actually realizing that this structure has been traversed. The rotator cuff can then be felt as a change of resistance as the needle passes into it. The injection should be made on a rather tangential basis to the tendon, which makes the needle lie at almost right angles to the long axis of the humerus. Again, it is preferable not to inject a great amount of material into the substance of the rotator cuff since this will lead to attritional changes and subsequent rupture. However, a small amount can be injected into the cuff at this level if done without a great amount of pressure; this is usually the site of most of the inflammatory reaction.

After thorough injection of the cuff with a series of forward thrusts of the needle and then withdrawal so that the material is disbursed through the substance of the tendon, the needle is usually then passed through the rotator cuff into the shoulder joint. This can, once again, be ascertained by a change in resistance as the needle passes from the tendinous area into the relative lack of resistance offered by the joint space. It may be possible to inject the anterior–superior aspect of the cuff through this same portal of entry through the skin. However, often it will be necessary to make a separate approach more directly over this location (which can be palpated and pinpointed usually by the tenderness to pressure over this specific area). A total of 40 to 60 mg of steroid diluted in 2 or 3 ml of anesthetic solution should be used for the injection, with at least half going into the tendon itself and half into the joint. There is no specific postinjection management routine necessary.

Shoulder Joint

The shoulder joint per se can usually be injected as described above in conjunction with the rotator cuff injection. It is possible to enter the joint anteriorly but this is sometimes harder to do. If done directly over the deltopectoral groove, this may result in an encounter with the cephalic vein that can cause rather massive soft tissue bleeding if it is punctured or torn. For this reason it is usually better to inject the shoulder joint lateral aspect as described by going through the rotator cuff.

INJECTIONS IN THE REGION OF THE ELBOW JOINT

The injections in the region of the elbow joint are done into one of four specific locations (Fig. 17-2): the lateral epicondyle at the point of attachment of musculature to bone, into the medial epicondylar area to the point of attachment of the forearm flexor group into bone, into the elbow joint per se, or into the olecranon bursa.

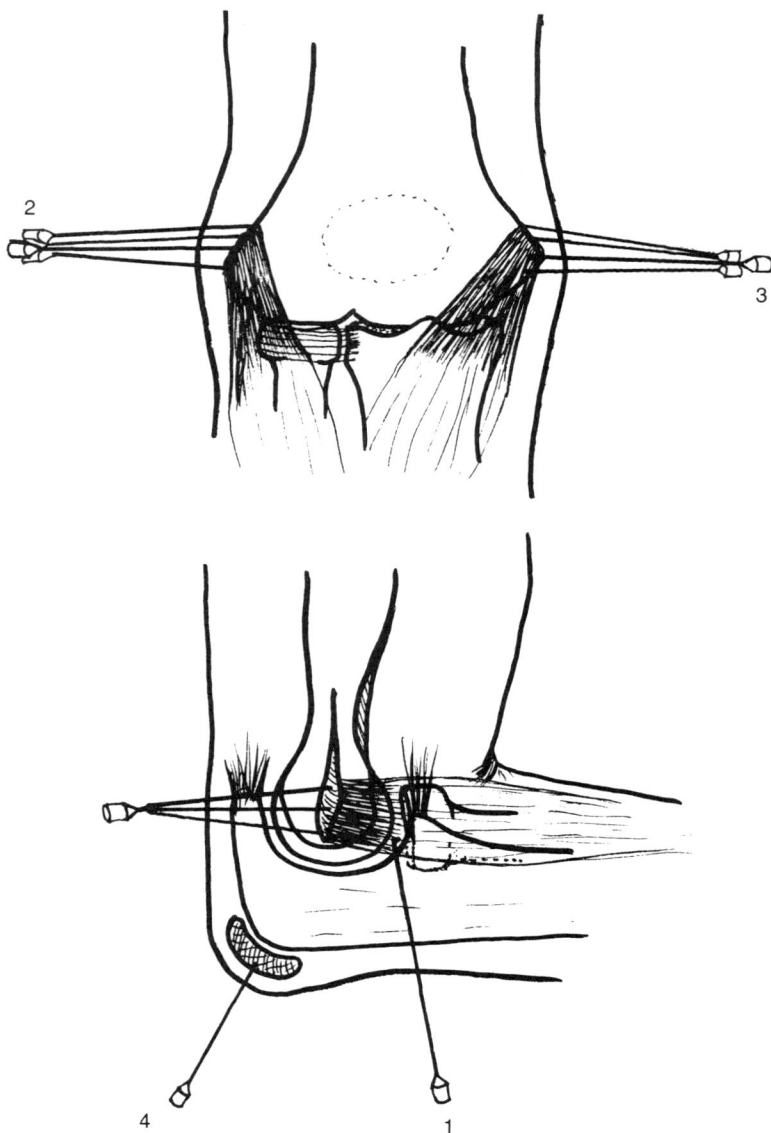

Fig. 17-2. Injection sites for the elbow: (1) elbow joint, (2) lateral epicondyle, (3) medial epicondyle, and (4) olecranon bursa.

Lateral Epicondyle

Injections into the regions of the lateral epicondyle are the most frequently used in the region of the elbow joint since they are ordinarily done for lateral epicondylitis or "tennis elbow." The injection into this area is often quite painful and care must be taken to anesthetize slowly and to progress slowly so that the patient will not have an agonizing amount of pain during the injection. The injection is usually done best with the patient lying down with the elbow up over the side of his chest wall, flexed at 90 degrees. In this position the extensor carpi radialis brevis muscle is relaxed and its attachment to the rim of bone just superior to the lateral epicondyle can be very easily palpated. It is into this general area that the injection is to be made. There will most likely be point tenderness of a greater magnitude just at the tip of the epicondyle, but often the pain extends up a distance of 2 or 3 cm from the tip of the epicondyle along this muscular attachment line. Since this is a purely soft tissue injection the steroid is diluted with several milliliters of local anesthetic. Since the area covered is sometimes relatively large a total of 80 mg is often necessary. The area first injected is just anterior to the epicondyle and from there the injection is carried proximally to insure inclusion of all of the area of expansion of the origin of the extensor carpi radialis brevis muscle.

The "needling" approach is usually used, with multiple thrusts and withdrawal of the needle during the procedure. A 25- or, at the very most, a 23-gauge needle is usually required. There is no postinjection procedure necessary except that patients will often have a considerable exacerbation of their pain once the anesthetic has worn off. This is thought to be due to the presence of insoluble crystals in this area of considerable inflammatory reaction, with resulting aggravation of the inflammation by irritation before the local effects of the steroids have had time to occur.

Patients should be warned about this occasional exacerbation and given sufficient medication to control their pain at home that night. It is also well to advise them to use warm moist compresses over the area if they do experience considerable pain, since heat tends to diminish the pain considerably. This warm compress is made by applying a wash cloth that has been squeezed out after being saturated with warm water to cover the area entirely. This cloth is covered with a layer of plastic, like that used to protect dry cleaned clothing. A thicker towel is then usually applied over this for insulation and then the heating pad is applied at low heat. The patient should be warned to avoid overheating with resultant soft tissue burn.

Medial Epicondyle

Injections into the medial epicondyle are much less often required but are done similarly to the more frequent lateral epicondylar injection. There is usually a single area to be injected which is about 1 or 1.5 cm in diameter. There usually is not the extension of the muscular attachment up the medial epicondylar as there is on the lateral side. The injection is done in a very similar manner to that described and postinjection care is the same.

Elbow Joint

Injections into the elbow joint are best made from the lateral approach since this is somewhat more accessible. The injection is best made into the radiocapitellar joint either from the posterior or perhaps from the straight lateral position.

In both instances the injection is made with the elbow flexed and if done from the posterior–lateral approach (usually preferred by most surgeons) the area of contract between the radius and distal humerus can be palpated and the needle introduced directly into the joint. Once the needle enters into the joint, you can be certain of its location by the sudden change in resistance, as previously described, and also by the fact that the adjacent joint surfaces can be gently palpated with the tip of the needle. Local anesthetic should be injected into the joint as soon as it is penetrated since this helps to anesthetize the entire synovial surface topically and makes the remainder of the injection much less painful. The amount of steroid usually injected is 40 to 60 mg diluted in 1 or 2 ml of local anesthetic. No post injection procedures are necessary.

Olecranon Bursa

Injections into the olecranon bursa are usually made only when there is swelling in the bursal wall, usually with the accumulation of fluid. When fluid is present the injection is quite simple since the bursa can easily be identified and the entrance into the bursa is signaled by a sudden evacuation of fluid. This fluid, however, is often quite viscous and a larger needle may be needed to evacuate the bursa in some cases. There is some difficulty in injecting a bursa that has no fluid accumulation, particularly when the bursal walls are thickened by inflammatory process. Usually, however, the needle can be introduced with care into the bursal cavity. The success of this introduction into the cavity can be determined by injecting local anesthetic, which will distend the bursa and then can be withdrawn back into the syringe.

INJECTIONS IN THE REGION OF THE WRIST JOINT

In the region of the wrist joint there are four primary points of injections of steroids (Fig. 17-3): the carpometacarpal joints, particularly between the first metacarpal bone and the trapezium; the radiocarpal joint; the radioulnar joint; and DeQuervain's canal.

There may be instances in which injections into the midcarpal joints are indicated. These should pose no real problems since the joints lie in a relatively subcutaneous position and should be injected from the dorsum of the wrist. Various of these injections may be necessary from time to time but the need is relatively rare compared with injections into the carpometacarpal joint of the thumb, the joint between the radius and the carpus per se, and the injections into the distal radioulnar joint.

Trapezio-First Metacarpal Joint Of The Thumb

The trapezium–first metacarpal joint of the thumb is often the site of degenerative disease, either from wear and tear changes or from trauma. Injections into this joint will quite often give remarkable relief for extended periods of time.

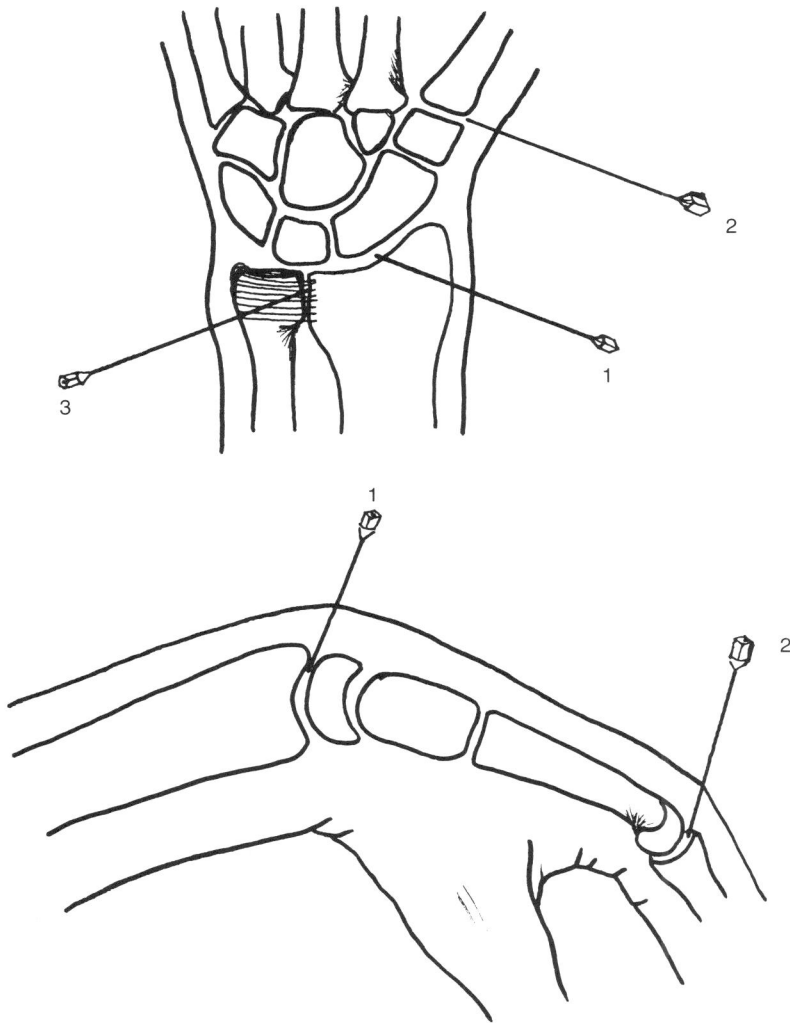

Fig. 17-3. Injection sites for the wrist: (1) radiocarpal joint, (2) carpometacarpal joint, and (3) radioulnar joint.

The injection should be made using 0.5 ml of 80 mg/ml preparation and the injection should be made from the radial side. It is probably best to dilute the steroid at least with equal parts of local anesthetic. At this point the first metacarpal base can be easily palpated and is often subluxated radially to the extent that it creates an obvious protrusion at the base of the thumb in the wrist area. The small joint has very little joint space as such but traction on the thumb by an assistant give a considerable distraction between the joint surfaces in most cases and makes it quite easy to slip a small 25-gauge needle into the joint. There occasionally will be an effusion in this joint which should be aspirated and in this case a larger case needle will be necessary. This should offer no problem once the area has been anesthetized, as previously described. The joint can quite easily be entered since it is relatively superficial and is protected on the radial side only by the tendons of the long abductor and short extensor of the thumb. While it is not necessary, nor really advisable, to inject through these tendons, there is no real harm in doing so; avoiding the tendon should not be any real objective when attempting to make the injection into this joint. Once the injection has been made, the traction is released after the needle has been withdrawn.

Radiocarpal Joint

The radiocarpal joint is easy to inject if one remembers that it lies somewhat further proximal than is usually realized. It is much easier to do this injection with the wrist flexed so that the radiocarpal articulation can be identified more easily. The needle should be slipped in at a slight angle so that actually it is inserted over the curve of the proximal carpal row. This is done with the wrist relatively acutely flexed. The joint can be entered without much difficulty with a 1 inch needle, usually 23- or 25-gauge. A total of 1 ml of 80 mg/ml steroid is used, usually diluted with an equal volume of anesthetic. There is no particular postinjection protocol.

Radioulnar Joint

The distal radioulnar joint is often the site of considerable inflammatory reaction degenerative joint disease, as well as rheumatoid disease. These are often manifested by swelling, hypermobility of the distal ulna, and pain, particularly on the extremes of supination and pronation. It is usually easier to do this injection from the dorsum using a 1 inch 23- or 25-gauge needle. A total of 40 mg can be injected, usually diluted with equal parts of local anesthetic solution. The injection is best made with the wrist in marked pronation since in this position there is normally some distraction of the joint. The joint in full supination is quite a tight fit and it is much more difficult to insert the needle between the two bones. Insertion of the needle through the extensor digiti quinti tendon poses no problem, but the fingers should be kept relatively still while the injection is being made in case the insertion is made through this tendon, since it lies in a small canal just dorsal to this joint. There is no particular postinjection protocol.

DeQuervain's Canal

Injections of steroids are often necessary into deQuervain's canal when a stenosing tenosynovitis has resulted in acute pain, swelling, and sometimes accumulation of fluid. The small canal, as will be remembered from the section on wrist anatomy, lies just at the radial styloid and extends about 2 cm proximal to this. The canal has a fibrous tissue roof and houses the tendon of the extensor pollicis brevis and the abductor pollicis longus, the latter of which is often reduplicated.

After the area has been anesthetized, a 25- or 23-gauge needle is inserted at somewhat of an angle from distal to proximal through the skin subcutaneous tissue. The fibrous tissue roof of the canal can be detected with the point of the needle. This can be traversed rather easily and a lack of resistance can then be felt as the needle enters the canal. If, however, the needle enters one of the tendons there will be continuing resistance and the needle should be withdrawn slightly and reinserted at somewhat more of an angle to try to miss direct injection into the tendon. Once the needle has been inserted, there should be only moderate resistance to the injection of local anesthetic into the canal. If the canal has been entered without entering the tendon there should be no problem. Occasionally, when adhesions exist in a canal there will be a small palpable snap or pop as adhesions are lysed and the material being injected will suddenly be felt to extend much more easily.

Once the canal has been irrigated with the local anesthetic solution a total of approximately 40 mg of steroid diluted in an equal volume of local anesthetic can be injected with ease. Usually the total volume of injection should not exceed 2 ml, since the material will tend to run out from under the roof of the canal and be dispersed away from the point of maximum need. No particular postinjection procedures are indicated.

INJECTIONS IN THE REGIONS OF THE HAND

Injections into the hand are usually made into one of three areas (Fig. 17-4): the metacarpophalangeal joints; the interphalangeal joints of the fingers, both middle and distal; and the flexor tendon sheath.

Metacarpophalangeal Joint

Injection into the metacarpophalangeal joint is relatively easy if it is done with the joint rather acutely flexed to near 90 degrees. In this position after the area has been thoroughly anesthetized the needle should be inserted at a slight angle from proximal to distal. This allows the needle to slip in over the curve of the metacarpal head into the joint. The capsule and extensor hood can be felt to give resistance which suddenly releases as the needle passes through them into the joint. If the other hand is used to palpate, the joint fluid can be felt to run into the joint quite readily since this results in a considerable distention. This joint will usually hold 1 ml of fluid with 0.5 ml of 80 mg steroid diluted with equal parts of local anesthetic agent.

Middle and Distal: Interphalangeal Joints

The middle joint will likewise hold a reasonable volume of solution, usually approximately 0.5 ml. Injection is made as with the metacarpophalangeal joint, with the joint flexed at 90 degrees and with an angled position for the needle

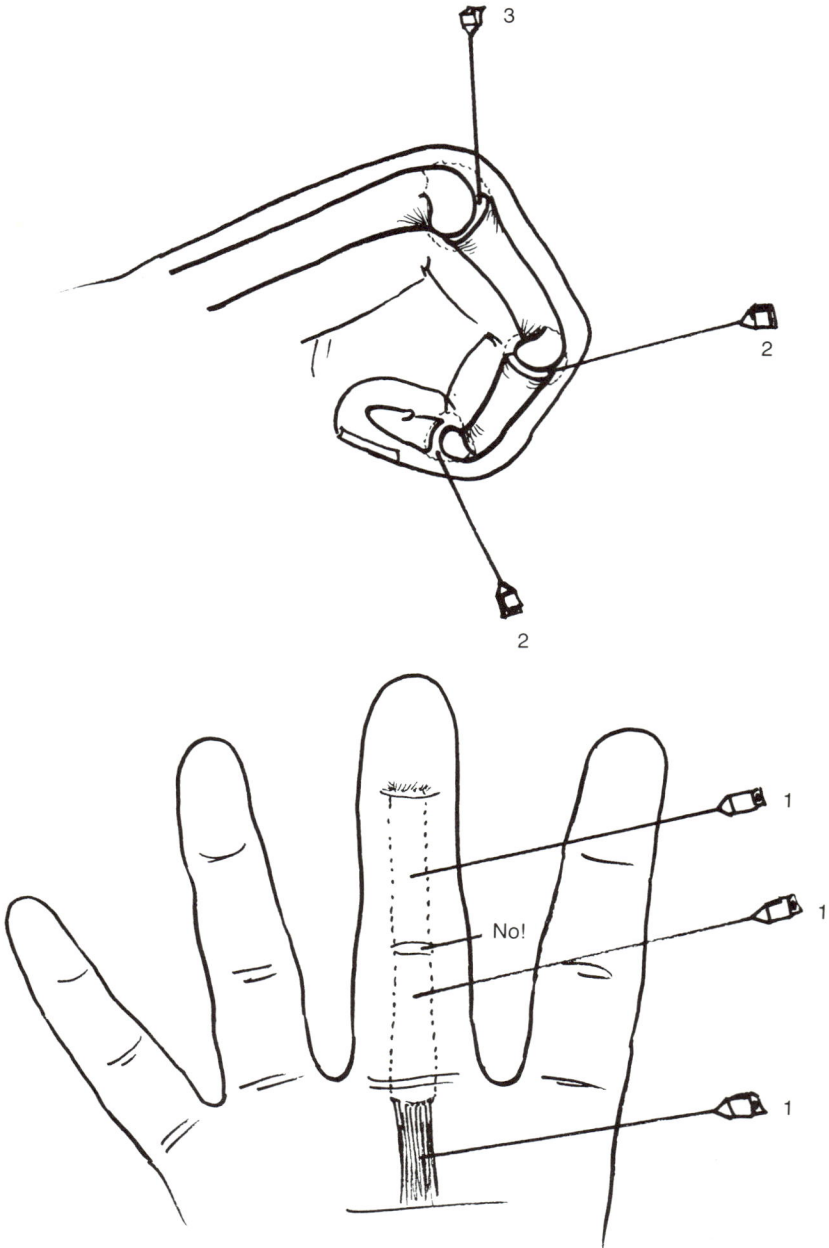

Fig. 17-4. Injection sites for the hand: (1) tendon sheaths, (2) interphalangeal joints, and (3) metacarpophalangeal joints.

from proximal to distal so that it actually curves over the condyles of the proximal phalanx into the joint. From 0.25 to 0.5 ml of steroid preparation with 80 mg/ml is injected, usually diluted with a very small amount of local anesthetic agent. The distal joint will not hold quite as much solution and usually two or three drops of concentrated steroid may be injected without much dilution. The injection is made, again, with the joint acutely flexed and is made over the curve of the condyle going from proximal to distal.

Flexor Tendon Sheath

Injections into the flexor tendon sheath are made for acute tendinitis or for stenosing tenosynovitis of the flexor tendon sheath with catching of the flexor tendon. Most of the time the catching occurs from slipping of the nodule underneath a stenotic band at the A1 pulley level, so that injection can be made into the flexor tendon sheath in the palm.

After the area is completely anesthetized a 23- or 25-gauge 1 inch needle can be used, usually inserted with a slight angle from proximal to distal. The tendon sheath can be felt and usually the needle will slip on into the flexor tendons and must be withdrawn slightly. One can tell if the tendon has been entered since the solution is very difficult to inject into the canal. By retracting it slightly one can feel very easy injection of solution into the canal. Often the palpating thumb or finger of the opposite hand will recognize a distention of the sheath as the material is injected. Usually the sheath is injected and even distended with localized anesthetic, then this is withdrawn and 40 mg of steroid is injected into the canal, usually undiluted since there will be some local anesthetic still present.

If the injection is made into the canal as it courses through the finger, either overlying the middle or proximal phalanx, the same procedure should be followed except that the injection must be made into the pad between the flexor creases. Under no circumstances should the injection be made through the flexion creases since there is no subcutaneous tissue in this area. Here, the skin lies directly on the flexor tendon sheath so that often a leak of material may occur after injection. If, on the other hand, the injection is made through the fatty pad the material will not leak out except into the pad where it causes no harm. There is therefore little chance of a fistula, as there is when injection is made into the flexion crease. Care should be taken at this level again to avoid injection directly into the tendon. The position of the needle should be ascertained by the ease of injection felt with the local anesthetic before the steroid solution is injected.

INJECTIONS IN THE REGION OF THE HIP

In the region of the hip there are three areas where injections are often successful in relieving symptoms of synovitis or tendinitis (Fig. 17-5): the iliac crest, the hip joint, and the trochanteric bursa.

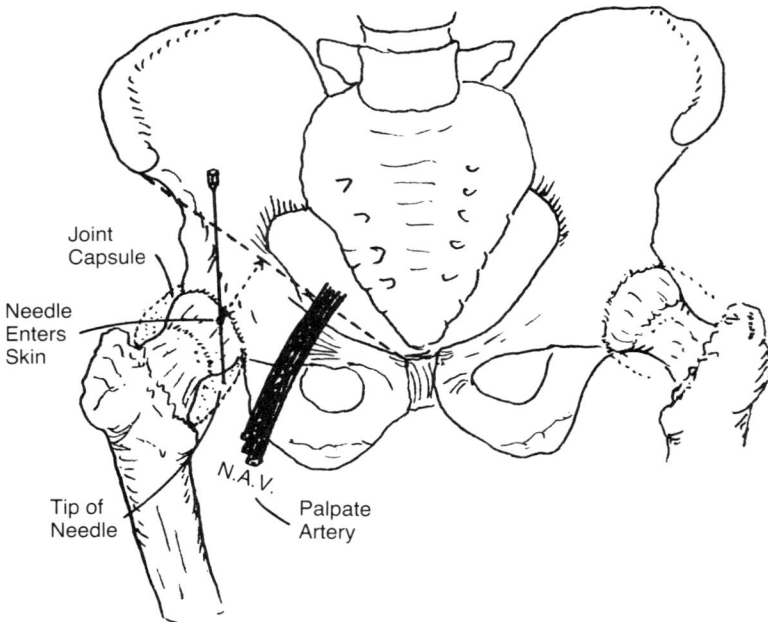

Fig. 17-5. Injection sites for the hip. (N.A.V. = nerve, artery, vein.)

Iliac Crest

Occasionally there are instances of severe pain and tenderness related to the muscular attachments along the iliac crest area. These are usually posttraumatic and represent the "hip pointer" that many football players receive from failure to wear properly fitting hip pads. These areas usually cause a discretely localized point of exquisite tenderness and can successfully be injected.

The patient usually lies down on the opposite side so that the skin can be stretched tightly over the iliac crest area. After the area is thoroughly anesthetized, the bony attachments of the musculature in the tender region are liberally infiltrated with approximately 80 mg of steroid preparation diluted in several milliliters of local anesthetic. It should be done with a relatively short needle to avoid penetration through the peritoneum. If carefully done, there should be no real danger. There is no specific postinjection procedure.

Hip Joint

The hip joint may be successfully injected. While the ball and socket portion of the joint provides relatively little space the rather voluminous capsule that extends from the rim of the acetabulum down to attach at the base of the neck provides a large joint space that may be injected quite easily.

The patient should be lying on his back with the leg free and in neutral position. A point is selected about midway along a line extending from the anterior superior iliac spine to the pubis. A point is then selected approximately

2 cm distal to this line and the needle is introduced here with the technique described earlier for anesthetizing the area. The femoral vein, artery, and nerve pass longitudinally in this region from medial to lateral. The point of injection should be lateral to the palpable pulsation in the femoral vessels. The area may be anesthetised with 1-1/2 or 2″ needles in the superficial levels but a 3″ spinal needle with a 21-gauge bore is better for approaching the joint. If the local anesthetic is injected carefully in front of the needle this can be done with relatively little pain.

If the needle is inserted from the point selected, slightly caudad and slightly medial, the wing of the ilium will be encountered by its tip. This area is then flooded with anesthetic solution. The needle can be "walked" down the wing of the ilium until the acetabular rim is encountered. The capsule of the hip joint in this level is relatively thick and the "Y" ligament of Bigelow, which amounts to the acetabular labrum, is quite thick and heavy so that an injection cannot be made into it without considerable pressure. If soft tissue resistance is encountered in the region where the acetabulum is felt to lie, the needle should be moved slightly further distal. At this point the capsule will be encountered with the usual feeling of the needle passing through the capsule. If local anesthetic solution can be injected with ease at this point, one is reasonably certain that the capsule has been entered. If, however, one again encounters a great amount of resistance to injection, the needle should be replaced. If there is no accumulation of fluid in the joint, the capsule will lie in close proximity to the neck or the margin of the head of the femur. Because of this, once the capsule has been traversed bone will be encountered once again. However, if the needle is gently impaled into the bone that is palpated the leg can then be rotated gently back and forth. If the needle is impaled in the bone of the femur, it will be seen to move as the leg is rotated. It can be withdrawn slightly then and the injection made in this location.

The injection is made into the joint at the level of the neck or the point of attachment of the neck to the head. No attempt is made to extend the needle into the small joint space existing between the femoral head and the acetabular wall, since this space is quite small and very difficult to hit. If material is placed into the hip joint cavity at the level of the neck, the objective will have been achieved since the material will be injected into the hip joint cavity and should disperse through the joint without difficulty.

Dilution of the 80 mg dose of steroid with several milliliters of local anesthetic agent should help to be certain that this dispersion occurs. There is no particular postinjection procedure. However, a word of caution again should be given concerning proximity of this injection to the femoral neurovascular structures. Care must be taken to be certain that these have not been encountered or injured at the time of injection.

Trochanteric Bursa

The "trochanteric bursa" is a rather nebulous structure and several have been described lying around the trochanteric area. Actually the term "trochanteric bursitis" probably represents a syndrome rather than an anatomical description, since some patients have inflammatory reaction in the interspace between the trochanter and the overlying facialata, while others seem to have pain in a more posterior location, probably from the fibrous tissue attachments to the posterior aspect of the trochanter.

An injection into the area overlying the point of maximum tenderness is usually effective. The patient should be lying on the opposite side and the anesthetization should be done, using needles of gradually increasing length up to the actual injection being done with a 3″ spinal needle. Usually, since there is a rather wide area of symptoms two or three wheals may be raised, one over the crest of the trochanter itself, one or two lying somewhat posterior, and possibly another one 2 or 3 cm down the shaft of the femur. With the patient lying on his side and the leg adducted the trochanter is quite prominent and the introduction of the needle is relatively easy. If one carefully injects the local anesthetic in front of the needle there usually is not a great amount of pain.

Three or four separate wheals are made, since it is seldom possible to make all of the injections through a single location. Once these are done the anesthetic is injected through each of these portals into the areas described. As the needle strikes the trochanter it is withdrawn slightly and injection made in this area. Posteriorly the injection is made into the heavy fibrous tissue elements that attach to the posterior trochanter. These can be determined by the amount of resistance met with the needle being introduced. Once the two or three needles are in place, 80 to 120 mg of methylprednisolone are diluted up to about 10 ml of solution with local anesthetic and are injected into these areas in a "needling" type of injection. Care should be taken to cover all of the tender areas.

There are no specific postinjection techniques, though the patient should be warned that, as with some other tissue injections, extreme exacerbation of pain may occur later in the day after the local anesthetic subsides. This will usually respond to heat and medication but sometimes it may last as long as 24 hours and be quite severe. The patient is not usually concerned about this as long as he has been warned of it.

INJECTIONS IN THE REGION OF THE KNEE

The knee is one of the most common sites for injections of steroids and the knee joint is probably the most common joint in which aspiration and/or injection is necessary. There are, however, four separate areas that may be injected in the region of the knee joint (Fig. 17-6): the knee joint proper, the prepatellar bursa, the anserine bursa, and popliteal cysts.

Knee Joint

The knee joint is best injected with the patient lying on the examining table with the knee completely extended. If the joint is filled with fluid, full extension may not be possible. The knee should be extended, however, as fully as possible for insertion of the needle. The point best suited for insertion of a needle into the

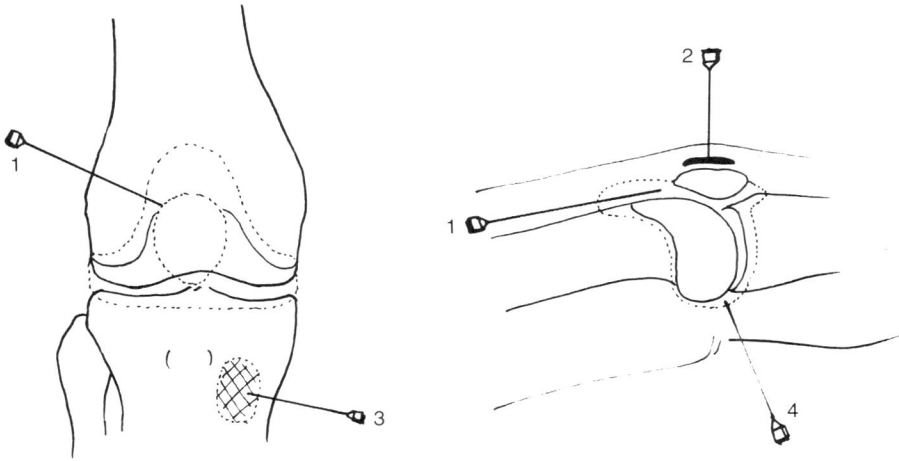

Fig. 17-6. Injection sites for the knee: (1) knee joint, (2) patellar bursa, (3) anserine bursa, and (4) popliteal cyst.

knee joint is the upper outward quadrant. This can be done only with the patient lying down and the knee straight. In this location, however, the needle must pass through only skin, joint capsule, synovium, and into the joint per se. In the upper medial quadrant the needle must go through the vastus medialis muscle, which inserts much lower than the lateralis, and in the lower quadrants on either the medial or lateral side the needle must pass through the prepatellar fat pad. Often this causes problems in getting the tip of the needle into the joint per se. Many people inject the knee joint with the patient sitting up and the knee bent at right angles over the edge of the examining table. In this position the lateral upper quadrant approach is impossible and one must insert the needle in either the medial or lateral inferior quadrant, passing through the fat pad into the joint. If the joint is distended with fluid this is not difficult to do. However, if the joint does not contain a great amount of excess fluid, it is difficult to know when one is in the cavity of the knee joint proper; the injection may be made into the extrasynovial tissue if one is not extremely careful. The best point, however, in the author's opinion, is the upper lateral quadrant and this will be described.

After the local anesthetic has been administered, the relatively large bore needle is introduced. Unless the patient is extremely obese it is easy to anesthetize the capsule quite well with a relatively small needle so that the introduction of an 18-gauge needle does not cause any pain. One must remember, however, that when the needle is first introduced into the joint there are still pain fibers present in the synovial lining on the opposite side of the joint. If one manipulates the needle within the joint the patient will experience rather acute pain. Therefore, once the needle has been felt to enter the joint through the heavy capsular tissue a small amount of local anesthetic can be instilled into the joint. One can tell by the lack of resistance that the fluid is going into an open, free cavity. If this is not the case one must assume that the point of the needle is in some soft tissue structure and it should be withdrawn and reinserted until one is certain that the knee joint has been entered.

A total of 80 mg steroid is injected in the knee joint diluted in 3 or 4 ml of local anesthetic to facilitate dispersion through the joint. As soon as the needle is withdrawn the knee is moved back and forth to ensure complete distribution of the solution before settling occurs in a localized area. The patient is ordinarily completely relieved immediately by the aspiration and injecting. Any postinjection pain is very rare. There are no specific postinjection restrictions.

Prepatellar Bursa

The prepatellar bursa is difficult to enter with a needle unless the bursa has fluid in it since it is quite flat when empty. It is then quite easy to enter and usually this is done with the point angling from distal to proximal after the area has been anesthetized. The needle is inserted directly into the bursa which is then aspirated and material is injected without moving the needle in order to be certain that the needle remains within the bursal sac itself.

Injection will not be met with any great amount of resistance but this is also true of the fatty tissue that surrounds the bursa and therefore this is not a particularly good sign. A good sign, however, is when local anesthetic is injected through the needle and a localizing accumulation of fluid is palpated, indicating that it is retained within a constrained limit of the bursal wall. The average prepatellar bursa should receive about 40 mg of steroid solution diluted with a small amount of local anesthetic. There are no specific postinjection precautions.

Anserine Bursa

The anserine bursa lies on the medial aspect of the upper tibia just to the medial side of the tibial tubercle in the region of the insertion of the gracilis and sartorius tendons. This is very difficult to enter since it does not form fluid ordinarily and one injects basically into the deeper structures just superficial to bone. The bursa lies in this area and since fluid accumulation seldom occurs it is difficult to tell when the bursa has been entered. However, if injection is made just superficial to the bone underneath the tendons and soft tissue structures in the area the patient will usually experience immediate relief of pain from the local anesthetic agent, indicating that the steroid has been injected in the proper location. In this location 40 mg of steroid diluted in 2 or 3 ml of local anesthetic is optimum for injection. This injection tends to cause a considerable amount of postinjection pain. The patient should be warned about this and proper provisions made for the administration of compresses and medication. Other than this there are no specific postinjection precautions.

Popliteal Cyst

Popliteal cysts occur on the medial side of the posterior capsule of the knee joint and practically never are seen laterally. Since the popliteal fossa is filled with fat, it is oftentimes difficult to palpate small bursae and therefore difficult to find the cyst for introduction of a needle. As indicated, the cyst should always be expected to be medial to the midcentral line of the knee joint and therefore medial to the neurovascular structures coursing through the popliteal space. The needle is ordinarily introduced with the patient lying prone and the knee extended as far as possible.

The usual technique for administration of local anesthetic is used, with the anesthetic injected in front of the advancing needle. If there is a considerable amount of fluid in the cyst, the identity will be easily confirmed and the fluid may be withdrawn with care being taken to hold the needle in exactly the same place for injection of the steroid and local anesthetic mixture. A total of 40 mg is usually sufficient, diluted with a small amount of local anesthetic.

If no fluid is encountered one must presume that the popliteal cyst does not exist. Unless the patient has symptoms that would suggest a capsulitis of the posterior joint capsule, an injection of steroid is not necessary if fluid is not obtained. Even when fluid is obtained, injection of steroid into the cyst is merely a temporizing measure that generally will not result in a complete eradication of the cyst. The patient should be told that ultimate surgical excision will be necessary for permanent relief of symptoms. Aspiration of fluid from the cyst and injection of steroids into it, however, are excellent temporizing measures and may give relief of symptoms of the cyst for a considerable length of time.

Injection into the popliteal space is somewhat more risky because of the presence of the femoral artery and vein in the general region. These can be easily palpated in most instances and the injection made considerably medial, so that the likelihood of encountering these structures is small. However, the patient should be observed and cautioned about the presence of marked swelling in the popliteal space during the immediate postinjection period.

INJECTIONS IN THE REGION OF THE ANKLE

In the region of the ankle and the hindfoot three specific areas often require injection of steroids (Fig. 17-7): the ankle joint per se, the peroneal canal, and the subtalar joint.

Injections into the collateral ligaments on either side are not often necessary since these ligamentous structures do not ordinarily continue to cause pain unless instability exists. When persistent pain does occur, particularly in the lateral collateral ligament, one should not hesitate to make a local injection into the area. As in the case of all ligaments and tendons, however, the injection should be made with relatively low pressure so as to not create attritional changes in the ligament that might result in its weakening and ultimate rupture. Much more commonly, however, injections into the ankle joint, peroneal canal, and subtalar joint are necessary.

Ankle Joint

Injection into the ankle joint is usually done with the patient lying down. The joint is approached from the anterior aspect, with the needle angled from the medial side of the joint line toward the central portion or from the lateral

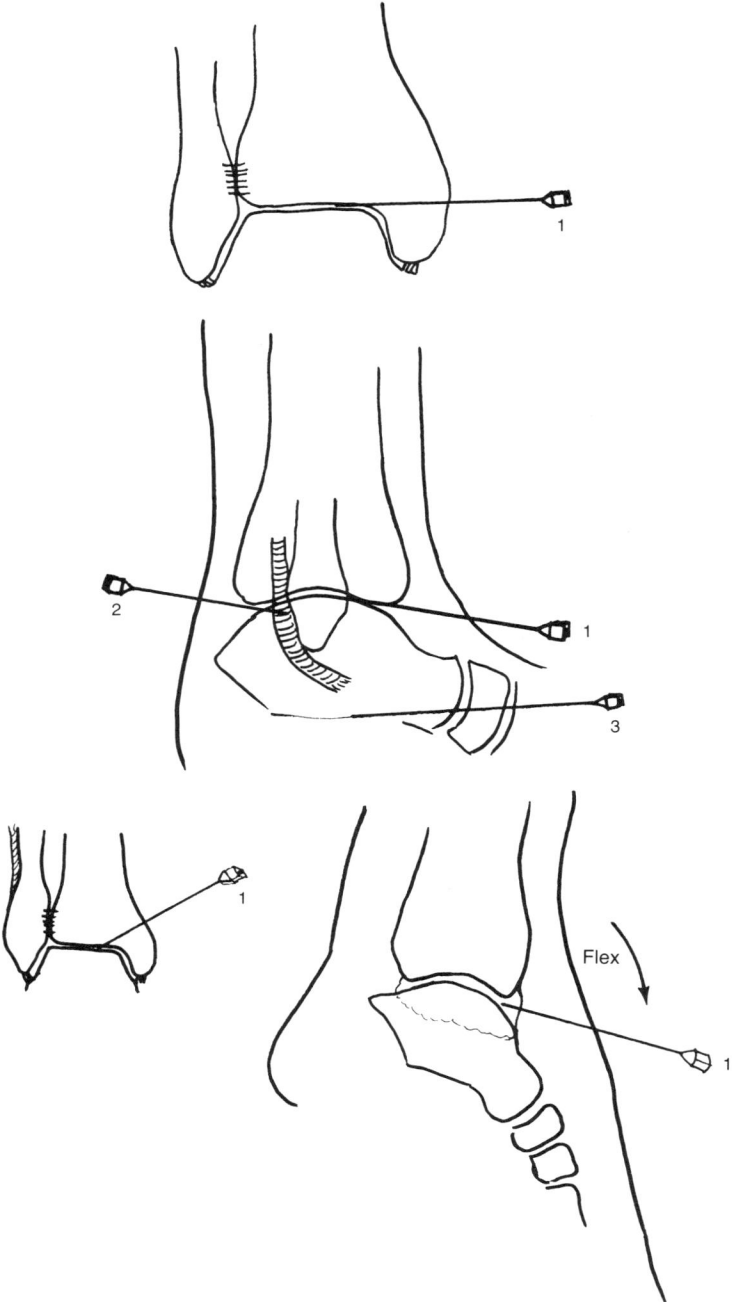

Fig. 17-7. Injection sites for the ankle: (1) ankle joint, (2) peroneal canal, (3) subtalar joint.

aspect of the joint line into the central portion of the joint. The needle should angulate slightly from distal to proximal so that it may slide over the rounded surface of the superior articular surface of the talus. The ankle should be plantar flexed during the beginning of the injection so that the needle may be introduced over this angle. Occasionally, if the joint surface has been narrowed by degenerative changes or trauma, application of traction to the foot by an assistant will help open up the joint so that it may be easier to enter. The standard technique for anesthetizing the area is used and the needle is then inserted. If the joint is not immediately entered, the needle may be "walked" down the tibia until the joint space is reached.

The best way to determine that the joint has been entered is that the needle can be introduced at least another centimeter. Usually the ankle joint will not hold a great amount of fluid, and 0.5 ml of 80 mg/ml preparation is used, diluted with an equal amount of local anesthetic solution. The ankle should be vigorously moved into flexion and extension after the injection to be sure that the fluid is dispersed. There are no specific postinjection precautions and there is usually not a great amount of postinjection pain in the ankle unless a tremendous amount of degenerative changes exist.

Peroneal Canal

The peroneal canal lies just posterior and inferior to the distal end of the fibula, through which the peroneus brevis and the peroneus longus tendons glide. It is a relatively closed canal and can be entered from the lateral and slightly posterior aspect. The patient should be lying on his back and tilted slightly to the opposite side for easier insertion of the needle. The needle can be felt to enter through the tough fibrous roof of the canal. If considerable resistance is met when attempts are made to inject the local anesthetic solution, the needle should be withdrawn slightly since the tip of the needle probably is within one of the peroneal tendons. Usually 0.5 ml of an 80 mg/ml preparation is used, diluted with only a small amount of local anesthetic. There are no specific postinjection precautions and the patient usually has very little postinjection pain.

Subtalar Joint

Injections into the subtalar joint are usually necessitated by degenerative changes that follow a fracture of the os calcis with extension up into the subtalar joint. This joint is best entered from the lateral position. A point approximately 1 cm distal to the tip of the fibula and slightly forward is selected in which the sinus tarsi can be palpated. The needle should go through the fat in the sinus tarsi to extend into the subtalar joint, which lies directly deep to the central portion of the sinus tarsi. The area should be anesthetized according to standard tecnhiques, and the needle introduced by aiming at the central portion of the sinus tarsi but probing slightly with the end of the needle until it is felt to enter the joint cavity. If the part has been anesthetized properly it should not cause a great amount of pain. The subtalar joint has a small volume and will hold only a

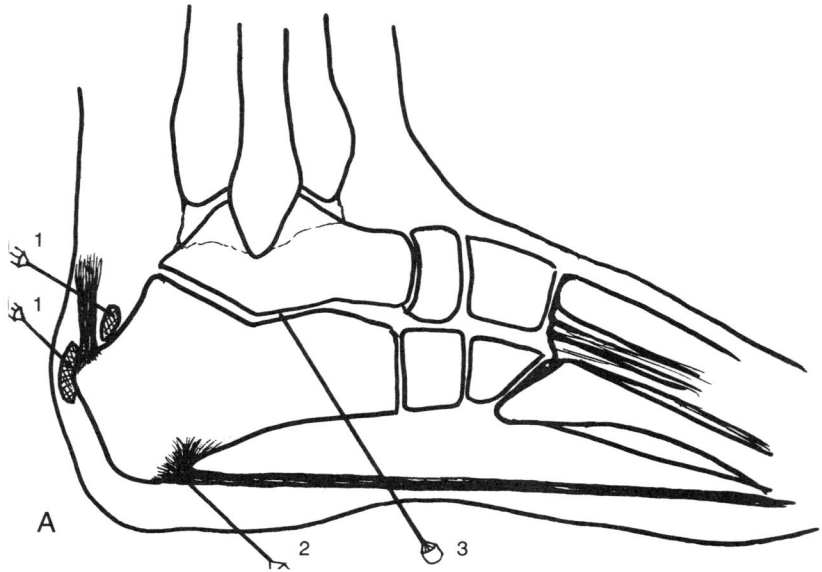

Fig. 17-8. Injection sites for the foot. (**A**): (1) os calcis bursa, (2) plantar fascitis, and (3) subtalar joint. (*Figure continues.*)

small amount of steroid, probably no more than 0.5 ml diluted with a minimal amount of local anesthetic solution.

INJECTIONS IN THE REGION OF THE FOOT

Injections into the foot are usually made into the metatarsophalangeal joints or the interphalangeal joints of the toes, or into structures in the region of the heel (Fig. 17-8A). Specific areas are metatarsophalangeal and interphalangeal joints, os calcis bursae, attachment of the plantar fascia to the os calcis in cases of plantar fasciitis, and the subtalar joint (previously described).

Metatarsophalangeal and Interphalangeal Joints

Injections into the metatarsophalangeal or interphalangeal joints should be made in a similar manner to that described for the fingers (Fig. 17-8B). Injections should be made with the joint in acute flexion and with the needle tilted from proximal to distal so that it slides over the metatarsal head or the condyles of the phalanges into the joints. The metatarsophalangeal joints are relatively large and will hold 0.5 ml of steroid solution diluted with the same amount of local anesthetic. However, the tiny interphalangeal joints will hold only a drop or two of solution and should be injected with pure steroid solution once the area has been thoroughly anesthetized according to standard techniques.

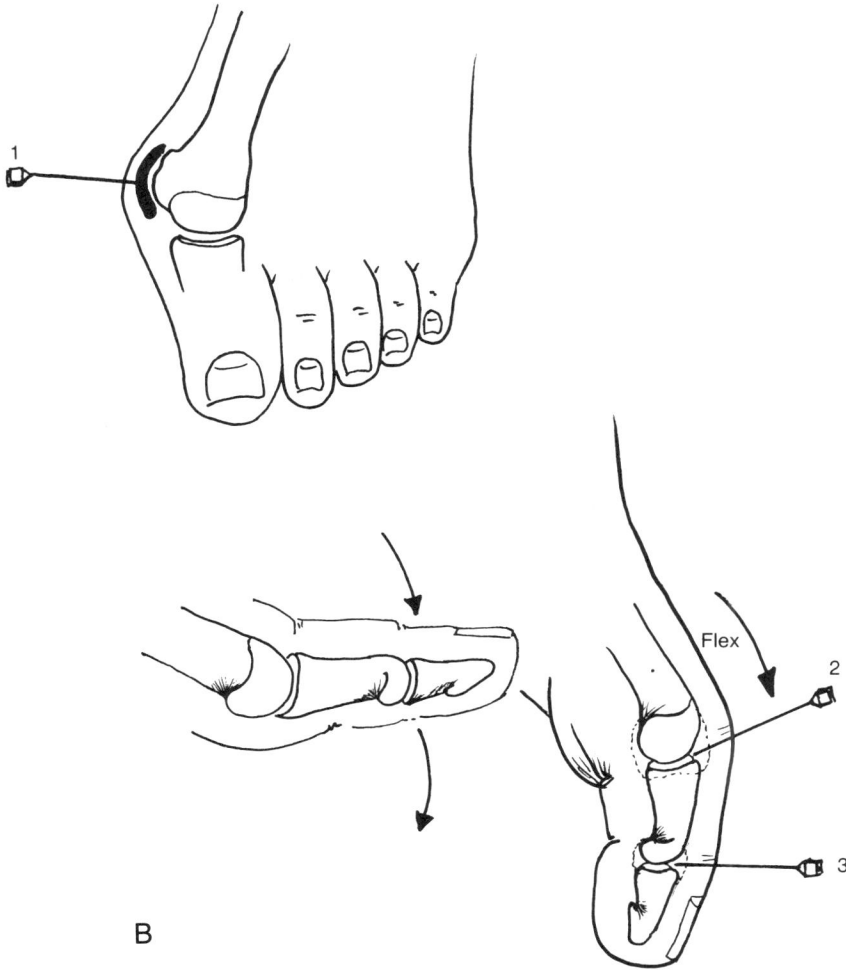

Fig. 17-8 (Continued). (B): (1) os calcis bursa, (2) metatarsophalangeal joint, and (3) interphalangeal joint.

Os Calcis Bursa

Injections into the os calcis bursa should be made in one of two locations. Either the bursa lies external to the point of attachment of the tendo Achilles to the os calcis and, therefore, is palpable underneath the skin, or it may lie internal to the attachment of the tendo Achilles to the os calcis, in which instance it lies in the small angular space between the tendon and bone. Since most ankles are relatively thin it is easy to palpate this point of attachment and make the injection accordingly.

Both of these bursae are quite small and will hold only 0.5 ml of steroid solution and perhaps a small dilution using local anesthetic solution.

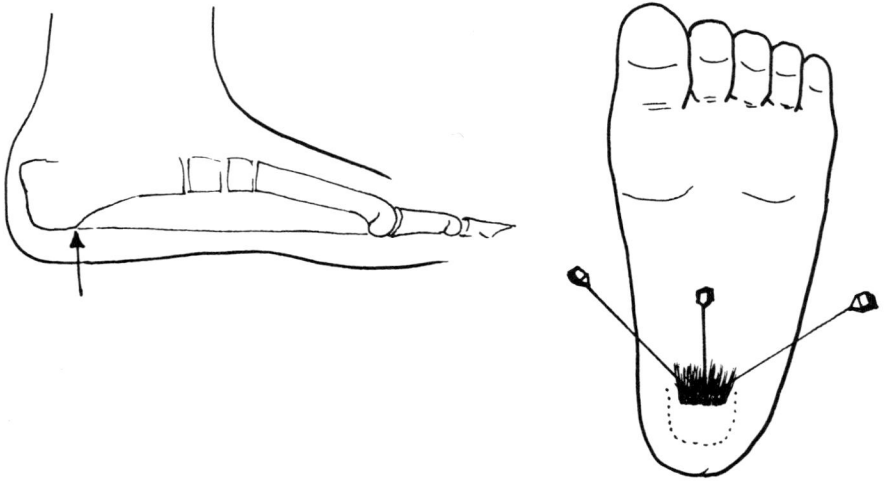

Fig. 17-9. Injection sites for the painful heel.

Plantar Fascia

Injections into the attachment of the plantar fascia of the os calcis are extremely difficult to do because the procedure is extremely painful, particularly when the patient already has a great amount of tenderness in this area (Fig. 17-9). The attachment of the plantar fascia to the os calcis is 3 or 4mm wide, from an anterior-posterior direction but about 1 cm or slightly more in the lateral extension. It is almost impossible to anesthetize this area with local anesthetic. For this reason it is often better to consider the administration of a small amount of sodium pentothal by the anesthesiologist for this injection. The injection should, therefore, be done in the operating room although it may well be done as an outpatient procedure since the duration of the anesthetic is extremely short and the recovery likewise very rapid.

The patient is placed on his back on the operating room table and the heel is prepared. Once the anesthesiologist gives a bolus of sodium pentothal or similar medication, the area can be injected within a minute or so. The injection is thus done without a local anesthetic. Eighty mg of steroid are diluted to about 4 or 5 ml total volume to allow good disperal. Once the patient is anesthetized, an assistant holds the foot in marked dorsiflexion so that the area of attachment can be rapidly "needled" with multiple injections through the attachment and the steroid anesthetic solution generously dispersed through the area. One should have no difficulty feeling the resistance as the needle passes through the plantar fascia into bone. This area should be thoroughly injected before the patient awakens.

It is surprising how little postinjection pain these patients have. They usually can be allowed to walk on the heel relatively soon after the injection.

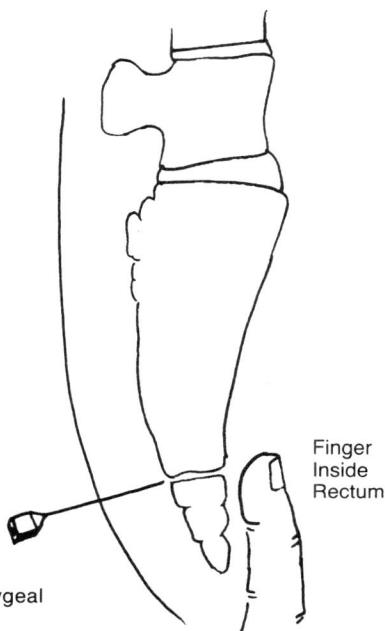

Fig. 17-10. Injection site for the sacrococcygeal joint.

INJECTIONS IN THE SACROCOCCYGEAL JOINT

Since the "painful tailbone" syndrome is generally related to degenerative changes in the sacrococcygeal joint, injection of a small amount of steroid into this joint often yields dramatic relief of symptoms that can be of long duration (Fig. 17-10). The joint is injected using a 25-guage needle with the patient lying on his side. If the operator is right-handed the patient should be lying on his right side so that the operator can insert his left index finger into the rectum in order to palpate the underside of the joint. The injection is otherwise difficult to do without penetrating the rectum, since the rectal wall lies directly on the sacrococcygeal articulation. The skin and subcutaneous tissues are then anesthetized with infiltration and then usually a 0.5 ml dose of steroid diluted with a small amount of local anesthetic can be injected directly into the joint. The needle can be felt to enter the joint by palpating it with the finger in the rectum and by gentle manipulation of the coccyx back and forth through the sacrococcygeal joint. The patient usually experiences immediate complete relief of pain. There is usually very little postinjection pain and, oftentimes, the relief of the pain is not only dramatic but of long duration. There are no postinjection precautions.

18

EPIPHYSEAL INJURIES IN CHILDREN AND ADOLESCENTS

Growth in the long bones in children and adolescents occurs in definite patterns that center around the epiphyseal centers. Basic activity involves the epiphyseal plate, which is made up of cells that by continuously dividing create new bone cells along the diaphyseal margin. They thereby add to the length of the bone by addition between the old diaphysis and the epiphyseal plate. The epiphysis itself is represented by the portion of bone that lies on the opposite side of the epiphyseal plate from the diaphysis. This so-called epiphyseal center often, but not invariably, extends into the joint at the end of that particular long bone. If the epiphyseal plate is healthy and if no abnormalities are involved in its normal growth pattern, an orderly longitudinal lengthening of the bone occurs with preservation of the long axis of the bone. In other words, the normal growth of the epiphysis is at right angles to the epiphyseal plate and normal growth results in a longitudinal growth of the bone along this line.

If constitutional or systemic alteration changes this normal growth pattern, either increased or decreased bone formation results in a change in the speed of growth along these longitudinal lines. If damage occurs to the epiphyseal plate in a localized area the remaining portion of the plate continues to grow at its normal rate but the injured area will often grow at a much slower rate, resulting in various deformities. These usually occur as angular deformities and may take a variety of forms. While there is a certain predicability related to the type of injury to the epiphyseal plate, one is often surprised that the amount and extent of change may not always follow the predicted course.

A certain capriciousness about the growth of these epiphyseal plates will occasionally defy prediction of the ultimate condition of bone growth. However, any great amount of damage to or disruption of the epiphyseal plate itself will result in abnormal bone growth. On the other hand, injuries near the epiphyseal plate that do no involve the plate will usually result in a stimulation of growth from the epiphyseal plate. Overgrowth of long bones near fractures has been noted and sometimes may be extreme, particularly if the injury is relatively near to the epiphyseal plate and if the patient is quite young. An example is fracture of the shaft of the femur in children under 7 years of age, in whom overgrowth of the femur will result in some leg length discrepancy in many cases. For this reason it is acceptable and often desirable to leave the bone ends in a fractured femur in these young children in up to 1 cm of overriding. With such "bayonet apposition" the overgrowth of the femur will be compensated in advance by this overriding. The ultimate result will be a restoration of the normal length of the bone compared with the opposite, uninjured, side.

INJURIES INVOLVING THE EPIPHYSEAL PLATE

Because of the rapid growth of its cells, the line of the epiphyseal plate often becomes the site of injury and the attachment of the plate to the adjacent diaphysis is a point of diminished strength. Injuries through the epiphyseal plate, the epiphysis itself, and the adjacent diaphysis often occur in children who are still experiencing active longitudinal bone growth. These injuries may assume a variety of configurations and each is related to a particular type of deformity that is usually predictable. In 1963 Salter and Harris presented a classification of these epiphyseal injuries with the implication that the growth disturbances predictable after healing could be related to classification of the epiphyseal injury present.

Figure 18-1 shows the basic configuration of the Salter–Harris classification. Type 1 results in a mere separation of the epiphysis that ordinarily occurs between the epiphyseal plate and the diaphysis. Type 2, on the other hand, occurs between the diaphysis and the epiphyseal plate but fractures up through the diaphysis so that a spike of bone is left attached, yet the epiphyseal plate remains intact for the most part. Type 3 is a fracture through the epiphysis itself, with a disruption of the epiphyseal plate and a separation of that portion of the plate from its diaphyseal attachment, leaving it attached to the displaced fragment of epiphysis. Type 4 results in a fracture through the epiphysis, the epiphyseal plate, and the diaphysis along a continuous line. These, of course, result in the disruption of the epiphyseal plate but without much detachment of the plate from the adjacent epiphysis or diaphysis. Finally, type 5 injuries result in a crushing of the epiphyseal plate without separation but with damage to the cell in the epiphyseal plate, resulting in diminution of their growth potential.

Salter and Harris point out that while any epiphyseal injury may result in growth disturbance, it is much more common following types 3, 4, and 5, in which there is actual disruption of the epiphyseal plate. Most injuries that are

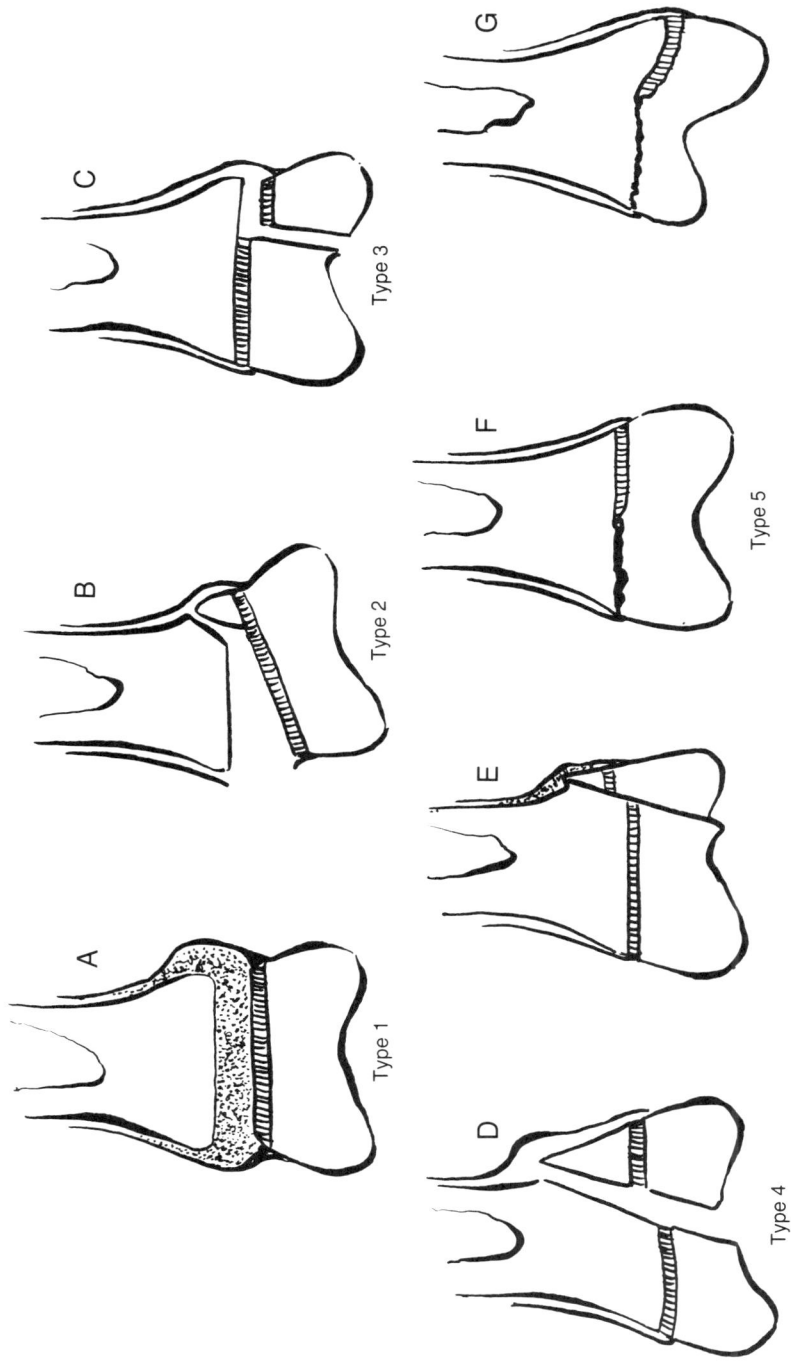

Fig. 18-1. Various types of epiphyseal damage included in the Salter-Harris classification. (See text for complete description of types 1, 2, 3, 4, and 5). Note that Figure E demonstrates the healed condition after a type 4 injury and Figure G demonstrates the type of deformity created by cessation of growth in a portion of the epiphyseal plate caused by type 5 injury.

Type 1

Type 2

Type 3

Type 4

Type 5

classified as type 1 or 2 may be treated by closed reduction and seldom present any growth disturbance unless there is localized damage to the plate. In types 1 and 2 the epiphyseal plate remains intact, with the fracture in type 2 occurring through the associated diaphysis. Type 3 and 4 injuries often require open reductions and internal fixation to position accurately and securely fix the fragments so that the epiphyseal plate is as nearly restored as possible to diminish the possibility of growth disturbances. In type 5 injuries damage to the cartilage cells of the epiphyseal plate has occurred. Regardless of the form of treatment, growth disturbance is extremely common but usually is not manifested for some time since it is related to equal growth between the normal cells and the damaged cells. As a general rule the development of deformities following epiphyseal injuries is slow and children or adolescents with injuries to the epiphyseal complex should be evaluated for at least 1 year after injury to be certain that growth deformity has not occurred.

In all instances of injuries involving the epiphysis the parents and the patient should be warned that growth disturbances may occur regardless of the type of treatment given. However, the physician can usually predict the greater likelihood of the occurrence of these disturbances in these certain types of injuries involving the disruption of the epiphyseal plate itself (Fig. 18-2A).

This should not be taken to mean that damage to the epiphysis in trauma to the extremities is always deleterious, since often, quite the opposite is true. It has long been recognized that children and adolescents have a tremendous ability for remodeling following fractures. This is useful in allowing the surgeon to accept somewhat less than total anatomical reduction of fractures and allow for this remodeling to correct the deformity. However, all remodeling does not necessarily result in relief of the contracture: if marked angulation of a fracture occurs near the midshaft of the bone, there is likely to be only an increase of longitudinal growth in the deformed position. However, if a fracture occurs near the epiphyseal plate, such as in fractures of the distal radius (Fig. 18-2B) in children, one can accept a relatively high degree of resulting angulation at the fracture site with the assurance that the remodeling effect of the epiphyseal plate will correct the angulation. In the extremely young child dorsal angulation of up to 30 or 40 degrees of the distal radius will almost invariably correct down to a normal functional degree. Most practitioners, however, are not willing to take the chance that correction of these marked angulatory deformities will occur since the capricious nature of the epiphyseal growth has been previously pointed out. Therefore, gross abnormalities of position should always be corrected.

TREATMENT

From the foregoing it would appear that the treatment of injuries to the epiphysis requires special judgment and a special level of care. These four specific points should be remembered when one is treating fractures of the epiphysis.

1. Reduce accurately and as nearly anatomically as possible. If damage to the growth center has occurred, reestablishment of as normal a relationship as

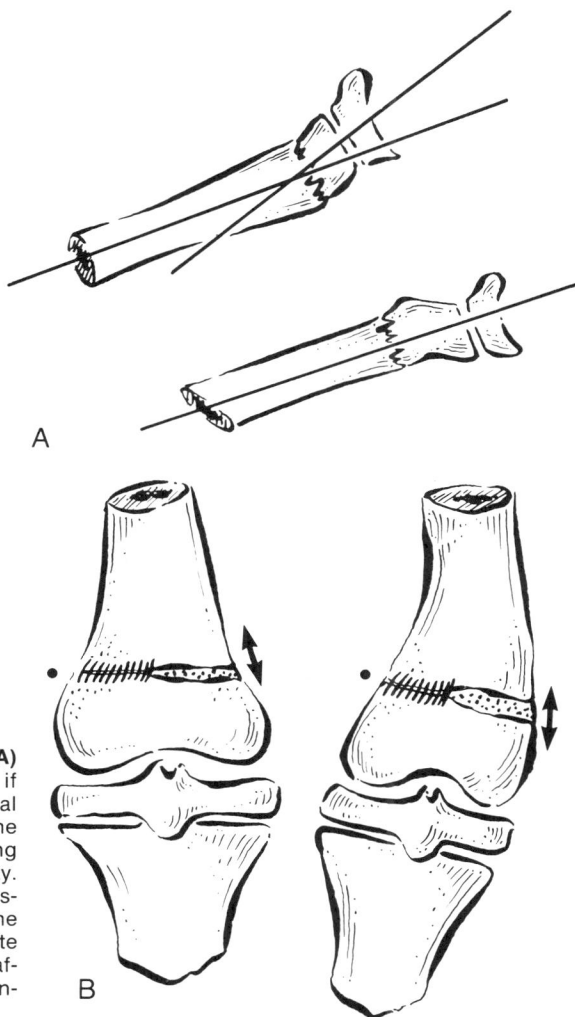

Fig. 18-2. The effect of growth. **(A)** The deformity may be corrected if the fracture is near the epiphyseal plate, so continued growth at the diaphysis may result in remodeling and straightening of the deformity. **(B)** Deformity may be created if cessation of growth of one side of the epiphyseal plate leaves the opposite side unaffected. Growth on the unaffected side will then result in an angular deformity.

possible between the epiphysis, the epiphyseal plate, and the diaphysis will result in the least damage to the growth potential. This is one instance in which anatomical reduction must be accomplished even if open operation is necessary. An open operation, however, should be very minimal and only the amount of manipulation absolutely necessary to secure an anatomical reduction should be done. From a practical standpoint injuries to the epiphysis, particularly those in which the diaphysis is separated from the epiphyseal plate, are extremely easy to reduce and usually anatomical reduction can be obtained.

2. Fixation with pins, if necessary, is advisable to maintain this anatomical reduction. These injuries usually are relatively stable and fixation devices will not often be required. However, in Salter classifications 3 and 4 the disruption of the epiphyseal plate itself demands anatomical reduction. Since this maintenance reduction is so important the use of percutaneous fixation pins for a short

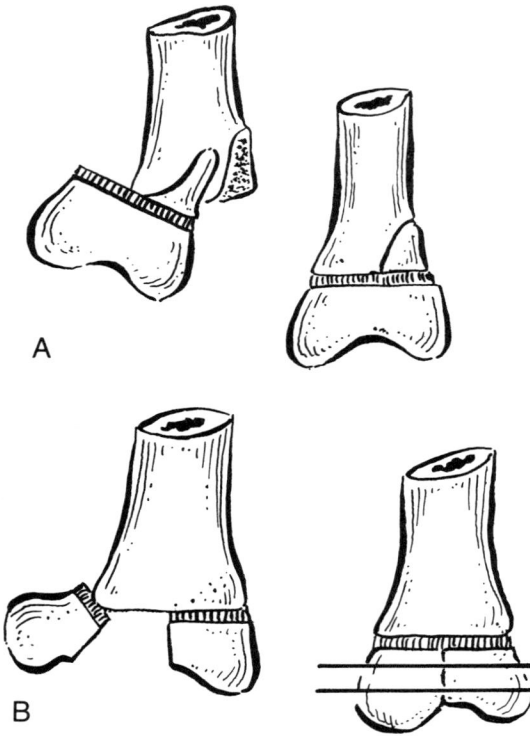

Fig. 18-3. Anatomical reduction. **(A)** Anatomical reduction is mandatory in the case of a Salter 2 injury. The small spike of diaphysis will serve as a guide and make anatomical reduction more stable. Likewise, it will result in some increased healing since bone healing will occur across the small disrupted spike. **(B)** A Salter 3 injury must be anatomically reduced and fixation by a pin is often necessary to maintain this reduction.

period of time (while early healing occurs) will often assure the surgeon that this anatomical reduction will be maintained (Fig. 18-3B). If done percutaneously, pinning should be done with the assistance of an image intensifier so that accurate reduction can be visualized as well as the accurate fixation of pins.

3. Since fixation is not provided by the irregular margins of a fracture in many of these cases it should be provided by external means for a somewhat longer period of time than with fractures through the bone. When a spike of diaphysis is contained within the fracture complex, such as in Salter 2 classifications, the spike itself will heal at its ordinary pace and fixation may not need to be maintained for as long (Fig. 13-3A). However, in Salter 1 fractures particularly, maintenance fixation for an extra 20 percent longer time will make certain that healing has been established across the interface between the epiphysis and the diaphysis so that migration will not occur once external fixation has been removed.

4. Children with injuries to the epiphysis of any degree should have rather long-term follow-up by x-ray studies to determine whether injury to the epiphyseal function has occurred. One year is usually considered the minimum time that these injuries should be evaluated, since enough growth should occur in this time to allow one to determine whether this growth is going to be in an orderly and normal pattern. The family practitioner should refer these cases relatively early if he or she suspects some alteration in normal growth.

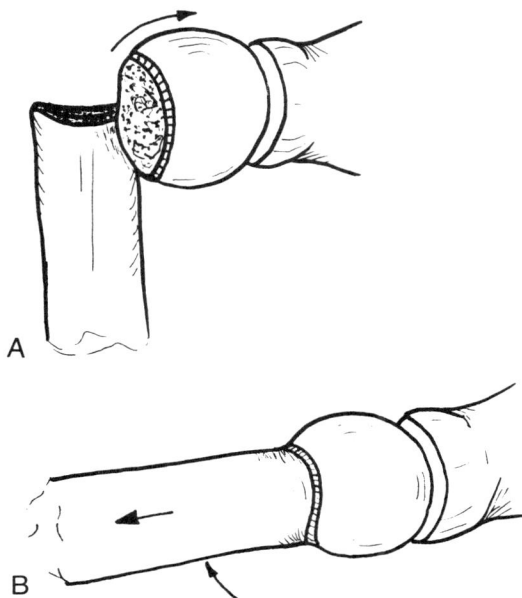

Fig. 18-4. Fracture–dislocation of the proximal humerus results in an abducted position of the proximal fragment with angulation of the shaft fragment as it is pulled down into alignment with the body. Reduction requires that traction be applied in the side-arm position so that the humerus can be brought up to the abducted proximal fragment.

With the above discussion concerning the general principles of the management of epiphyseal fractures as a foundation, the following sections will discuss characteristics of most major epiphyseal injuries seen in the child or adolescent. This discussion will not include relatively rare injuries to epiphyseal centers that are not related to longitudinal bone growth or to proper development of periarticular structures but will be limited to those most common injuries in which the factors discussed above are most applicable.

Region of the Shoulder Joint

The most common injury to the shoulder joint is separation of the epiphysis at the proximal end of the humerus. This is generally a Salter 1 injury, though occasionally a small spike of diaphysis may be included, making it a Salter 2 fracture. For the most part, however, the injury occurs with an actual slipping off of the upper epiphysis, with separation through the interface between the epiphyseal plate and the diaphysis. The upper or small epiphyseal fragment will immediately be drawn into abduction while the humeral or shaft fracture fragment is brought downward by the force of gravity. When the amount of slippage is incomplete, it can sometimes by reduced and held out into a reasonable position until a spica-type cast can be applied. However, most of these separations, when complete, require the patient to be treated with side arm traction for a few days (Fig. 18-4) until reduction has been obtained. Once this has occurred the patient can be taken to the operating room and a spica cast applied in the "pivotal" position. If the shoulder spica cast is applied with the arm out to the side, a buckling will often occur at the site of the separation and loss of position will occur. The pivotal position means that the arm is brought upward so that the hand and arm are held above the head (usually with the elbow flexed). In this position the separation will be stable and reduction can be maintained.

The cast is left on for about 6 weeks after which it is removed; several days are required to bring the arm down to the side. Some degree of angulation can be accepted at this particular location. If an incomplete separation occurs in which the epiphysis has slipped and is angulated slightly but is stable, the patient can be treated with a sling and swathe type of immobilization. Frequent radiographs should be taken both in the anteroposterior (AP) and axillary (or transthoracic lateral) views to be certain that the position is maintained. If there is any question about the adequacy of the position, the patient should be referred to the orthopedist for a more experienced opinion.

Region of the Elbow (Fig. 18-5)

Fractures involving the epiphysis of the bones comprising the elbow usually can be classified into those involving the medial condyle, those involving the lateral condyle, those involving the medial epicondyle, and those involving the neck of the radius (Fig. 18-6). While other epiphyseal injuries may occur in this region, these constitute the vast majority of injuries seen.

Fracture of the lateral humeral condyle is much more common than of the medial condyle or medial epicondyle. It usually results from a fall on the outstretched arm and is usually Salter type 4. Therefore accurate anatomical reduction must be maintained until the fracture unites or growth disturbance will result. Moreover, maintenance of reduction is often difficult due to the pull of

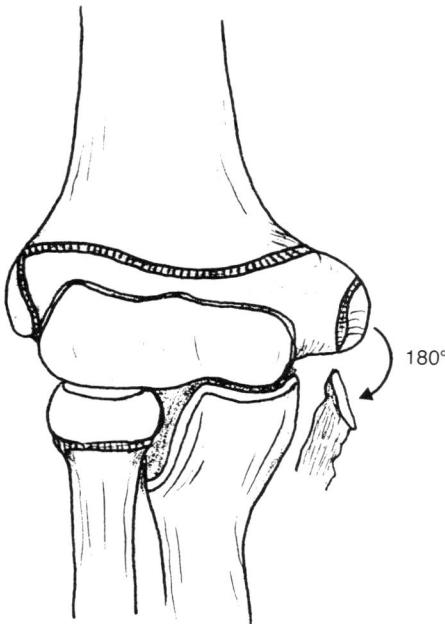

180°

Fig. 18-5. The epiphyses surrounding the elbow are shown. These include the transverse epiphysis at the distal humerus, both epicondylar epiphyses, and the epiphysis at the radial head. Avulsion of the medial epicondyle is shown with the typical 180 degree rotation deformity caused by the pull of the flexor musculature.

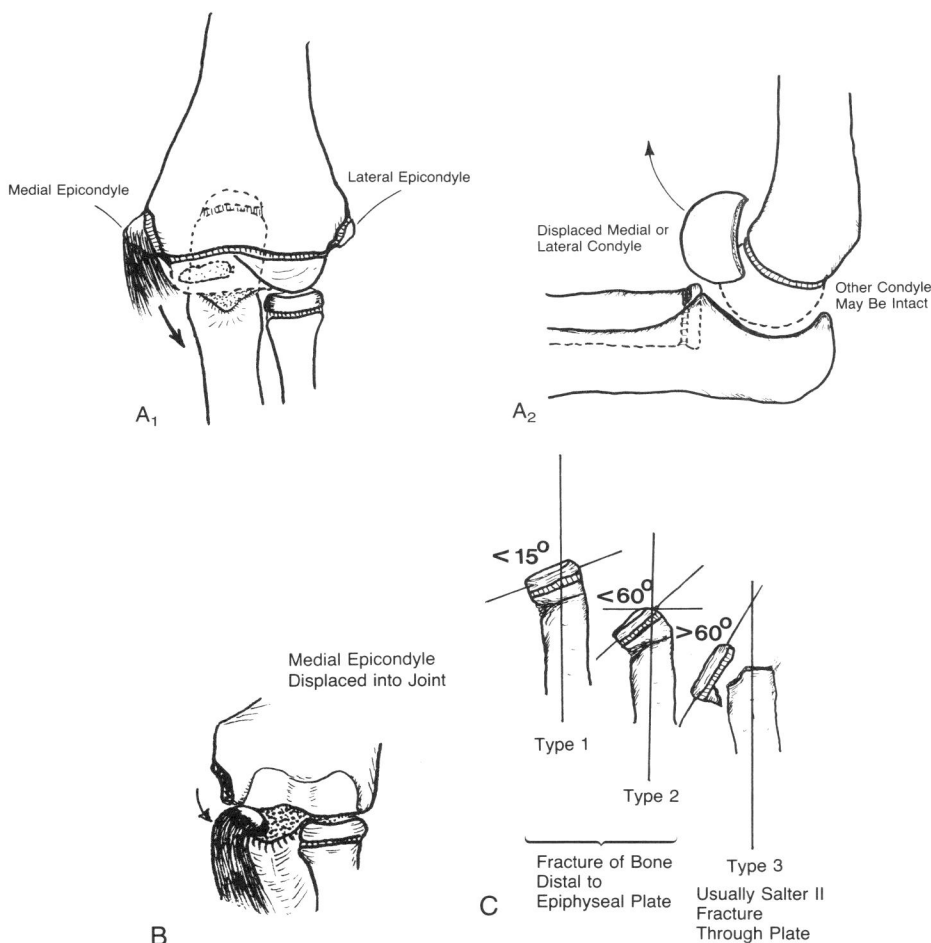

Fig. 18-6. Fracture–dislocation of epiphyseal centers about the elbow. **(A)** Fracture–dislocation of the lateral or medial condyles must be reduced anatomically, even if open reduction is required, and stabilized with fixation pins. **(B)** Avulsion of the medial epicondylar epiphysis requires open reduction and fixation in most instances. **(C)** Fracture–dislocation of the proximal radial epiphysis. Angulation of less than 15 degrees is probably acceptable but more than this should be corrected by either manipulation or open reduction, if necessary.

the extensor musculature originating from the lateral epicondyle. This tends to result in rotation of the fragment and makes it extremely difficult to control. For the most part, fractures of the lateral epicondyle should be referred to the orthopedic surgeon for open reduction and internal fixation by pinning.

Fractures of the medial humeral condyle are likewise often Salter type 4. Similarly to those of the lateral condyle, they must be opened for an anatomical reduction and internal fixation with multiple pins. While these are rarer than those of the lateral epicondyle, the likelihood of injury to the ulnar nerve is greater because of the close proximity to the bone posterior to the condyle.

Almost all of these fractures, however, do involve the epiphyseal plate along with the epiphysis and the diaphysis. Anatomical reduction is therefore mandatory if one is to avoid growth disturbance with the resulting deformity.

Avulsion of the medial epicondyle is seen relatively commonly in children and represents an actual avulsion by the flexor mass, which attaches to this region and pulls the epiphysis off by sudden contracture or a sudden valgus force to the elbow. There is considerable difference in opinion as to whether anatomical reduction of the epiphysis is necessary. Most orthopedic surgeons will usually leave a medial epicondyle that is displaced less than 1 cm from its bed. Even this amount of displacement occasionally will cause disturbances, particularly from abnormal growth of the epiphysis in its faulty location. If there is displacement further than 1 cm, open reduction is usually definitely indicated. As mentioned, even those with any displacement at all will be treated by anatomical reduction and pinning by many orthopedic surgeons. The greatest problem concerning the medial epicondyle avulsion injuries is that if the joint has been opened by the force that resulted in the avulsion, the epiphysis may often dislocate into joint. If the epicondyle has been displaced into the joint, removal is mandatory since failure to do this will result in a devastating amount of damage to the joint and permanent consequences. When open reduction is accomplished, fixation with one or two small Kirschner wires is usually adequate.

Fractures of the radial head usually involve the neck just on the diaphyseal side of the side of the epiphyseal plate and result ordinarily in marked angulation of the proximal radius.

Most orthopedic surgeons believe that angulation of less than 15 degrees is probably acceptable since some correction will occur with epiphyseal growth. However, any angulation greater than this is unacceptable and correction must be obtained either by manipulation or by open reduction, if necessary. Excision of the radial head in children is contraindicated because of the severe valgus deformity that will result. While the corrected radial head fracture is usually stable enough that no fixation is necessary, the use of fixation pins for a short time is acceptable.

The Wrist

Epiphyseal separations at the distal radius are ordinarily at the diaphyseal–epiphyseal plate interface and are ordinarily a Salter 2 separation with a spike of diaphysis avulsed dorsally. The entire epiphyseal fragment is dorsal and reduction can only be obtained by placing the distal radius in marked flexion, as described in the section on treatment of distal radius fractures. The small diaphyseal spike will ordinarily reduce anatomically with pressure and serves to maintain the reduction of the entire distal radial epiphysis (Fig. 18-7).

Epiphyseal Separation in the Hand

The hand has an unusual distribution of epiphyseal centers in the small bones. All of the phalanges have only a single epiphysis at the base while the metacarpal epiphysis lies at its distal end in the region of the neck. The metacar-

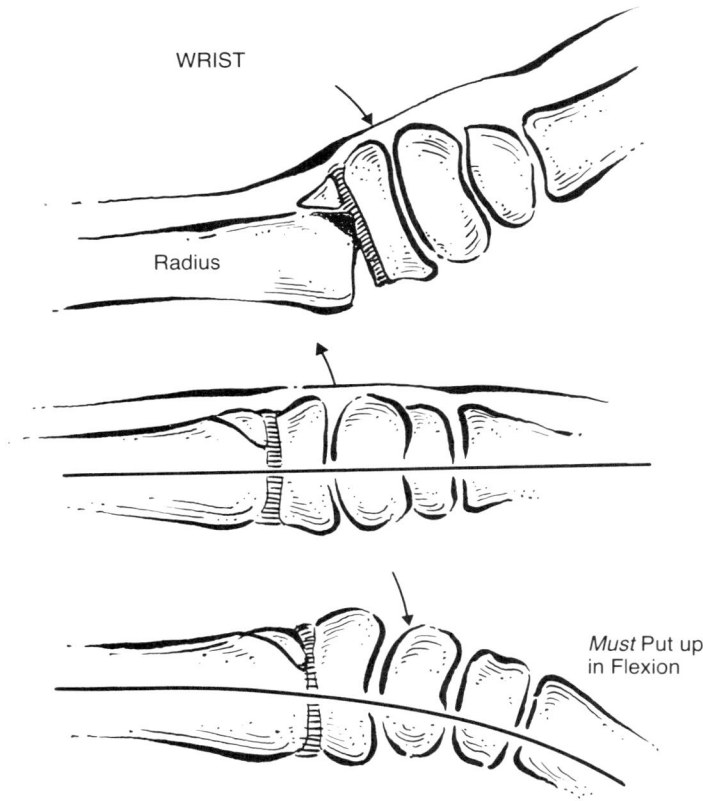

Fig. 18-7. Fracture–dislocation of the distal radial epiphysis usually involves a dorsal spike of bone (Salter 2) that must be drawn down into anatomical alignment with reduction of the epiphysis and held in this position by immobilization and in flexion.

pophalangeal joint therefore has two epiphyseal centers involved in the adjacent bones, as do most other joints in the body, but the interphalangeal joints have only one. The first metacarpal bone has epiphyseal centers at both ends.

Most epiphyseal separations in the hand are at the distal metacarpal epiphysis with a separation of the metacarpal head. These fractures are ordinarily drawn into flexion of the distal fragment because of intrinsic pull and are usually displaced enough that reduction is mandatory. Once reduction has been accomplished these are usually reasonably stable and can be maintained by external fixation alone. Near-anatomical reduction, however, should be established and maintained even if fixation with percutaneous pins is necessary.

Injuries to the epiphyseal centers at the base of the phalanges may take the form of either a complete separation of the epiphyseal plate from the diaphysis of the proximal phalanx with angulation of the shaft fragment in relationship to the small epiphyseal fragment, or a fracture through the epiphysis itself due to the pull of the strong collateral ligament that attaches to the epiphysis (Fig. 18-8). The complete separation is usually a Salter 1 or 2, can be reduced by manipu-

HAND

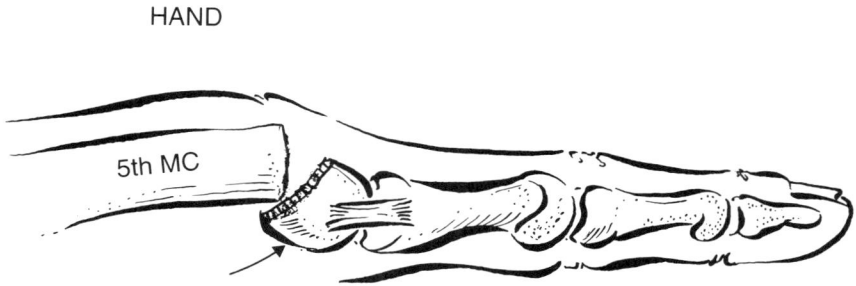

Fig. 18-8. Fracture–dislocation of the distal epiphysis of the metacarpal shafts. The deformity is maintained by the ligamentous attachments of the proximal joints of the fingers and pin fixation is often necessary to obtain stability.

lation, and is ordinarily quite stable with external fixation alone. The fracture occurring through the epiphysis itself, however, is ordinarily markedly displaced and, of course, as is characteristic of Salter 3 fractures, usually results in a defect in the epiphyseal plate. These small fractures must be reduced anatomically; this is usually impossible to accomplish without open reduction. Internal fixation with small Kirschner wires is ordinarily satisfactory and renders the fracture stable. Fractures of the other epiphyses in the phalanges are not often seen and usually constitute no problem from the standpoint of treatment. An exception is the Salter 3 injury to the proximal phalangeal epiphysis, which is held off by ligament attachment and must often be reduced by open operation (Fig. 18-9).

Region of the Hip

The slipped capital femoral epiphysis has been described in some detail in Chapter 12, The Hip. It occurs in adolescents, usually boys. The patient is usually of a Frölich-type body build and is almost invariably overweight. The biggest

HAND

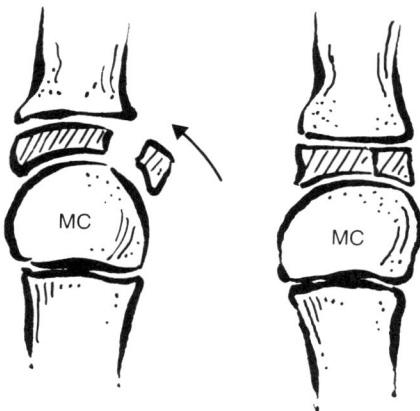

Fig. 18-9. Fractures occurring at the proximal epiphysis of the proximal phalanx. Fractures here at the metacarpophalangeal joint usually result from ligament attachment. As with all Salter 3 injuries, an anatomical reduction must be obtained even if open reduction is necessary.

problem for the family practitioner in dealing with slipped capital femoral epiphysis is recognition. The index of suspicion should be high in a youngster who
complains of gradually increasing pain in the hip with a sudden acute exacerbation following a relatively trivial injury. Often the pain is referred almost entirely
to the knee so that the hip is not suspected as the origin of the pain and the knee
is exonerated after radiographs show negative findings. The epiphyseal separation at the capital femoral epiphysis is invariably a Salter 1 and the radiographic
findings are very subtle in the early stages of the condition. Since the slip is
always into varus and is posterior, the condition is first identified on the lateral
films as a posterior migration of the head. Later on the deformity appears more
dramatic and, of course, the complete separation is very dramatic, with severe
pain and deformity. All instances of slipped capital femoral epiphysis should be
referred to the orthopedic surgeon as soon as the diagnosis is made so that
adequate care, usually operative, can be given.

Region of the Knee

The upper tibial epiphysis is usually not the site of separation or slip. The
only condition of importance concerning this epiphysis is Osgood-Schlatter's
disease, which has been discussed in great detail in Chapter 13, The Knee.
Almost all of the epiphyseal separations and injuries in the region of the knee
joint involve the distal epiphysis of the femur. All five of the Salter classification
groups may be seen but by far the most common are types 1 and 2 (Fig. 18-10).
Closed reduction is usually possible in both of these instances and therefore
operative intervention is seldom necessary unless reduction cannot be obtained.
Even when perfect reduction is obtained, however, some damage to the epiphyseal plate may occur so that growth abnormalities are relatively common. When
Salter type 3 or 4 injuries occur to the distal femoral epiphysis, reduction and
accurate maintenance of this reduction are, of course, mandatory. This can
almost never be accomplished by closed means and invariably open reduction
with internal fixation using pins is necessary. Transverse fixation pins are relatively easy to apply and are not likely to cause or accentuate epiphyseal damage.

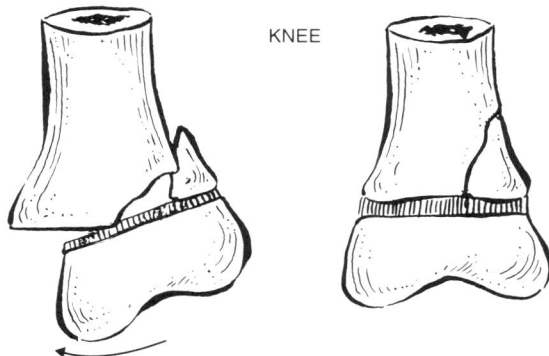

KNEE

Fig. 18-10. Fracture–dislocations of the distal epiphysis of
the femur generally occur as a
Salter 2 fracture with marked
dislocation. They are usually
easy to reduce by closed methods and are ordinarily quite stable with plaster immobilization.

As in many instances of Salter 3 or 4 injuries, however, even with the most meticulous reduction and fixation, growth abnormalities occur and patients and their families should be advised of this possibility.

Even after fixation has been accomplished by open means, additional external immobilization is necessary. It has been well documented that long leg casts do not provide adequate immobilization of these injuries because of the shear force provided by the remainder of the extremity in relationship to the trunk. Therefore, immobilization in a spica cast is necessary. One should not tempt fate by depending upon a long leg cast alone.

Injuries to the epiphyseal centers at the upper tibia and fibula are not common since a force great enough to cause damage to these centers will have already resulted in disruption of the distal femoral epiphysis. When damage to the upper tibial center does occur it is usually in combination with massive damage to the knee. In the relatively young patient Salter 1 and 2 dislocations may occasionally occur, but tibial epiphyseal injuries must be associated with fibular epiphyseal injuries for positional loss to occur. Reduction of these type 1 or 2 injuries is usually relatively simple by closed means. Immobilization with a long leg cast is ordinarily acceptable as long as the knee is flexed.

The injury to the anterior lip of the upper tibial epiphysis resulting in Osgood-Schlatter's disease has been discussed in detail in the section on conditions involving the knee.

Region of the Ankle

Since ankle injuries are relatively common, and since the distal tibia and fibula have very little muscular support with tremendous strains placed on them by alterations in body position, it is reasonable to expect injuries to the distal epiphyses of the tibia and fibula to be relatively common. Salter type 1 and 2 injuries form the majority of these epiphyseal injuries, particularly in the younger patient (Fig. 18-11). However, the very fact that the medial malleolus is included within the distal epiphysis of the tibia makes the occurrence of Salter 3 injuries much more common: a fracture of the medial malleolus must of necessity break through the epiphysis into the epiphyseal plate. Salter type 4 injuries, however, are extremely uncommon and occur only as a result of severe massive trauma to the ankle.

As is the case with injuries to the upper fibular epiphysis, those to the lower epiphysis almost invariably are Salter 1 or 2 and are related to injuries to the tibia. One exception occurs in Salter 1 injuries resulting from "ankle sprain," which reduce spontaneously so that they cannot be identified on the radiograph. A child with a "turned ankle" who has a negative x-ray finding but exquisite tenderness over the epiphyseal plate level and less tenderness over the lateral collateral ligaments should be considered to have a Salter 1 epiphyseal separation and treated by casting. Many of these youngsters are seen and radiographs taken, and are treated without immobilization when the x-ray studies are found to show no evidence of bony damage. Later radiographs will show damage around the epiphysis and many of these children will develop a chronically

ANKLE

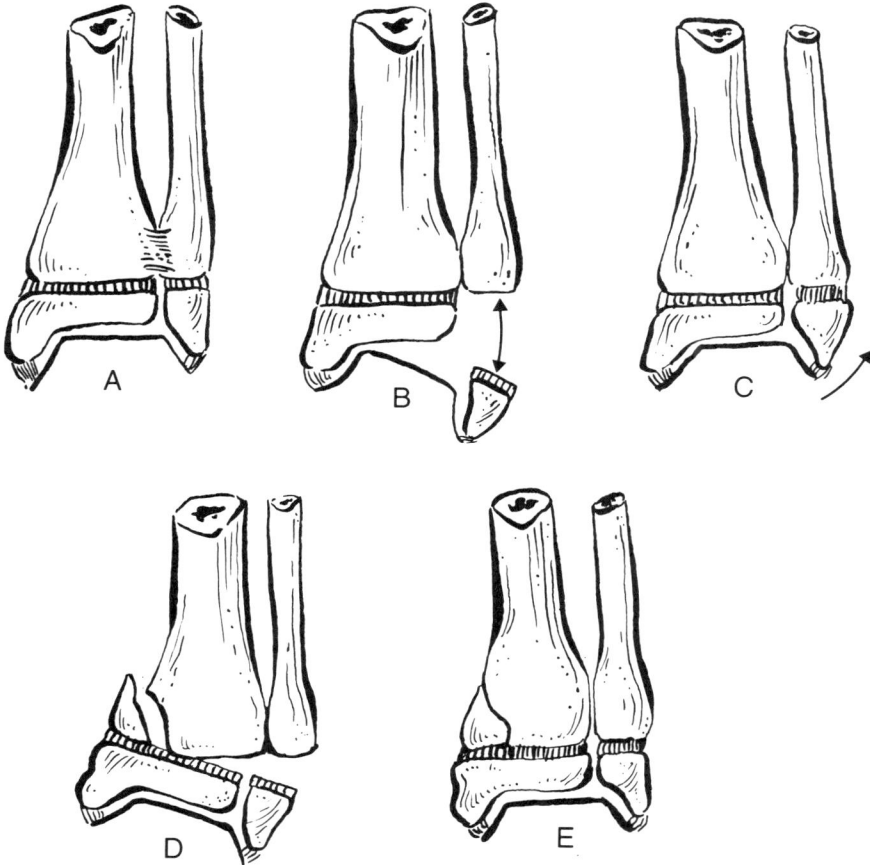

Fig. 18-11. Fracture–dislocations at the ankle may take one of several courses. **(A)** Normal anatomy. **(B)** The mechanism by which a disruption of the distal epiphysis of the fibula may result in lateral stability with marked dislocation of the ankle being possible. **(C)** Appearance after closed reduction by manipulation: the original injury can hardly be seen. **(D)** When the distal tibial epiphysis is included, a Salter 2 fracture–dislocation usually occurs since the foot segment invariably dislocates medially, knocking off a piece of bone from the diaphysis. Again, closed reduction can result in complete restoration of normal anatomical features of the ankle and immobilization with a plaster cast is usually sufficient.

painful distal fibula as a result of poor healing of the epiphyseal separation. For this reason exquisite tenderness over the epiphyseal plate, particularly when greater than the tenderness over the collateral ligaments, should constitute a presumptive diagnosis of Salter 1 separation of the distal fibular epiphysis; immobilization in a plaster cast should be carried out.

As with the other epiphyseal injuries described above, epiphyseal disruptions in the distal tibia should be treated with accurate reduction, secure immobilization, and continuation of immobilization for long enough to allow for certain healing of the soft tissue elements. Many times in Salter 1 or 2 injuries this can be accomplished by closed means and immobilization in a short leg cast. In the Salter 3 injuries involving the medial malleolus, however, open reduction and internal fixation with pins are almost invariably necessary. These shuld be done by someone experienced in procedures of this type.

Epiphyseal Separation in the Foot

Injuries to the epiphyses of the foot are relatively uncommon. The inflammatory reaction occurring in the apophysis of the os calcis has been described in detail in Chapter 15, The Foot. However, the other epiphyseal centers of the tarsal bones are quite stable and injuries seldom occur unless they are the result of violent trauma. Somewhat more common are injuries to the tarsometatarsal area, which will occasionally result in disruption of the proximal epiphyses of the metatarsal bones. Even these are not seen without relatively violent trauma and are then associated with other more serious injuries to the foot. The simple Salter 1 separation of the distal metatarsal epiphysis occasionally occurs but it is much less common than the similar injury seen in the hand and ordinarily responds to local infiltration and closed reduction. These injuries are quite stable once reduced since they are invariably Salter 1 or 2. Epiphyseal injuries to the phalanges are generally Salter 1, can be reduced under a local anesthetic without difficulty, and are quite stable.

INDEX

Page numbers followed by *f* indicate figures; those followed by *t* indicate tables.